South Asian Perspectives in Mental Health and Psychology

Series Editors

S. M. Yasir Arafat, Bangladesh Specialized Hospital Limited, Dhaka, Bangladesh

Sujita Kumar Kar, Department of Psychiatry, King George's Medical University, Lucknow, Uttar Pradesh, India

This series of books is an endeavor to gather and present a comprehensive understanding of the various aspects of mental health that are relevant to people living in South Asia. The books aim to provide in-depth guidance and practical solutions to the mental health challenges that are unique to these areas. The content covers a wide range of topics, including but not limited to, climate change and its impact, prison mental health, perinatal mental health, social psychiatry, mental health and disorder among the elderly population, psychiatry education and training, suicide, SDGs and mental health, trauma, addiction, and social isolation. The books also emphasize the importance of early intervention and provide resources for seeking help. The ultimate goal of this series is to empower individuals and communities to take proactive steps toward enhancing their mental wellbeing. The proposed books will fill the existing unmet need in the region with huge populations in low and middle-income country (LMIC) settings.

South Asia, home to about 2 billion people, is a region of diverse cultures, languages, and religions. It caters to about 25% of the global population. This densely populated region faces a myriad of challenges, both natural and man-made. The frequent occurrence of natural disasters, such as earthquakes, floods, and landslides, threaten the lives and livelihoods of millions of people. War, terrorism, and political instability have caused significant disruptions to the region's socio-political fabric. Poverty, migration, and tropical infectious diseases remain major challenges that hinder progress towards sustainable development. Climate change exacerbates these challenges, causing widespread environmental degradation, food insecurity, and water scarcity. Despite these obstacles, South Asian people have shown remarkable resilience and strength in the face of adversity.

Mental health issues in the South Asian region significantly contribute to the global burden of mental illnesses. However, the region faces plenty of challenges such as high stigma, low mental health literacy, poor budgetary allocation, high out-of-pocket expense for mental health services, lack of adequate infrastructure, and limited human resources are significant barriers in mental healthcare. The majority of research on mental health issues is produced by the western countries which may not fit all in the South Asian culture, albeit evidence is needed to test. There is a paucity of research and evidence-based strategies that are region-specific. This series of books is an attempt to compile the important dimensions of mental health that will benefit the regional people.

Nilamadhab Kar · Sujita Kumar Kar ·
S. M. Yasir Arafat
Editors

Geriatric Psychiatry in South Asia

Current Status and Ways Ahead

Springer

Editors
Nilamadhab Kar
Black Country Healthcare NHS
Wolverhampton, UK

Sujita Kumar Kar
Department of Psychiatry
King George's Medical University
Lucknow, Uttar Pradesh, India

S. M. Yasir Arafat
Bangladesh Specialized Hospital
Dhaka, Bangladesh

ISSN 3059-3646 ISSN 3059-3522 (electronic)
South Asian Perspectives in Mental Health and Psychology
ISBN 978-981-96-7468-8 ISBN 978-981-96-7469-5 (eBook)
https://doi.org/10.1007/978-981-96-7469-5

This Springer imprint is published by the registered company Springer Nature Singapore Pte Ltd.
The registered company address is: 152 Beach Road, #21-01/04 Gateway East, Singapore 189721, Singapore

Dedicated to ladies, we are growing old with
Sasmita Kar
Sarvodaya Tripathy
Asma Khatun

Foreword by Femi Oyebode

This is a unique and impressive book. It is a deep and profitable exploration of the current state of geriatric psychiatry in South Asia and a call to action to clinicians, scientists, policy makers, and politicians. The editors have brought together a knowledgeable group of clinicians and academics who summarise what is already known, identify the scale of the problems the countries under examination face, and scope the range of solutions that should ameliorate the difficulties that they describe.

A quarter of the world's population lives in this region. The demographic transition in which there is reduced infant mortality coupled with increasing life expectancy means that for a period there is an increasing population of young people with all the social and economic advantages of that. But soon this is accompanied by an increase in the population of people over 65 years and the exponential growth of diseases associated with ageing including Alzheimer disease and other dementias. This book addresses these issues in a thorough and informed manner, focusing attention on the social and structural facts of each country, so that what is general and what is determined by local factors can be fully grasped.

The issues that are dealt with in this book have relevance for other low to middle-income countries. The dilemmas and potential solutions are important, also, for countries in South Asia, Sub-Saharan Africa, the Sahel, and the Middle East. There is richness and depth in these analyses. There are profound insights and thoughtful conclusions.

I am very pleased to be associated with this book.

Femi Oyebode MBBS, MD, PhD,
FRCPsych. Honorary FRCPsych.
Institute of Mental Health, School
of Psychology
University of Birmingham
Birmingham, UK

Foreword by Subodh Dave

South Asia is home to more than a quarter of the world's population. Traditionally, seen as a "young continent", with a small percentage of the population over the age of 60 years, rapid rises in life expectancy in recent years has meant that the geriatric population is estimated to rise over a fifth of the population over the next two decades. This will mean that the current "ageing" population (>7% of the population) as defined by Asian Development Bank will become "super-aged" (>20% of the population) in the near future.

This demographic "time-bomb" has important health and social care implications not to mention financial consequences given the high prevalence of mental illness in this age group. Recognition and acknowledgement of the issues is the first step towards building preventive strategies. This is especially important because geriatric psychiatry is underfunded and often sidelined, as evident from the paucity of specialist training in Old Age Psychiatry in this part of the world.

This was one of the reasons, why, as Dean of the Royal College of Psychiatrists (and incidentally a psychiatrist trained in South Asia—Mumbai, India), I launched the College's first ever Diploma Programme in Old Age Psychiatry.

It is therefore, a pleasure to write the foreword for this dedicated resource on Geriatric Psychiatry in South Asia. Featuring eminent and respected academic clinicians from across the world, this book provides an in-depth review of the prevalence of psychopathology in South Asia with specific chapters devoted to each of the larger/most populous nations. A focus on gaps in services for the elderly with mental illness will provide policy makers and health and social care providers with a roadmap for solution-focused planning.

Public mental health is a particular passion of mine, having launched new curricula for postgraduate training in Psychiatry with a focus on public mental health and the College's first ever certification course on Public Mental Health Leadership; so it is heartening to see the focus on public mental health in this volume. Prevention at all levels—primary, secondary, and tertiary is the key to addressing the rising.

The breadth and depth of the topics covered makes it an essential read for not only psychiatrists, psychologists and other healthcare professionals but also for policy planners, health economists, social care professionals, and other cross-sector workers involved in the care of the elderly in South Asia. And it is a particular pleasure to see many of my colleagues from the Royal College of Psychiatrists' Old Age Faculty contributes to this volume. I congratulate congratulating the editors for producing a very timely academic resource aimed at resolving the real-world problem of the ageing population of South Asia.

Prof. Subodh Dave FRCPsych. MMed (Clinical Education)
Dean, Royal College of Psychiatrists
Consultant Psychiatrist and Deputy Director of Undergraduate Medical Education, Derbyshire Healthcare Foundation Trust
Professor of Psychiatry
University of Bolton
Bolton, UK

Preface

Matching improved longevity, the geriatric population has increased fast in recent years in South Asian countries. Along with this, the mental health burden of older adults is increasing. Considering the sheer number, South Asia is home to a large proportion of the world's older adults. It is well known that the resources are limited, and most of the older adults in these areas are not recognised or treated.

Given the current trend, it is highly probable that the older adult population and the burden associated with their care will increase. There is a critical need to anticipate and prepare for this, not only through policy and strategies but also by enhancing multidisciplinary resources, professional manpower, and sociocultural readiness for demographic changes.

There has been significant progress in the care of older adults in high-income countries, which is not reflected in the low- and middle-income countries (LMIC) for various reasons, including the health and social care structure and economic resources. Additionally, socioeconomic and cultural changes in LMIC are leading to nuclear family systems, with an increasing number of older adults living alone and the number of care homes rising in many areas. These are rapidly changing times for older adults, and their ability to cope with these changes has been challenged, impacting their mental health. These factors influenced the conception of this project, focusing on the issues in South Asia, where a significant proportion of the world's elderly reside and reflecting on their support systems. There is an urgent need to explore the services available, assess their appropriateness and effectiveness, and consider region-specific, economically viable solutions that can be implemented promptly.

However, mental health care for older adults in South Asia is a neglected area. Little is known about the burden of mental disorders and available mental health services specific for the older adult population in South Asia and other LMICs. We did not find any volume compiling the scenario from South Asian countries. Therefore, this book will be the first of its kind to address these concerns.

The book starts with a chapter with an overview of the burden of geriatric mental health in South Asia. Then there are country-wise chapters. Each of these country chapters, discuss various areas such as the population pyramid and proportion of the elderly population, epidemiology and burden of geriatric mental disorders, current status of services, neuropsychiatry, end-of-life care, legal and ethical aspects of relevant to practice of geriatric psychiatry, digital services in old age mental health care, specialist course and training opportunities in geriatric psychiatry, available research and gaps, current challenges in geriatric mental health and ways out.

The book also covers the public mental health aspects of geriatric mental health in the region. The practical preventive aspects of age-related mental illnesses are suggested for these populations. A specific focus would be on how the suggestions can be integrated into the existing system of health and social care in these countries.

The book explores the evidence to mention the current status of services and highlights the potential unmet need for services in South Asia. This book is helpful for multidisciplinary health professionals, family caregivers, academics, researchers, staff in nongovernmental organizations, and state authorities working for older adults. This book highlights the areas for further research and gives recommendations for culturally appropriate interventions that can be adapted for geriatric populations in South Asia.

Wolverhampton, UK — Nilamadhab Kar
Lucknow, Uttar Pradesh, India — Sujita Kumar Kar
Dhaka, Bangladesh — S. M. Yasir Arafat

Contents

Disease Burden and Services Gap in Geriatric Psychiatry in South Asia: An Overview 1
Mani Santhanakrishnan, Suvarna Jyothi Kantipudi, and Jiann Lin Loo

Geriatric Psychiatry in Bangladesh: Current Status and Ways Ahead 19
S. M. Yasir Arafat and Atiqul Haq Mazumder

Geriatric Psychiatry in India 37
K. L. Vidya and Prerak Kumar

Geriatric Psychiatry in Nepal 53
Pawan Sharma, Rika Rijal, and Omkar Dhungel

Geriatric Psychiatry in Pakistan 67
Osamah Khan, Saima Sheikh, and Saeed Farooq

Geriatric Psychiatry in Sri Lanka 89
Anuprabha Wickramasinghe and Malsha Gunathilake

Geriatric Psychiatry in Other South Asian Countries: Afghanistan, Bhutan, the Maldives 113
Sujita Kumar Kar and S. M. Yasir Arafat

Substance Use in Old Age in South Asia 125
Amit Singh, Shreya Shukla, and Arpit Parmar

Social Determinants and Cultural Aspects of Geriatric Mental Health in South Asia 147
Hitesh Khurana and Sujata Sethi

Public Mental Health Aspects of Geriatric Psychiatry in South Asia 185
Abhinav Tewari, Aditya Agrawal, and Anuranjan Vishwakarma

Preventing Mental Illnesses in Old Age: Strategies and Evidence 207
Sarmishtha Bhattacharyya, Susan Mary Benbow,
and Sathyan Soundararajan

Policies, Programs, and Action Plans in Geriatric Mental Health in South Asia 235
Nilamadhab Kar, Sanhita Bhattacharya, and Shreyan Kar

Correction to: Geriatric Psychiatry in South Asia C1
Nilamadhab Kar, Sujita Kumar Kar, and S. M. Yasir Arafat

About the Editors

Prof. Nilamadhab Kar, MD, DNB, DPM, FRCPsych is a consultant psychiatrist in the Black Country Healthcare NHS Foundation Trust, Wolverhampton, UK. He is the college tutor for undergraduate and postgraduate psychiatry training and the lead for the International Clinical Fellowship Programme in Psychiatry for the Trust. He is an honorary professor of psychiatry at the University of Wolverhampton, UK, and is a visiting honorary professor in the Faculty of Contemplative and Behavioral Sciences, at the Sri Sri University, India. His research contributions have been in the fields of geriatric psychiatry, stress-related mental health disorders, preventive psychiatry, disaster mental health, clinical psychopharmacology, and quality of life. Besides journal articles and book chapters, he has written and edited a few medical books which include Handbook of Dementia, Comprehensive Textbook of Sexual Medicine and Handbook for Disaster Workers.

Dr. Sujita Kumar Kar is currently working as an Additional Professor of Psychiatry at King George's Medical University, Lucknow, Uttar Pradesh, India. He is the editor-in-chief of *Indian Journal of Health, Sexuality and Culture.* He is also the editorial board member and reviewer of various national and international journals. He had written 74 book chapters and more than 500 articles in various national & international journals and made 70 presentations at various national and international conferences. He has been included in the global 2% researcher list released by Stanford University in 2021, 2022, 2023, and 2024. His research interests include brain stimulation, neuropsychiatry, and suicide prevention.

Dr. S. M. Yasir Arafat is currently working as an Associate Consultant of Psychiatry at Bangladesh Specialized Hospital, Dhaka, Bangladesh. He is affiliated with Frontier University Garowe, Somalia as an Associate Professor, Dnet as an Honorary Research Fellow and with the Biomedical Research Foundation, Bangladesh as a Senior Research Fellow. He was affiliated with the University of Bristol, UK as a Visiting Senior Research Associate (August 2021–2023). He completed his MD in Psychiatry from Bangabandhu Sheikh Mujib Medical University, Dhaka, and his MBBS from the Dhaka Medical College, Dhaka, Bangladesh. He also did an MPH in Health Economics and an MBA in Marketing. Dr. Arafat has (co)authored more than 350 peer-reviewed articles and 50 book chapters, and (co)edited more than 10 books with Springer. He has been included in the global 2% researcher list in 2021, 2022, and 2023. He is an editorial member of more than 10 leading journals in mental health, published by Elsevier, Wiley, Springer, and Taylor and Francis. His research focused on mental health, suicidal behaviour, psychometrics, panic buying, and psycho-sexual disorders.

List of Figures

Geriatric Psychiatry in Sri Lanka

Fig. 1 Relative size of children (< 15 years), youth (15–29 years) and older adults (60 + years) populations in Sri Lanka, 2012–2042 (*Source* de Silva and De Silva, 2023) 90

Preventing Mental Illnesses in Old Age: Strategies and Evidence

Fig. 1 The individual and their mental health shown at the centre of multiple levels of influence—Interventions to promote mental health can be designed for each, some, or all of these levels 215

Policies, Programs, and Action Plans in Geriatric Mental Health in South Asia

Fig. 1 A comprehensive structure of levels and domains for supporting positive mental health in old age 237

List of Tables

Disease Burden and Services Gap in Geriatric Psychiatry in South Asia: An Overview

Table 1 Challenges and strategies for advancing geriatric mental health services in south Asian nations 12

Geriatric Psychiatry in Bangladesh: Current Status and Ways Ahead

Table 1 Epidemiology of geriatric mental illnesses in Bangladesh 22
Table 2 Suicidal behavior among older adults in Bangladesh 27

Geriatric Psychiatry in India

Table 1 Programmes policies and action plans in relation to geriatric mental health in India 45

Geriatric Psychiatry in Nepal

Table 1 Important programs for geriatric population in Nepal (NHSSP: Nepal Health Sector Support Programme, 2022) 59

Substance Use in Old Age in South Asia

Table 1 Percentage of adults aged 65 and above who are current tobacco users 128

Social Determinants and Cultural Aspects of Geriatric Mental Health in South Asia

Table 1 Epidemiological studies of prevalence of mental disorders among older adults in South Asia (other than India) 151
Table 2 Epidemiological studies of prevalence of mental disorders among older adults in India (2014–2024) 155

Public Mental Health Aspects of Geriatric Psychiatry in South Asia

Table 1 Challenges of public mental health in South Asia 194

Preventing Mental Illnesses in Old Age: Strategies and Evidence

Table 1 Some of the factors that increase risk of poor mental and cognitive health outcomes in later life 210
Table 2 Publications that support national and international level interventions 217
Table 3 Publications that support individual, family, and community-level interventions 224

Policies, Programs, and Action Plans in Geriatric Mental Health in South Asia

Table 1 Policies, programs, and laws for older adults in Afghanistan 241
Table 2 Policies, programs, and laws for older adults in Bangladesh 242
Table 3 Policies, programs, and laws for older adults in Bhutan 243
Table 4 Policies, programs, and laws for older adults in India 244
Table 5 Policies, programs, and laws for older adults in Maldives 247
Table 6 Policies, programs, and laws for older adults in Nepal 248
Table 7 Policies, programs, and laws for older adults in Pakistan 250
Table 8 Policies, programs, and laws for older adults in Sri Lanka 251

Disease Burden and Services Gap in Geriatric Psychiatry in South Asia: An Overview

Mani Santhanakrishnan, Suvarna Jyothi Kantipudi, and Jiann Lin Loo

Abstract The global population is ageing. 25% of the global ageing population live in eight countries in the Asian continent. They are experiencing accelerated demographic transition. Risk factors such as physical disability, chronic illnesses, social isolation, poverty and inequality contribute to mental health burden of these elderly population in South Asia. The authors have tried to review the published literature from the region to address some of these issues. The authors highlight importance of psychiatric conditions like depression, anxiety, psychosis, dementia and substance use as well as impact of elder abuse within the context of local resources and cultural diversity in access to services. Despite these burden, mental health services for the elderly remain inadequate. Barriers such as stigma, lack of trained professionals, rurality and lack of national policies and infrastructure play a role. The authors highlight an urgent need to address these issues to develop policies and infrastructure and train professionals to bridge this gap and to improve the population mental health of elderly population in South Asia.

Keywords Old age psychiatry · Geriatric psychiatry · Older adults mental health · Dementia · Delirium · Depression · Frailty · Aging

M. Santhanakrishnan · S. J. Kantipudi
Department of Psychiatry, SRMC and RI, Sri Ramachandra Institute of Higher Education and Research (SRIHER), Chennai, India
e-mail: suvarna@sriramachandra.edu.in

M. Santhanakrishnan (✉)
Mental Health Services for Older People, Tees Esk and Wear Valleys NHS Foundation Trust, Stockton On Tees, United Kingdom
e-mail: mani.krishnan@nhs.net

J. L. Loo
Betsi Cadwaladr University Health Board, Bangor, Wales
e-mail: jiann.loo@wales.nhs.uk

N. Kar et al. (eds.), *Geriatric Psychiatry in South Asia*, South Asian Perspectives in Mental Health and Psychology , https://doi.org/10.1007/978-981-96-7469-5_1

1 Introduction

We live in an aging world with demographics rapidly changing. By 2050 nearly 80% of older people will be living in low and middle-income countries (LMIC) economies. While it took around 150 years for a demographic transition in Europe to double the percentage of population older than 60 years but it would take only 20 years in developing countries like India (World Health Organization, 2015).

South Asia is a geographically distinctive region in the southern part of the Asian continent that comprises around 25% of the global population and one-fifth of the world's psychiatric morbidity. Although there is no uniform definition for the phrase South Asia, it is generally referring to countries that form the South Asian Association for Regional Cooperation (SAARC), i.e., Afghanistan, Bangladesh, Bhutan, India, Maldives, Nepal, Pakistan, and Sri Lanka (Arafat & Kar, 2024).

This region is experiencing accelerated aging relative to the rest of the world because of advancements in healthcare, hygiene, lifestyle, sanitation, and infection control. The demographic landscape in South Asia is seeing a notable transformation due to a rising geriatric population. This alteration introduces distinct cultural, social, and economic issues for senior care, encompassing mental health factors (Arafat & Kar, 2024).

Therefore, we need to have demographic preparedness to address the needs of the aging population in South Asia as we currently are grappling with the same issue in the western world.

In this chapter, we will discuss the prevalence and risk factors of geriatric mental health disorders and explore relevant social cultural determinants that play a role in effective delivery of mental health services for the geriatric population in South Asian countries.

2 Cultural Context of Aging

In South Asian countries, mental health issues and the needs of older adults are often under-recognized, unnoticed. Even though depression remains the most prevalent condition other conditions like anxiety, psychotic disorder and delirium are also prevalent. The effect and impact of depression in older adults are exacerbated by factors such as social isolation, poverty, chronic medical condition and bereavement as well as physical comorbidities like diabetes and cardiovascular diseases.

Dementia awareness continues to remain low. There is a lack of structures diagnostic services for dementia. There is a misconception of symptoms of dementia as part of aging which prevents access to diagnosis and professional intervention. An important socio-cultural aspect to consider in South Asia is the pivotal supportive role to care for elderly played by the extended family structures. The traditional joint family system, which historically provided social and emotional support to older adults, is disintegrating due to urbanization and economic pressures. This shift leaves many elderly individuals vulnerable to neglect, loneliness, and elder abuse. Furthermore, cultural stigma around mental illness often prevents families from seeking psychiatric help, further marginalizing older adults with mental health conditions.

Social determinants such as poverty, illiteracy, and gender disparities significantly influence mental health outcomes among the elderly. Older women face higher risks of depression and anxiety due to widowhood, lower socioeconomic status, and limited access to healthcare.

3 Geriatric Psychiatric Disorders in South Asia

3.1 Epidemiology

Compared to western literature, there are very few studies published on the epidemiology of mental health in older adults in South Asia. Using a literature search, we found under 50 papers that have discussed various aspects of mental health in older adults. Nevertheless, the prevalence studies are mainly spread across India, Pakistan, Bangladesh, and Nepal (Hossain et al., 2020; Vidyasagaran et al., 2023). Other countries have published one or two papers indicating a clear need for more research in this field, especially in the rural population.

Dementia, particularly Alzheimer's disease, is a growing concern. Alzheimer's Disease International (ADI) estimates that over 9 million people in South Asia live with dementia, a figure projected to double by 2050 (Dementia in the Asia Pacific Region, 2014). Depression is the most prevalent mental health disorder, with prevalence estimates ranging from 21 to 42% (Vidyasagaran et al., 2023), (Edwards et al., 2023). Anxiety disorders are next most common with prevalence rates between 4 to 29% (Vidyasagaran et al., 2023), (Edwards et al., 2023). Dementia, particularly Alzheimer's disease, has a reported pooled prevalence of 2% (Vidyasagaran et al., 2023). The findings suggest inadequate epidemiological research among the elderly in South Asia. Most of the research is focused on urban areas with an underrepresentation of the rural population. There are gaps in understanding of the mental health burden among older adults. The variability and inconsistencies in prevalence rates across the region could be due to multiple factors including under representation of the rural population in research, variability in diagnostic methods, cultural stigma, and lack of mental health infrastructure. The details of disorder-specific prevalence and risk factors will be discussed in the disorder-specific subsections below.

3.2 Depression

Geriatric depression is an emerging public health problem in South Asia. Depression is the most common mental illness among older adults globally. Findings from global burden of disease 2017 indicates that depression will become the leading cause of disease burden by 2030 (Liu et al., 2020).The prevalence of depression among Indian elderly population as 34.4% (95% CI: 29.3–39.7). In sub-group analysis, the pooled prevalence was higher among females, rural populations, and in the eastern part of the country (Pilania et al., 2019). In Nepal, the prevalence of geriatric depression is 52% of the (95% CI: 44%–59%) (Khanal et al., 2024). The pooled prevalence in the subgroup analysis was higher in the central region and among elderly individuals residing in senior living facilities. Chronic diseases, age $\geq$ 70 years, female gender, illiteracy, limitations in Instrumental Activities of Daily Living (IADL), and feelings of loneliness were identified as independent predictors of geriatric depression (Khanal et al., 2024). Even though there may be other factors that could explain the results like culture, genetics and study methodology and geographical variability we can still conclude that there an urgent need for more research, national strategies to detect and treat depression.

Geriatric population is at higher risk of suffering from depression. The key risk factors include social isolation, physical comorbidity, restricted mobility, bereavement, loss of employment/income, and elder abuse. From western literature it is evident that when older adults suffer with chronic illness and frailty depression is commonly under-detected (Katon, 2011; Lenze et al., 2001).

Lack of nationwide studies and public health strategies to detect depression in older adults is an important factor in under detection and under treatment of depression in older adults. Stigma about mental illness is another factor that deters people from accessing help. Depression in older adults may not be typically present like the core symptoms—low mood, lack of energy and lack of enjoyment. This can impact early identification. Older adults with depression may not have formal help in South Asian countries due to their cultural beliefs, lack of support, and stigma.

The mainstay of treatment of depression in older adults in South Asian countries remains pharmacological. Psychological intervention has evidence base for treating depression for older adults, even in western countries there is variable uptake and availability of formal psychological therapies (Muhammad & Meher, 2021; Murray and GBD 2021 Collaborators, 2024).

3.3 Anxiety Disorders

Anxiety disorders frequently co-occur in the elderly population of South Asia, with research indicating differing prevalence rates influenced by geographical and demographic variables. A study in Bangladesh indicates that 72.7% of urban elderly individuals experience varying degrees of anxiety, attributed to risk factors such as financial instability and chronic health conditions (Any et al., 2021). The prevalence of anxiety among the elderly in India was approximately 10% (Subramanyam et al., 2018). Late-life anxiety is frequently underdiagnosed, under-researched, and under-treated in South Asia, despite its high prevalence (Hossain et al., 2020).

Anxiety disorder in older adults is under-recognized and subthreshold anxiety symptoms are more common than threshold anxiety disorder. We postulate that similar presentation may be seen in South Asian population with sub threshold anxiety symptoms that are not brought to attention for health and care professionals to assess and treat (Miloyan et al., 2015). An editorial by Chong et al. from Australia highlights the need for more work and attention on anxiety disorders in older adults (Twh et al., 2020).

3.4 Psychosis

There is limited literature on psychotic disorders in older adults in South Asia, with much of the existing literature focusing on non-Western conceptualizations of psychosis. Cohen (2024), in a commentary on Devanand et al.'s review of late-onset psychosis, highlights the significant variation in understanding and interpreting psychotic phenomena across cultures, emphasizing the need to consider variable presentations in older adults (Cohen, 2024; Devanand et al., 2024).

The nomenclature for psychosis in older adults has also evolved, with terms such as "primary psychotic disorder," "late-onset schizophrenia," and "very late-onset schizophrenia-like psychosis" (VLOSP) being used to describe distinct subtypes. Howard et al. (2000) published an international consensus outlining the classification criteria for these conditions. According to this guidance, psychotic symptoms with an onset between the ages of 40 and 60 should be termed "late-onset schizophrenia," whereas symptoms beginning after age 60 are classified as "very late-onset schizophrenia-like psychosis" (Howard et al., 2000).

Late-onset psychosis in the elderly presents unique clinical characteristics and challenges. Studies have shown that delusions and hallucinations are common symptoms, with persecutory delusions being the most prevalent (Ramasamy & Bharath, 2017). While traditionally viewed as independent of psychopathology, recent research suggests that insight in psychosis may be an explanatory model influenced by cultural and social factors (Jacob, 2014). Late-life psychosis in elderly could be caused by many conditions, including chronic conditions like schizophrenia, dementia-related psychosis, and organic causes and the management is complex, with limited evidence for the efficacy of atypical antipsychotics and concerns about their use in dementia patients (Nebhinani et al., 2014). Understanding indigenous beliefs about mental illness among community health workers is crucial, as these often differ from biomedical models (Joel et al., 2003).

3.5 Dementia

The number of people living in Asia Pacific region will triple by 2050 as per the Alzheimer's Disease International report on dementia in the Asia–Pacific region and the report highlights four major challenges; the limited awareness of dementia, false perception of dementia as a part of natural aging, lack/inadequate resources (human and financial) resources to meet the care needs of people with dementia, inadequate training of professional carers (Dementia in the Asia Pacific Region, 2014). Unlike developed countries where there are well formed national strategies for south Asian countries have not caught up to making dementia a national priority (Sun et al., 2020).

A multinational study, which included south Asian countries such as India and Pakistan, examined the diverse pathways individuals with dementia follow to access specialized care. It revealed significant delays, with a median time of 56 weeks from symptom onset to specialist consultation and highlighted the role of general practitioners as the primary point of access. Psychotropic medications were commonly prescribed, but psychosocial interventions were rarely offered (Volpe et al., 2020).

The Lancet Commission on dementia prevention, intervention, and care, led by Gill Livingston et al., highlights the modifiable risk factors for dementia. Among these, diabetes, obesity, and vascular risk factors, such as elevated LDL cholesterol levels, require urgent attention due to their strong association with cognitive decline. Other critical factors include hearing and visual impairments, excessive alcohol intake, and low educational attainment, all of which play a significant role in increasing the risk of dementia later in life. Addressing these modifiable factors through targeted interventions and public health initiatives is essential to reducing the global burden of dementia (Livingston et al., 2024).

The key factors that are highlighted as modifiable risk factors the following will be more relevant to South Asian Countries, which are:

- Diabetes
- Hypertension
- Obesity
- Smoking
- Excessive Alcohol
- Hearing Loss
- Physical Inactivity

Detailed discussion on dementia in South Asia will be beyond the scope of the chapter however learning from countries like UK, Europe, and USA we may want to look at the model of care for tackling dementia. The key priorities are:

- Prevention
- Consistent early accurate diagnosis
- Validated diagnostic tools that are culture/region specific.
- Use of technology to aid diagnosis (rural remote areas difficult to reach population)
- Embedding research to get high quality data.
- Post diagnostic support and care in the community.

3.6 Substance Use Disorders

The problem of substance use disorder increases with the growing of aging population, which is not unique to the South Asian population. Commonly used substances include tobacco, alcohol, prescribed medications, and other illicit drugs, which are used by younger patient groups, e.g., cannabis and opioids. The data from the Study on Global Ageing and Adult Health (SAGE) study in India indicates that a higher rate of alcohol consumption among age group of 60–64 years, especially those at the lower social-economic status (Gupta et al., 2024). There is limited published literature on substance use disorder from other South Asian countries. Some of the addiction issues may be perceived as socially acceptable among older men, e.g., tobacco chewing or alcohol use. However, the issue of underdiagnosis and limited health-seeking behavior may be fueled by cultural taboos around discussing substance use, especially among the elderly (Sarkar et al., 2015). Given the higher rate of medical comorbidities, pain management and other medical conditions can lead to prescription drug dependence, especially opioid type analgesia. Health professionals' prescription practice sometimes overlook substance use as a health issue in older adults given the complex interaction of multiple medical comorbidities. Rural areas often lack specialized addiction treatment centers or geriatric care. Learning from the SAGE study, the way forward includes improving awareness and strengthening public health facilities through creation of policies and programs that focus on prevention (Gupta et al., 2024). Community-Based Programs, integrated care approach using the existing primary healthcare setting, and harnessing social support are viable options to improve the care for elderly struggling with substance use disorder.

3.7 Elder Abuse and Its Impact on Older Adults Mental Health

Abuse of older adults is an important public health problem. A 2017 review of 52 studies from 28 countries indicated that 1 in 6 people older than 60 were subjected to some form of abuse (Gulland, 2017). The World Health Organization defines elder abuse as any act, either one-time or recurring, or a failure to take necessary action, that occurs in a relationship where trust is expected and causes injury or suffering to an older person. This kind of violence, which includes financial and material abuse, desertion, neglect, physical, sexual, psychological, and emotional abuse, as well as a significant loss of respect and dignity, is a violation of human rights (World Health Organization, 2025).

The WHO has emphasized the importance of this through United Nations Decade of Healthy Ageing (2021–2030), by offering a chance to significantly advance the fight against elder abuse. The decade is a global endeavor to concentrate resources on strengthening older persons' quality of life, which includes preventing and responding to abuse, promoting their health and well-being, and making sure their rights and dignity are respected (World Health Organization, 2022).

In South Asia, there are cultural contexts where there may be paucity of published literature on elder abuse, probably due to under-reporting of such occurrences. In many cases the main caregivers may be the abusers resulting in older adults not reporting any abuse due to fear of abandonment or other harm as well as social stigma. Due to their physical restrictions and co-morbidities, socioeconomic constraints and lack of support network put older adults in a vulnerable position to be subjected to various forms of abuse and neglect. Elder abuse can result in people suffering from fear, anxiety, distress, and depression. Mohammed et al. describe the Association of elder abuse, crime victimhood, and perceived neighborhood safety with major depression among older adults in India (Muhammad et al., 2021).

3.8 Other Mental Illness of Elderly

Obsessive compulsive disorder (OCD) can occur as a diagnostic entity on its own or as part of comorbid symptoms in depression. A recent meta-analysis indicates higher prevalence of OCD among older adults in Asia 3.5% compared to worldwide prevalence of 2.4% (Heydarikhayat et al., 2024).Late onset OCD presentation could be an indication to look at underlying neurodegenerative disorders like frontotemporal dementia, Lewy body dementia or Huntington's disease (Frileux et al., 2020), (Scicutella, 2000). Cultural norms, gender roles, and societal expectations commonly influence the presentation of OCD symptoms in South Asian nations. For example, in Bengali society, symptoms manifest as compulsive washing in women, popularly known as "such Bhai," is societally reinforced and limits seeking treatment help (Chakraborty & Banerji, 1975).

Sleep problems are highly common in older adults living in South Asian countries and associated with poorer general well-being and quality of life, and psychiatric comorbidities (Stranges et al., 2012). REM sleep behavior disorder, specifically encountered in older adults with underlying Parkinson's disease or Lewy body dementia (Sixel-Döring et al., 2023).Screening for RBD may help with identifying underlying cause of dementia. RBD is listed as one of the core clinical features for diagnosis of Lewy Body Dementia (Chan et al., 2018).

Geriatric sexual health is often influenced by changing sexual needs with increasing age and family structure, cultural norms/expectations around sexuality, and hormonal changes, that can reduce decreased libido in women and erectile dysfunction in men. A community study done in India, reported in only 27.4% of individuals over 60 years are sexually active and none beyond 75 years. Among those who are sexually active, 43.5% experienced erectile dysfunction, 10.9% had premature ejaculation, while females reported 28% arousal disorder, 16% hypoactive sexual desire disorder, and 20% anorgasmia (Sathyanarayana Rao et al., 2015). In most of the South Asian nations, cultural beliefs dictate the acceptability of discussing geriatric sexuality, leading to stigma in seeking help. In most of the South Asian nations, cultural beliefs dictate the acceptability of discussing geriatric sexuality, leading to stigma in seeking help. Furthermore, conditions like paraphilias, sexuality in special population like LGBTQ + individuals, widowed elderly, and the impact of psychotropics on sexual function are under explored (Lodha et al., 2021).

Stress-related disorders in South Asia are influenced by complex interplay between socio-cultural factors and mental wellbeing. The WHO SAGE data from India reveals that higher work and social participation enhances cognitive performance in older adults, emphasizing the need for financial security and social engagement (Chanda & Mishra, 2019). Retirement from work, bereavement, comorbid chronic illnesses, social isolation are significant risk factors that can adversely impact mental health of the elderly (Mukku et al., 2018). However, more research is needed to understand the potential impact of socio-economic adversities on cognition and mental health.

Somatic presentations of depression and anxiety are common in South Asian contexts. A hospital-based study in India, reports that 98.8% of elderly have moderate to severe somatization (Grover et al., 2019).There is a possible role of heightened somatic awareness and cultural acceptance of somatic symptoms in determining somatic presentations of depression and anxiety (Ma-Kellams, 2014).

Suicide in older adults is commonly reported in the news with emphasis on economic, social, and cultural factors rather than psychiatric illness. A community study from India, reports average annual suicide rate of 189 per 100,000 for individuals over 55, with a male-to-female ratio of 1:0.66 and an age-related increase in suicide rates (Abraham et al., 2005). Another study from India, analyzed national and state-wise suicide rates in relation to macroeconomic indices, finding significant association between suicide rates and per capita gross domestic product, consumer price index, foreign exchange, trade balance, total health expenditure as well as literacy rates (Rajkumar et al., 2015).

4 Health Care Systems and Policies—Challenges and Opportunities

South Asia's rapidly aging population and rising life expectancy necessitate addressing older adults' mental health issues at a system level. South Asia has many mental health specialists, but 90% of mental illnesses go untreated (Shidhaye et al., 2015). The problem of mental health stigma, poor funding from government, and insufficient specialized training worsen this gap (Murad & Siraj, 2024; Shaji et al., 2004).

Cultural stigma plays a significant role deterring those with mental health conditions getting treatment. Depression, for example, is frequently undiagnosed and untreated (Dhoot, 2020). Furthermore, the region's diverse socioeconomic and geopolitical situations have resulted in fragmented policies for health funding and social care provision for older individuals.

Most South Asian countries allocate less than 1% of their healthcare budgets to mental health, resulting in a dearth of resources and services tailored to older adults. Primary care physicians and healthcare workers, often the first point of contact for elderly patients, receive minimal training in geriatric psychiatry. Specialized services, such as memory clinics and dementia day-care canters, are scarce and largely confined to urban areas, leaving rural populations underserved (Arafat et al., 2024; Mazumder et al., 2020).

In India, the most populated country in the world, the elderly population are projected to grow from 8.6% in 2011 to 19.5% by 2050, which could potentially pose a significant challenge to the nation's healthcare system (Ravindranath & Sundarakumar, 2021). Limited public governance, inadequate policymaking focus, and a fragile primary healthcare infrastructure exacerbate these issues (Kafczyk & Hämel, 2024). Fragmented family structures and pervasive loneliness further strain mental health among older adults, leading to higher rates of depression and dementia (Kaur et al., 2023). Despite the alarming statistics, 30% of the elderly experiencing depression and 7.4% diagnosed with dementia—treatment gaps persist, with only 0.7% of dementia cases being self-reported (Rangarajan et al., 2021). Initiatives like *Ayushman Bharat*, the Mental Healthcare Act, and the National Programme for Health Care of the Elderly (NPHCE) have been introduced but have faced inconsistent implementation, especially in rural areas, where healthcare resources remain scarce. Ageism, stigma, and societal biases have also hindered the recognition and treatment of mental health issues in older adults (Kaur et al., 2023).

In Bangladesh, the elderly population constitutes 9.3% of the total, with 15.7 million people aged over 60 (Arafat et al. 2024). Despite the growing aging population, geriatric psychiatry is in its infancy. Since the retirement of the country's first and only geriatric psychiatrist in 2020, no new specialists have been recruited. The absence of postgraduate programs in geriatric psychiatry, limited access to mental health care, and a focus on physical health over mental health exacerbate the challenges. High out-of-pocket medical expenses and the lack of social security measures further restrict access to care (Tanira et al., 2022). To address these gaps, policymakers must prioritize funding for geriatric psychiatry training, expand mental health services, and implement social pension plans to support the aging population (Mazumder et al., 2020).

In Nepal, geriatric population is projected to rise from 9% in 2015 to 18.6% by 2050, driven by increased life expectancy (Risal et al., 2024). Rural elderly populations face significant barriers, including poverty, isolation, and inadequate healthcare infrastructure. Financial support provisions, such as the Older Citizen Act of 2006, exist but are often insufficient, with many elderly individuals relying on family members for caregiving. Migration of younger generations to urban areas has left elderly individuals without adequate support. The prevalence of depression is alarmingly high, reaching 53.1% in some rural communities. Contributing factors include chronic illnesses, illiteracy, loneliness, and verbal or physical abuse (Kamholz et al., 2022). Nepal has only five geriatric physicians and limited training for healthcare professionals in geriatric care. While there are about 100 private aged care facilities in urban areas, government-run facilities remain scarce, underscoring the geriatric mental health treatment gap in Nepal.

Pakistan too faces considerable challenges arising from its swiftly aging population, anticipated to reach 43.3 million by 2050 (Noreen et al., 2021). Despite the pressing necessity to confront this demographic transition, there is a lack of specialized care, exacerbated by low government financing and poor mental health training for healthcare personnel (Murad & Siraj, 2024). Moreover, societal transformations, like the emergence of nuclear families and modernity, exacerbate elder abuse, social isolation, and loneliness (Ahmad et al., 2018; Noreen et al., 2021). Although constitutional measures for the welfare of the elderly are established, their execution is inadequate, and the absence of a comprehensive support network intensifies the difficulties encountered by older persons (Table 1).

In Sri Lanka, the older adults constitute 12.3% of the total population, adding a significant burden to the mental health care system. Despite recent reforms aimed at community-based treatment and enhancements in psychiatric facilities, it faces challenges related to inadequate human resources and inadequate physical infrastructure for mental health care (Kathriarachchi et al., 2019). Additional challenges include limited community mental health literacy, inadequate multi-sectoral collaboration, and a shortage of geriatric specialists (Minas et al., 2017).

There is not much literature on the system specific challenges in other South Asian nations. Afghanistan faces significant mental health challenges due to ongoing conflict, community violence, and malnutrition, particularly impacting the elderly vulnerable population., While there is some progress in integrating mental health services into primary care, access remains limited in conflict areas (Bragin et al., 2018; Kovess-Masfety et al., 2022). Bhutan also faces significant challenges in delivering mental health services, including limited accessibility due to geographical barriers, a shortage of mental health professionals, and insufficient funding (Gyeltshen et al., 2025). Maldives mental health system faces challenges such as governance issues, limited access to health services, lack of integration of tradition faith healing system with modern medicine, health care manpower shortages, and lack of preventive models and research in mental health (Mohamed & Mansoor, 2024).

5 Emerging Initiatives and the Way Forward

Despite the challenges, there are promising developments in geriatric psychiatry in South Asia. Non-governmental organizations (NGOs) and community-based initiatives play a critical role in bridging gaps in care. For instance, organizations like Help-Age India and the Alzheimer's and Related Disorders Society of India (ARDSI) focus on raising awareness, providing caregiver support, and advocating for policy changes.

Studies have explored various interventions, including traditional practices like yoga and meditation, behavioral therapies, technology-based solutions, and music therapy. While most evidence comes from India, there's a notable lack of research

Table 1 Challenges and strategies for advancing geriatric mental health services in south Asian nations

Theme	Challenges	Strategies
Human resources	• Shortage of trained geriatric mental health specialists and allied healthcare professionals (Occupational therapists, speech and language therapists, physiotherapists, psychological therapists etc.) • Limited postgraduate training programs • Limited professional development opportunities	• Expand training opportunities for geriatric care professionals • Increase the number of geriatric specialists • Integrate geriatrics into medical education and continuous professional development
Health financing	• Insufficient government funding for mental health services, • Excess reliance on out-of-pocket expenses leading to financial burden on elderly individuals and families	• Increase public investment in mental health services • Strategic investments in social security and healthcare services • Social pension plans to reduce the financial burden
Integration with primary care	• Primary healthcare providers lack sufficient training in geriatric psychiatry, limiting their ability to treat mental health issues in older adults	• Integrate geriatric psychiatry into primary healthcare training • Strengthen the capacity of primary care professionals to address elderly mental health • Improve service delivery at the community level
Governance and policy	• Inconsistent implementation of government programs (e.g., Ayushman Bharat, Mental Healthcare Act) • Lack of unified policy • Inconsistent non-governmental support for mental health initiatives	• Ensure seamless and effective implementation of government programs • Facilitate collaborative efforts among governments, NGOs, and community stakeholders can help close service delivery gaps • Promote greater participation from non-governmental organizations
Access to care	• Stigma surrounding mental health and aging • Lack of targeted policies for geriatric mental health care	• Public awareness campaigns and community-based interventions are essential to combat stigma surrounding mental health and aging • Develop comprehensive geriatric-specific mental health policies

from other South Asian countries, indicating a need for more comprehensive studies in the region (Mazumder et al., 2023). Cultural factors and stigma in South Asian communities contribute to underreporting of depression among the elderly, necessitating culturally sensitive screening methods (Dhoot, 2020). To address the growing mental health needs of the aging population, task-shifting strategies have been proposed, such as training community health workers in geriatric mental health care and integrating mental health services. Telemedicine and digital health platforms are emerging as innovative solutions to address geographic and resource barriers. These tools enable elderly patients in remote areas to access psychiatric consultations and counseling services (Sivakumar et al., 2020).

To address the growing mental health needs of the elderly, South Asian governments must prioritize investment in geriatric psychiatry. This includes training healthcare professionals, integrating mental health services into primary care, and implementing national dementia strategies. Increasing public awareness and combating stigma are equally crucial to ensure that older adults receive timely and compassionate care.

A wellness model that emphasizes preventive measures could be a solution given the uncertainty around future resource allocation and the potential scarcity. Preventive measures can reduce the disease burden and increase longevity in the older population. Healthy aging, i.e., maintaining and developing abilities that enable physical, mental, and social well-being in the process of growing older should be incorporated while drafting the public health policy (World Health Organization, 2015). The existing preventive measures, i.e., promoting physical exercise, cultivating healthy eating patterns, preventing and managing chronic diseases, staying mentally engaged, and fostering strong social connections, are all essential components to healthy aging. Additionally, governmental policies supporting this concept are critical to improving outcomes in an aging population, which has been outlined as one of the sustainable goals in UN Decade of Healthy Ageing: Plan of Action 2021–2030 (World Health Organization, 2022).

6 Conclusion

Geriatric psychiatry in South Asia is at a critical juncture, facing the dual challenges of a rapidly aging population and inadequate system preparedness. There is an urgent need for a holistic and multipronged approach to enhance mental health service delivery for older adults in this region. Given these nations' unique cultural context, there is a need for the development of culturally sensitive mental health screening tools and interventions. Current challenges, including limited research, underdiagnosed conditions, stigma, mental health treatment gap, lacunae in healthcare infrastructure, and resource scarcity, underscore the urgent necessity for a paradigm shift in healthcare system. It is important that health care leaders and policymakers to give mental health of older adults a priority to develop strategic national program to address the gaps. For health care academics, (psychiatrists, geriatricians, and allied health professionals) there is a need to look at bespoke training and education to the workforce to tackle the needs of older adults in coming decades.

For health and social care services in these countries there is a need for strengthening cultural sensitivity, family support systems and health care infrastructure to meet the need of this vulnerable population. To address these challenges, South Asia nations must prioritize strengthening mental health infrastructure, integrate geriatric psychiatry into primary care, and adopt task shifting models of care. Promotion of public–private partnerships, enhancing professional training, increasing community awareness to reduce stigma, utilizing technologies to improve access to care, public funding of health care services, social pension schemes and fostering health aging are crucial to improving geriatric mental health in south Asia.

References

Abraham, V. J., Abraham, S., & Jacob, K. S. (2005). Suicide in the elderly in Kaniyambadi block, Tamil Nadu, South India. *International journal of geriatric psychiatry, 20*(10), 953–955. https://doi.org/10.1002/gps.1385

Ahmad, R., Mi, H., Keyao, R., Khan, K., & Navid, K. (2018). Aging and social security system in Pakistan: policy challenges, opportunities, and role of China–Pakistan Economic Corridor (CPEC). *Educational Gerontology 44*(99), 537–550. https://doi.org/10.1080/03601277.2018.1488382

Any, O. H., Moin, S., Akter, M., Afreen, K. N., & Mazumder, M. K. (2021). Status of anxiety disorders among elderly people in a selected urban area in Bangladesh. *Journal of National Institute of Neurosciences Bangladesh, 7*, 137–141. https://doi.org/10.3329/jninb.v7i2.58108.

Arafat, S. M. Y., & Kar, S. K. (2024). Epidemiology of psychiatric disorders and overview of access to mental health care in South Asia. In *Access to mental health care in South Asia* (pp. 1–15). Springer. https://doi.org/10.1007/978-981-99-9153-2_1

Arafat, S. M. Y., Mazumder, A. H., & Maruf, M. M. (2024). Geriatric psychiatry in Bangladesh. In S. M. Yasir Arafat (Ed.), *Mental health in Bangladesh: From bench to community* (pp. 311–322). Springer Nature. https://doi.org/10.1007/978-981-97-0610-5_18

Bragin, M., Akesson, B., Ayubi, B., & Tankink, M. (2018). From the editors … An introduction to a special issue: A focus on mental health and psychosocial support in Afghanistan. *Intervention Journal of Mental Health and Psychosocial Support in Conflict Affected Areas, 16*, 197. https://doi.org/10.4103/INTV.INTV_64_18

Chakraborty, A., & Banerji, G. (1975). Ritual, a culture specific neurosis, and obsessional states in Bengali culture. *Indian Journal of Psychiatry, 17*, 273.

Chan, P. C., Lee, H. H., Hong, C. T., Hu, C. J., & Wu, D. (2018). REM Sleep Behavior Disorder (RBD) in Dementia with Lewy Bodies (DLB). *Behavioural Neurology, 2018*, 9421098. https://doi.org/10.1155/2018/9421098

Chanda, S., & Mishra, R. (2019). Impact of transition in work status and social participation on cognitive performance among elderly in India. *BMC Geriatrics, 19*, 251. https://doi.org/10.1186/s12877-019-1261-5

Chong, T. W., Lautenschlager, N. T., Anstey, K. J., & Bryant, C. (2020). Anxiety disorders in late life-Why are we not more worried? *International journal of geriatric psychiatry, 35*, 955–961. https://doi.org/10.1002/gps.5300

Cohen, C. I. (2024). Putting late-onset psychosis into context. *International Psychogeriatrics, 36* (Issue theme: Schizophrenia and other psychotic disorders in later life), 13–17. https://doi.org/10.1017/S1041610223004490

Dementia in the Asia Pacific Region. (2014). Alzheimer's disease international and Alzheimer's Australia. https://www.alzint.org/u/Dementia-Asia-Pacific-2014.pdf

Devanand, D. P., Jeste, D. V., Stroup, T. S., & Goldberg, T. E. (2024). Overview of late-onset psychoses. *International Psychogeriatrics, 36*, 28–42. https://doi.org/10.1017/S1041610223000157

Dhoot, V. (2020). New insights for old age: Developing new practices for screening and treating depression in geriatric patients. *International Journal of Social Science and Economic Research, 5*, 2355–2360. https://doi.org/10.46609/IJSSER.2020.v05i08.017

Edwards, N., Walker, S., Paddick, S.-M., Prina, A. M., Chinnasamy, M., Reddy, N., Mboya, I. B., et al. (2023). Prevalence of depression and anxiety in older people in low- and middle- income countries in Africa, Asia and South America: A systematic review and meta-analysis. *Journal of Affective Disorders, 325*, 656–674. https://doi.org/10.1016/j.jad.2023.01.068

Frileux, S., Millet, B., & Fossati, P. (2020). Late-onset OCD as a potential harbinger of dementia with Lewy bodies: A report of two cases. *Frontiers in Psychiatry, 11*, 554. https://doi.org/10.3389/fpsyt.2020.00554

Grover, S., Sahoo, S., Chakrabarti, S., & Avasthi, A. (2019). Anxiety and somatic symptoms among elderly patients with depression. *Asian Journal of Psychiatry, 41*, 66–72. https://doi.org/10.1016/j.ajp.2018.07.009

Gulland, A. (2017). One in six elderly people is subjected to abuse, study finds. *British Medical Journal Publishing Group, 357*, j2927. https://doi.org/10.1136/bmj.j2927

Gupta, M. K., Nagdeve, D. A., Mahata, D., & Chaurasia, H. (2024). Substance abuse among elderly in India: Evidence based on study on global ageing and adult health (SAGE) Wave 1. *Global Social Welfare, 11*, 77–83. https://doi.org/10.1007/s40609-023-00307-5

Gyeltshen, K., Chhetri, B., & Gyeltshen, D. (2025). Delivery of mental health services in Bhutan: Challenges and way forward. *Public Health Challenges, 3*(3), e211. https://doi.org/10.1002/puh2.211

Heydarikhayat, S., Kazeminia, M., Heydarikhayat, N., Rezaei, M., Heydarikhayat, N., & Ziapour, A. (2024). Prevalence of obsessive-compulsive disorder in the older person: A systematic review and meta-analysis. *BMC Geriatrics, 24*, 874. https://doi.org/10.1186/s12877-024-05440-0

Hossain, M. M., Purohit, N., Sultana, A., Ma, P., McKyer, E. L. J., & Ahmed, H. U. (2020). Prevalence of mental disorders in South Asia: An umbrella review of systematic reviews and meta-analyses. *Asian Journal of Psychiatry, 51*, 102041. https://doi.org/10.1016/j.ajp.2020.102041

Howard, R., Rabins, P. V., Seeman, M. V., & Jeste, D. V. (2000). Late-onset schizophrenia and very-late-onset schizophrenia-like psychosis: An international consensus. The international late-onset schizophrenia group. *The American Journal of Psychiatry, 157*, 172–178. https://doi.org/10.1176/appi.ajp.157.2.172

Jacob, K. S. (2014). Insight in psychosis: An independent predictor of outcome or an explanatory model of illness? *Asian Journal of Psychiatry, 11* (This Issue Includes a Special Section on Classification of Psychiatric Disorders), 65–71. https://doi.org/10.1016/j.ajp.2014.06.001

Joel, D., Sathyaseelan, M., Jayakaran, R., Vijayakumar, C., Muthurathnam, S., & Jacob, K. S. (2003). Explanatory models of psychosis among community health workers in South India. *Acta Psychiatrica Scandinavica, 108*, 66–69. https://doi.org/10.1034/j.1600-0447.2003.01327.x

Kafczyk, T., & Hämel, K. (2024). Challenges and opportunities in strengthening primary mental healthcare for older people in India: A qualitative stakeholder analysis. *BMC Health Services Research, 24*, 206. https://doi.org/10.1186/s12913-024-10622-y

Kamholz, B., Marahatta, K., & Magar, S. T. (2022). The implications of accelerated aging in Nepal. *The American Journal of Geriatric Psychiatry: Official Journal of the American Association for Geriatric Psychiatry, 30*, 854–858. https://doi.org/10.1016/j.jagp.2022.01.003

Kathriarachchi, S. T., Seneviratne, V. L., & Amarakoon, L. (2019). Development of mental health care in Sri Lanka: Lessons learned. *Taiwanese Journal of Psychiatry, 33*, 55. https://doi.org/10.4103/TPSY.TPSY_15_19

Katon, W. J. (2011). Epidemiology and treatment of depression in patients with chronic medical illness. *Dialogues in Clinical Neuroscience, 13*, 7–23. https://doi.org/10.31887/DCNS.2011.13.1/wkaton
Kaur, H., Sivakumar, T., Manikappa, S. K., & Sarkar, S. (2023). The conundrum of geriatric public mental health in India: Initiatives and the road ahead. *Indian Journal of Social Psychiatry, 39*, 312. https://doi.org/10.4103/ijsp.ijsp_276_23
Khanal, G., Selvamani, Y., Thapa, S., & Chinnaiyan, S. (2024). Prevalence and covariates of depression among older adults in Nepal: A systematic review and meta-analysis. *PLOS Mental Health, 1*, e0000112. https://doi.org/10.1371/journal.pmen.0000112
Kovess-Masfety, V., Karam, E., Keyes, K., Sabawoon, A., & Sarwari, B. A. (2021). Access to care for mental health problems in Afghanistan: A national challenge. *International Journal of Health Policy and Management, 11*, 1442–1450. https://doi.org/10.34172/ijhpm.2021.46
Lenze, E. J., Rogers, J. C., Martire, L. M., Mulsant, B. H., Rollman, B. L., Dew, M. A., & Reynolds III, C. F. (2001). The association of late-life depression and anxiety with physical disability: A review of the literature and prospectus for future research. *The American journal of geriatric psychiatry, 9*(2), 133–135.
Liu, Q., He, H., Yang, J., Feng, X., Zhao, F., & Lyu, J. (2020). Changes in the global burden of depression from 1990 to 2017: Findings from the global burden of disease study. *Journal of Psychiatric Research, 126*, 134–140. https://doi.org/10.1016/j.jpsychires.2019.08.002
Livingston, G., Huntley, J., Liu, K. Y., Costafreda, S. G., Selbæk, G., Alladi, S., Ames, D., Banerjee, S., Burns, A., Brayne, C., Fox, N. C., Ferri, C. P., Gitlin, L. N., Howard, R., Kales, H. C., Kivimäki, M., Larson, E. B., Nakasujja, N., Rockwood, K., Samus, Q., Shirai, K., Singh-Manoux, A., Schneider, L. S., Walsh, S., Yao, Y., Sommerlad, A., & Mukadam, N. (2024). Dementia prevention, intervention, and care: 2024 report of the lancet standing commission. *The Lancet, 404*, 572–628. https://doi.org/10.1016/S0140-6736(24)01296-0
Lodha, P., Perumal, D., & De Sousa, A. (2021). Geriatric sexual health: The challenges in the Indian context. In M. K. Shankardass (Ed.), *Ageing issues in India: Practices, perspectives and policies* (pp. 193–210). Springer. https://doi.org/10.1007/978-981-16-5827-3_11
Ma-Kellams, C. (2014). Cross-cultural differences in somatic awareness and interoceptive accuracy: A review of the literature and directions for future research. *Frontiers in Psychology, 5*, 1379. https://doi.org/10.3389/fpsyg.2014.01379
Mazumder, H., Faizah, F., Gain, E. P., Sharmin Eva, I., Ferdouse Mou, K., Saha, N., Rahman, F., Das, J., Islam, A. M. K., Nesa, F., Hossain, M. M. (2023). Effectiveness of mental health interventions for older adults in South Asia: A scoping review. *PLOS ONE, 18*, e0287883. https://doi.org/10.1371/journal.pone.0287883
Mazumder, H, Murshid, M. E., Faizah, F., & Hossain, M. M. (2020). Geriatric mental health in Bangladesh: A call for action. *International Psychogeriatrics, 32*, 667–668. https://doi.org/10.1017/S1041610220000423
Miloyan, B., Byrne, G. J., & Pachana, N. A. (2015). Threshold and subthreshold generalized anxiety disorder in later life. *The American Journal of Geriatric Psychiatry, 23*, 633–641. https://doi.org/10.1016/j.jagp.2014.08.010
Minas, H., Mendis, J., & Hall, T. (2017). Mental health system development in Sri Lanka. In H. Minas & M. Lewis (Eds.), *Mental health in Asia and the Pacific: Historical and cultural perspectives* (pp. 59–77). Springer US. https://doi.org/10.1007/978-1-4899-7999-5_4
Mohamed, A., & Mansoor, S. (2024). Challenges and opportunities in the mental health landscape of the Maldives. *Australasian Psychiatry, 33*(2), 195–196. https://doi.org/10.1177/10398562241289879
Muhammad, T., & Meher, T. (2021). Association of late-life depression with cognitive impairment: Evidence from a cross-sectional study among older adults in India. *BMC Geriatrics, 21*, 364. https://doi.org/10.1186/s12877-021-02314-7

Muhammad, T., Meher, T., & Sekher, T. V. (2021). Association of elder abuse, crime victimhood and perceived neighbourhood safety with major depression among older adults in India: A cross-sectional study using data from the LASI baseline survey (2017–2018). *British Medical Journal Open, 11*, Article e055625. https://doi.org/10.1136/bmjopen-2021-055625

Mukku, S. S., Reddy, V. H., & Sivakumar, P. T. (2018). Psychological morbidity after job retirement: A review. *Asian Journal of Psychiatry, 37*, 58–63. https://doi.org/10.1016/j.ajp.2018.08.003

Murad, S., & Siraj, S. (2024). Bridging the void: Unraveling mental health policies for the older adults in Pakistan's tapestry—A literature review. *Journal of Clinical Psychology and Neurology, 2*(2), 1–4. https://doi.org/10.61440/JCPN.2024.v2.17

Murray, C. J. L., & GBD 2021 Collaborators. (2024). Findings from the global burden of disease study 2021. *Lancet (London, England), 403*, 2259–2262. https://doi.org/10.1016/S0140-6736(24)00769-4

Nebhinani, N., Pareek, V., & Grover, S. (2014). Late-life psychosis: An overview. *Journal of Geriatric Mental Health, 1*, 60. https://doi.org/10.4103/2348-9995.152424

Noreen, N., Abdullah, M., & Lalani, N. (2021). Geriatric care in Pakistan: Current realities and way forward. *Pakistan Journal of Public Health, 11*(4), 214–219. https://doi.org/10.32413/pjph.v11i4.872

Pilania, M., Yadav, V., Bairwa, M., Behera, P., Gupta, S. D., Khurana, H., Mohan, V., Baniya, G., & Poongothai, S. (2019). Prevalence of depression among the elderly (60 years and above) population in India, 1997–2016: A systematic review and meta-analysis. *BMC Public Health, 19*, 832. https://doi.org/10.1186/s12889-019-7136-z

Rajkumar, A. P., Senthilkumar, P., Gayathri, K., Shyamsundar, G., & Jacob, K. S. (2015). Associations between the macroeconomic indicators and suicide rates in India: Two ecological studies. *Indian Journal of Psychological Medicine, 37*, 277–281. https://doi.org/10.4103/0253-7176.162917

Ramasamy, S., & Bharath, S. (2017). Clinical characteristics of patients with non-affective, non-organic, late onset psychosis. *Asian Journal of Psychiatry, 25*, 74–78. https://doi.org/10.1016/j.ajp.2016.10.017

Rangarajan, S. K., Sivakumar, P. T., Manjunatha, N., Kumar, C. N., & Math, S. B. (2021). Public health perspectives of geriatric mental health care. *Indian Journal of Psychological Medicine, 43*, S1–S7. https://doi.org/10.1177/02537176211047963

Ravindranath, V., & Sundarakumar, J. S. (2021). Changing demography and the challenge of dementia in India. *Nature Reviews. Neurology, 17*, 747–758. https://doi.org/10.1038/s41582-021-00565-x

Risal, A., Kunwar, D., & Shrestha, B. (2024). Mental health among the elderly in Nepal: Special emphasis on depression. *OBM Geriatrics, 8*, 268. https://doi.org/10.21926/obm.geriatr.2401268

Sarkar, S., Parmar, A., & Chatterjee, B. (2015). Substance use disorders in the elderly: A review. *Journal of Geriatric Mental Health, 2*, 74. https://doi.org/10.4103/2348-9995.174271

Rao, T. S., Ismail, S., Darshan, M. S., & Tandon, A. (2015). Sexual disorders among elderly: An epidemiological study in south Indian rural population. *Indian Journal of Psychiatry, 57*, 236–241. https://doi.org/10.4103/0019-5545.166618

Scicutella, A. (2000). Late-life obsessive-compulsive disorder and Huntington's disease. *The Journal of Neuropsychiatry and Clinical Neurosciences, 12*, 288–289. https://doi.org/10.1176/jnp.12.2.288

Shaji, K. S., Arun Kishore, N. R., Praveen Lal, K., Pinto, C., & Trivedi, J. K. (2004). Better mental health care for older people in India. *Indian Journal of Psychiatry, 46*, 367–372.

Shidhaye, R., Sikander, S., Jordans, M., De Silva, P., & Chatterjee, S. (2014). Mental health programs and policies in South Asia: Initiatives and obstacles. In J. K. Trivedi & A. Tripathi (Eds.), *Mental health in South Asia: Ethics, resources, programs and legislation* (pp. 95–111). Springer Netherlands. https://doi.org/10.1007/978-94-017-9017-8_7

Sivakumar, P. T., Mukku, S. S. R., Kar, N., Manjunatha, N., Phutane, V. H., Sinha, P., Kumar, C. N., & Math, S. B. (2020). Geriatric telepsychiatry: Promoting access to geriatric mental health care beyond the physical barriers. *Indian Journal of Psychological Medicine, 42*(5_suppl), 41S–46S. https://doi.org/10.1177/0253717620958380

Sixel-Döring, F., Muntean, M.-L., Petersone, D., Leha, A., Lang, E., Mollenhauer, B., & Trenkwalder, C. (2023). The increasing prevalence of REM sleep behavior disorder with parkinson's disease progression: A polysomnography-supported study. *Movement Disorders Clinical Practice, 10*, 1769–1776. https://doi.org/10.1002/mdc3.13908

Stranges, S., Tigbe, W., Gómez-Olivé, F. X., Thorogood, M., & Kandala, N.-B. (2012). Sleep problems: An emerging global epidemic? Findings from the indepth who-sage study among more than 40,000 older adults from 8 countries across Africa and Asia. *Sleep, 35*, 1173–1181. https://doi.org/10.5665/sleep.2012

Subramanyam, A. A., Jahnavi Kedare, Singh, O. P., & Pinto, C. (2018). Clinical practice guidelines for geriatric anxiety disorders. *Indian Journal of Psychiatry, 60*, S371. https://doi.org/10.4103/0019-5545.224476

Sun, F., Chima, E., Wharton, T., & Iyengar, V. (2020). National policy actions on dementia in the Americas and Asia-Pacific: Consensus and challenges. *Revista Panamericana de Salud Pública, 44*, 1. https://doi.org/10.26633/RPSP.2020.2

Tanira, S., Shahriah, S., Amin, R., Sharmin, S., Shaikh, M. A. K., & Taha, S. F. (2022). Mental healthcare of elderly population of Bangladesh: Current situation and challenges. *Journal of Psychiatrists' Association of Nepal, 11*, 32–36. https://doi.org/10.3126/jpan.v11i1.53868

Vidyasagaran, A. L., McDaid, D., Faisal, M. R., Nasir, M., Muliyala, K. P., Thekkumkara, S., Wright, J., Huque, R., Benkalkar, S., & Siddiqi, N. (2023). Prevalence of mental disorders in South Asia: A systematic review of reviews. *Cambridge Prisms: Global Mental Health, 10*, Article e78. https://doi.org/10.1017/gmh.2023.72

Volpe, U., Amin, H., Ayinde, O. O., Burns, A., Chan, W. C., David, R., Dejanovic, S. D., et al. (2020). Pathways to care for people with dementia: An international multicentre study. *International Journal of Geriatric Psychiatry, 35*, 163–173. https://doi.org/10.1002/gps.5223

World Health Organization. (2015). World report on ageing and health.

World Health Organization. (2022). *Tackling abuse of older people: Five priorities for the United Nations decade of healthy ageing (2021–2030).*

World Health Organization. (2025). Violence info—Abuse of older people. http://apps.who.int/violence-info/abuse-of-older-people. Accessed 6/January.

Geriatric Psychiatry in Bangladesh: Current Status and Ways Ahead

S. M. Yasir Arafat and Atiqul Haq Mazumder

Abstract Bangladesh is one of the most populated countries in the world and caters to more than 15 million aged 60 years and above with a proportion of more than 9% of the total population. Among the age groups, psychiatric disorders were most prevalent in the geriatric age in Bangladesh. However, mental illness among this group remains under-diagnosed, and geriatric psychiatry is a neglected entity in the country. There is a lack of academic attention, research, and specialized mental health services for geriatric populations in Bangladesh. In this chapter, we discuss the proportion of the geriatric population, the burden of mental health problems among the elderly, available mental health services, existing programs and policies on geriatric mental health, available evidence and research gaps, enduring challenges, and ways ahead in Bangladesh.

Keywords Geriatric psychiatry · Old age psychiatry · Bangladesh · Psychiatry · Mental health · Psychiatric services

1 Introduction

There are more than 1 billion people with 60 years and above, which will rise to 1.4 billion in 2023. Among this elderly population, about 14% people are living with a psychiatric disorder (World Health Organization, 2023). The psychiatric disorders attributed to 10.6% of the global disability estimated by *disability-adjusted life years*

S. M. Y. Arafat (✉)
Bangladesh Specialized Hospital, Dhaka, Bangladesh
e-mail: arafatdmc62@gmail.com

Biomedical Research Foundation, Dhaka, Bangladesh

A. H. Mazumder
University of Oulu, Oulu, Finland

N. Kar et al. (eds.), *Geriatric Psychiatry in South Asia*, South Asian Perspectives in Mental Health and Psychology , https://doi.org/10.1007/978-981-96-7469-5_2

(DALYs) in the elderly group. Among the disorders, depression, and anxiety disorders are the most common psychiatric illnesses in the geriatric populations. Additionally, more than one in four suicides (27.2%) happen in this age group (World Health Organization, 2023).

Bangladesh is an Islamic country located in South Asia with a lower-middle income category. It has an area of 147,570 km^2 that caters to about 170 million populations (Bangladesh Bureau of Statistics, 2024). According to the latest census (2022, adjusted population), about 70% of the population lives in rural areas and 9.3% of the population is aged 60 years and above. Likewise, the global trend, the proportion of the elderly population has been increasing day by day in Bangladesh from 5.7–9.3% [5.7% in 1974, 6.4% in 2001, 7.5% in 2011, and 9.3% in 2022] (Bangladesh Bureau of Statistics, 2024; Barikdar et al., 2016). This can be attributed to the population pyramid of Bangladesh, success in attaining health-related *Sustainable Development Goals* [cutting down maternal and child mortality] (GBD 2019 Bangladesh Burden of Disease Collaborators, 2023). Therefore, the life expectancy of people has increased from < 50- > 73 years [<50 years in the 1970s, and < 60 years in the 1980s] (Macrotrends, 2024; Statista, 2024).

Geriatric psychiatry is a neglected domain of psychiatric services in Bangladesh. It has been poorly studied as evidenced by the number of available published articles. We published a recent chapter focusing on the country's demography, epidemiology, and available mental health services (Arafat et al., 2024). In the current chapter, we discuss the proportion of the geriatric population, the burden of mental health problems among the elderly, available mental health services, existing programs and policies on geriatric mental health, available evidence and research gaps, enduring challenges, and ways ahead in Bangladesh. Additionally, there are variations in categorizing older adults in different times and different cultures. It was considered 55 years in the literature of the 1950s and 1960s. However, in recent days 65 years has been frequently considered old age (Fischer et al., 2013). In this chapter, we considered 60 years as the geriatric group (Ates Bulut et al., 2018; Barikdar et al., 2016).

2 Mental Health Burden Among Older Adults in Bangladesh

2.1 Findings from National Mental Health Surveys

The first nationwide community-based survey in Bangladesh was performed between 2003 and 2005 to determine the prevalence of psychiatric disorders (Firoz et al., 2006). The study identified the prevalence of psychiatric disorders was 16.1% and those over 60 years were more vulnerable to psychiatric disorders (Firoz et al., 2006).

The latest (2021) nationwide mental health survey revealed the rate of mental disorders was 18.7% (Alam et al., 2024). The survey found the highest (20.2%)

prevalence of psychiatric disorders among the geriatric age group (60 years and above).

2.2 *Findings from Empirical Studies*

Multiple cross-sectional studies in Bangladesh assessed mental health among older adults (Table 1). The studies assessed mostly depression and dementia as outcome variables. The prevalence indicates a higher rate than the adult population in the country. Co-occurrence of physical and mental disorders was commonly noted among older adults visited at a geriatric clinic in a super specialized mental hospital (Jesmin et al., 2022).

A cross-sectional study in rural Bangladesh examined 471 individuals over 60 (Palmer et al., 2014). It included physical exams, interviews about socio-demographic and related factors, and blood tests to evaluate nutrition and clinical health. The number of dementia cases, assessed using DSM-IV standards, was 11.5% for questionable and 3.6% for definite dementia. Dementia risk increases with age and decreases with educational attainment. Malnourishment markedly raised the likelihood of developing dementia by almost six-fold, while participation in social activities lowered this risk. The study highlights the need for further research on malnutrition and dementia in low-income countries.

Another study conducted in a rural area included 130 healthy participants aged 40 and older, who did not have hypertension, cardiovascular diseases, liver or kidney diseases, or diabetes (Das et al., 2014). Utilizing the *Geriatric Depression Scale* (GDS-30), the study found that 42% of participants exhibited mild depression, while 17% experienced severe depression. Depression was 2.8 times more prevalent among females and individuals aged 60 and older. Higher risk factors included a vegetable-based diet, low income, and poor wealth index. These results remained consistent after adjusting for vitamin B_{12}, folic acid, hepatic function, and hemoglobin. This research emphasizes the occurrence of depression in healthy older adults and the impact of factors such as gender, age, diet, and socioeconomic status on the risk of depression.

A sampling study by Uddin et al. (2019) assessed dementia risk, including mild cognitive impairment (MCI) and Alzheimer's, in 390 adults aged 60–70. The *Takeda Three Colors Combination (TTCC)* test and *Clinical Dementia Rating* were used. Among 60–65 year-olds, 154 had MCI, 76 had mild dementia, and 4 had severe dementia. For 66–70 year-olds, 75 had MCI, 36 had mild dementia, and 2 had severe dementia. The TTCC test demonstrated 75% sensitivity for subtle dementia and 58% sensitivity for mild cognitive impairment, along with a specificity of 52%. Another study found behavioral problems were more prominent among persons with severe dementia than mild and moderate forms (Tarannum et al., 2014).

A study (Wahlin et al., 2015) used the *Self-Reporting Questionnaire (SRQ 20)* to assess depressive symptoms in 625 individuals, with 471 also evaluated for depression and suicidal ideation. Depressive symptoms were found in 45% of participants,

Table 1 Epidemiology of geriatric mental illnesses in Bangladesh

Study	Population	Assessment tools	Key Findings
Islam et al. (2024)	420 (case 210, control 210) rural geriatric persons (60 +)	GDS-15	It assessed the association between social capital and depression and revealed that geriatric depression was associated with sex, nuptiality, educational attainment, occupation, family dynamics (type, size, monthly income, interpersonal trust, and reciprocity
Palmer et al. (2014)	471 individuals aged 60 + in rural Bangladesh	DSM-IV standards, physical exams, interviews, blood tests	Dementia prevalence: 11.5% questionable, 3.6% definite. Increased risk with age, decreased with higher education. Malnutrition raised dementia risk nearly six-fold
Das et al. (2014)	130 healthy individuals aged 40 + (60 + persons 44) in rural Mirzapur	GDS-30	42% had mild depression, 17% severe. Depression 2.8 times more common in females and those aged 60 + . Risk factors: vegetable-based diet, low income, poor wealth index
Uddin et al. (2019)	390 older adults aged 60–70	TTCC test, Clinical Dementia Rating	Among 60–65 year-olds: 154 had MCI, 76 mild dementia, 4 severe dementia. Among 66–70 year-olds: 75 had MCI, 36 mild dementia, 2 severe dementia. TTCC test: 75% sensitivity for mild dementia, 58% for MCI
Wahlin et al. (2015)	625 individuals, with 471 evaluated for depression and suicidal ideation	SRQ 20	45% had depressive symptoms, highest rate (70%) in older females. Suicidal ideation in 23%. Risk factors: female gender, low education, living without partners. Protective factors: living with children, good social support
Uddin et al. (2017)	280 participants aged 60–75 from 10 villages in Lakshmipur and Noakhali	QOL assessment, depression evaluation	84.6% of participants had a perception of having moderate QOL, and 13.9% had low QOL in the psychological area. Significant moderate negative correlation between QOL and depression
Islam (2019)	2425 adults (1249 women) aged 18–90 in Narail upazilla	Kessler 10-item questionnaire	Moderate and severe distress was found among older adults (60–90 years) than adults (18–59). Females had more severe distress than males

(continued)

Table 1 (continued)

Study	Population	Assessment tools	Key Findings
Disu et al. (2019)	168 participants (Female-100, Male-68 males)	GDS-15	Geriatric depression prevalence: 36.9%. Higher rates in the 71–80 (41.4%) and 60–65 (38.5%) age groups compared to 66–70 (31.3%). Lower overall prevalence due to the exclusion of those with current illnesses
Mistry et al. (2021)	1032 elderly individuals (aged 60 +)	GDS-15 via telephone interviews	40.1% had depressive symptoms. The highest prevalence was noted in the oldest age group (52.7%), women (48.9%), widowed (51.6%), illiterate (43.9%), poor income (62.1%), living isolated (68.4%), and those with COVID-19 infection (62.5%)
Rahman et al. (2020)	400 individuals aged 65 +	Assessment of depressive symptoms	55.5% had depressive symptoms: 23% mild, 19% moderate, 13.5% severe. Risk factors: advanced age, gender, living situation, marital status, medical conditions, visual problems, past falls, loneliness, fear of falling
Islam et al. (2021)	600 elderly participants (aged ≥ 60) from three rural communities	GDS-15, MNA Short-Form	No significant gender difference. Malnutrition higher in depressed group (56%) vs. non-depressed (18%). Malnourished 3 times more likely to experience depression. Depression more common among unemployed, lower/middle class, poor diet, single, tobacco users
Alam et al. (2021)	400 participants (aged 60 +)	MNA, GDS	84% had depressive symptoms. Higher rates of malnutrition and depression among males. Malnourished individuals had a higher likelihood of depressive symptoms
Naheed et al. (2023)	2795 individuals aged 60 + in Bangladesh	MMSE	Dementia prevalence: 8.0%. Twofold increased rate in females than males, nine-fold increased rates among aged 90 + than 60–69. No education three times more likely than primary education
Akter et al. (2023)	200 elderly individuals (aged 60–80) in old homes in Dhaka	MMSE, GDS	43%, 36%, and 19.5% had moderate, mild, and no cognitive impairment respectively. Severe depression in 56% of participants
Alam et al. (2023)	430 geriatric Rohingyas	MNA Short-Form, GDS Short-Form	Malnutrition in 25.3%, 29.1% at risk of it. GD in 57.9%. Higher GD rates among malnourished. Recommends prioritizing geriatric malnutrition and GD

(continued)

Table 1 (continued)

Study	Population	Assessment tools	Key Findings
Tabassum et al. (2023)	230 elderly outpatients (aged 60–80) in Dhaka city	GDS-15 via in-person interviews	81.7% prevalence of depression: 52.6% mild, 25.2% moderate, 3.9% severe. Higher rates among divorced, separated, never married, widowed, retired, or jobless. More prone: those with education below primary level, socially isolated. Regular coffee drinkers were less likely to have depressive symptoms
Harun et al. (2022)	old care home residents	SCID	The prevalence of psychiatric disorder was 41.3%, depression 15.9%, anxiety 18.1%, and dementia 6.5%. Residents living in a private setting had more depressive and anxiety disorders
Haq et al. (2015)	Geriatric outpatients	DSM-5	Dementia was present in 5.1% of respondents

with higher (70%) prevalence in elderly women. The idea of suicide was present in 23%. Risk factors included female gender, low education, and living without partners; while living with children and having good social support were protective factors.

In 2017, a cross-sectional study (Uddin et al., 2017) assessed the quality of life (QoL) and its association with depressive disorder among older adults in Bangladesh. It included 280 participants aged 60–75 from 10 villages in Lakshmipur and Noakhali, excluding those with severe chronic diseases or needing assisted living. The study revealed that 84.6% of participants rated their psychological QoL as moderate, while 13.9% rated it as low. Additionally, there was a moderate negative association between QoL and depressive symptoms which was statistically significant.

A study in Narail Upazilla included 2425 adults (1249 females) with 18–90 years of age (Islam, 2019) and used the Kessler 10-item questionnaire to assess mental agony. Of the participants, 1,278 were aged 18 to 59, while 1,147 were between 60 and 90. The older adults exhibited significantly higher levels of moderate and severe mental stress compared to their younger counterparts. An intense problem was more common in females, with the gender disparity increasing with age.

A 2019 sampling study evaluated geriatric depression among 168 participants (Female-100, Male-68) in Patuakhali town and villages from its outskirts using the GDS-15 (Disu et al., 2019). The prevalence of depression among the elderly population was 36.9%. Higher rates were observed in the 71–80 (41.4%) and 60–65 (38.5%) age groups compared to that of 66–70 (31.3%). The lower overall prevalence rate may be attributed to the exclusion of elderly individuals with existing health conditions.

In 2020, a study involving 1,032 elderly individuals (aged 60 and older) was carried out through interviews over telephone using the GDS-15 (Mistry et al., 2021). Depression was found in 40.1% of the study population. The highest prevalence was among the oldest age group (52.7%), women (48.9%), widowed individuals (51.6%), illiterate participants (43.9%), those with the lowest family income (62.1%), those dwelling independently (68.4%), and those who received information on COVID-19 (62.5%).

One study by Rahman et al. (2020) examined depressive symptoms in 400 individuals aged 65 + . The prevalence rate was 55.5%, among which 23% was experiencing mild depression, 19% moderate depression, and 13.5% severe depression. Significant risk factors included advanced age, gender, living situation, marital status, general medical conditions, visual problems, loneliness, and history or fear of fall.

Another 2019 cross-sectional comparative study (Islam et al., 2021) involved 600 elderly participants (aged $\geq$ 60 years) from three rural communities. It included 300 patients with depression (cases) and 300 normal elderly individuals (controls), adjusted with age and dwelling area. Data collection involved a semi-structured questionnaire, using the GDS-15 to assess depression and the *Mini Nutritional Assessment* (MNA)-Short-Form to evaluate nutritional status. There were no significant gender differences observed between the depressed group (44% men, 56% women) and the non-depressed group (46% men, 54% women). The depressed group suffered significantly more from malnutrition compared to the non-depressed group. Participants who were malnourished were approximately three times more likely to suffer from depression. Depression was more prevalent among unemployed individuals, those from lower and middle socioeconomic status, and those with poor dietary habits, single, and smokers.

One community-based transactional study with 400 participants aimed to determine the prevalence and intensity of depression and malnourishment among the geriatric population (Alam et al., 2021). The average age of the participants was 72.1 $\pm$ 7.0 years, with an equal distribution of males and females. Excluded were those institutionalized or with terminal illnesses. The MNA was used to assess nourishment and GDS was used to assess depression. About 84% showed depressive symptoms, with higher rates of malnutrition and depression among males. Malnourished individuals had higher risks to develop depression. Maintaining good physical health, adopting a healthy lifestyle, and having a supportive family environment can contribute to lowering depression among the geriatric populations.

Another study involving 2795 individuals aged 60 years or more in Bangladesh found an 8.0% dementia prevalence (Naheed et al., 2023). Dementia was measured using the *Mini Mental State Examination (MMSE)*, with scores below 24 indicating dementia. The prevalence of dementia was influenced by age, sex, educational attainment, and profession, but not by dwelling in a city or village or by socioeconomic conditions. Twofold increased rate in females than males, nine fold increased rates among aged 90 + then 60–69. Additionally, individuals without any education were three times more likely to develop dementia than those who attended primary school. Another study found that age (positively) and social engagement (negatively) were associated with cognitive impairment (Hossain et al., 2023). Engagement with outdoor activities was associated with positive mental health outcomes (Tohan et al., 2024).

A 2019 cross-sectional survey was conducted on 200 older adults (aged 60–80) living in old age homes in Dhaka (Akter et al., 2023). MMSE and GDS were used to assess cognition and depression respectively. The study found that 43%, 36%, and 19.5% had moderate, mild, and no cognitive impairment respectively. Severe depression was found in 56% of participants. Another study found that depression was more common among females than males (Tithy et al., 2022).

A community-based transactional study was conducted among elderly Rohingya populations in Bangladesh, from November 2021 to March 2022. The study involved 430 participants aged 60 and above (Alam et al., 2023). Using the MNA Short-Form and GDS Short-Form, the study found malnutrition in 25.3% of the study population, and risk of malnutrition in 29.1% of the study population. Geriatric depression (GD) was present in 57.9%, with 17.5% also experiencing malnutrition. Depression rates were significantly higher among malnourished individuals. The finding recommends prioritizing geriatric malnutrition and GD in Cox's Bazar.

A cross-sectional study in Dhaka city involved in-person interviews with 230 older adults in outpatients (aged 60–80) to assess depressive disorder using the GDS-15 (Tabassum et al., 2023). The study found an 81.7% prevalence of depression, with 52.6% mild, 25.2% moderate, and 3.9% severe. Higher rates of depression were observed among those who were divorced, separated, never married, widowed, retired, or jobless. People with less than primary education and those who were socially isolated were more susceptible to depression. Regular coffee drinkers were less likely to have depressive symptoms, due to the association with higher socioeconomic status.

A case–control study with 420 geriatric persons assessed the association between social capital and depression in rural areas (Islam et al., 2024). It revealed that geriatric depression was associated with sex, nuptiality, educational attainment, occupation, and family dynamics (type, size, monthly income, interpersonal trust, and reciprocity.

DSM- Diagnostic and Statistical Manual for Mental Disorders, SCID- structured clinical interview for DSM-IV, GDS- Geriatric Depression Scale, GD- Geriatric depression; MMSE- Mini Mental State Examination, MNA- Mini Nutritional Assessment, SRQ- Self-Reporting Questionnaire, TTCC- Takeda Three Colors Combination; QoL- Quality of Life.

2.3 Suicidal Behavior Among Geriatric Population

It is an extremely under-studied entity in Bangladesh. One study assessed suicidal ideation among 471 older adults and found the prevalence of suicidal ideation was 23% (Wahlin et al., 2015). It was significantly higher among females, illiterate, and single persons. We did not find any other studies on geriatric suicidal behavior and we do not have any national data-base of suicidal behavior with age distribution (Kabir et al., 2023).

Studies with suicidal behavior among general populations revealed a lower rate among the older adults. The proportion of suicides in old age ranges from 0.1–11.5% with wide variations in sample size, characteristics, and study method (Table 2). One study with 403 suicidal behavior (attempt and suicide) collected reports from six daily newspapers and found 3 cases (0.7%) in the geriatric age group (Arafat et al.,

Table 2 Suicidal behavior among older adults in Bangladesh

Study	Sample size	Sample	Suicidal behavior	Number of suicidal behavior > 60 years	% of Suicidal behavior
Arafat et al. (2020a)	403	Reports of 6 print newspapers	Suicidal attempt and suicide	3	0.7%
Arafat et al. (2020b)	199	Reports of 4 online news portals	Suicidal attempt and suicide	5	2.5%
Shah et al. (2018)	56	1 year data of a suicide prevention clinic	Suicidal thought and attempt	2	3.6%
Arafat et al. (2018)	358	Reports of 8 Bangla online news portals	Suicidal attempt and suicide	5	0.1%
Shah et al. (2017)	271	News reports of 6 national daily newspapers	Suicidal attempt and suicide	7	2.6%
Salam et al. (2017)	95	Household census of seven sub-districts	Suicidal attempt and suicide	4	4.2%
Reza et al. (2013)	113	A community-based case–control study	Suicidal attempt and suicide	6	5.3%
Mashreky et al. (2013)	61	Cross-sectional study with multistage cluster sampling	Suicide	7	11.5%

2020a, 2020b). The maximum proportion was noted in an epidemiological study with 61 suicides where the proportion of geriatric suicide was 11.5% (Mashreky et al., 2013). However, it is important to consider the methodology and potential under-reporting of suicidal behavior due to being a criminal offense (Kabir et al., 2023).

3 Available Services in Geriatric Psychiatry in Bangladesh

Bangladesh lacks adequate resources and specialized services for geriatric psychiatry. Available services are inadequate, disperse, and inequitably distributed.

3.1 Conventional Services

Psychiatrists are not available in Bangladesh's health delivery services system at the primary and secondary levels as there is no post (Arafat, 2024; Government of The People's Republic of Bangladesh, 2022). They are only available at tertiary care level hospitals and institutions. Additionally, geriatric psychiatry has not been considered a separate entity. Therefore, geriatric psychiatry services in primary and secondary care are literally absent.

There is a department at the *National Institute of Mental Health (NIMH)*, Dhaka, the premier mental health services provider in the capital, the *Department of Geriatric and Organic Psychiatry* which was started in 2001. Currently, there are 24 inpatient beds for males and 20 beds for female old age psychiatric patients (Arafat et al., 2024). There are some specialized clinic activities and out-patient services at NIMH.

Pabna Mental Hospital (PMH) is the earliest establishment of mental health services in Bangladesh, which contains 500 inpatient beds and regular outpatients services (Arafat, 2024). However, it has no specialized unit for geriatric psychiatry. Also, likewise other medical colleges, the *Bangabandhu Sheikh Mujib Medical University* (BSMMU) has no specialized services for geriatric populations. The *National Institute of Neuroscience (NINS)* runs a dementia clinic on Thursday of the week. There is a geriatric medicine unit at the *Dhaka Medical College Hospital* with 28 inpatient beds which was started in 2014 (Kahhar, 2015; Nayak, 2018). However, there are no specialized geriatric psychiatric services there.

Old Rehabilitation Centre (Boyoshko Punorbashon Kendro), is the largest old home established in 1987 in Gazipur (Ferdous et al., 2022). It accommodates and provides support to about 1200 geriatric people (Nayak, 2018). It is important to mention that mental health services are not available in old home settings in Bangladesh. There are some other Non-Government Organizations (NGOs) working in the sector like *Bangladesh Association for the Aged and Institute of Geriatric Medicine (BAAIGM)* (popular as *Probin Hitoishi Sangha (PHS)*, started in 1960), *Shailan Probeen Nibash, Subarta Trust, Sir William Beveridge Foundation, Senior Citizen Hospital, Parents lounge, Retired officers Welfare Association* and *Retired Police Officers Welfare Association, Rehabilitation Center for Aged and Child, Service Center for Elderly People,* and *Elderly Development Initiative* (Arafat et al., 2024; Kabir et al., 2016; Nayak, 2018).

3.2 Digital Services in Old Age in Psychiatry

There are no specialized tele-psychiatry services for elderly populations in Bangladesh. However, with the expansion of modern technology and smartphones, telemedicine and generic tele-psychiatric services are available in the country. WhatsApp, Messenger, IMO, FaceTime, and Skype are the popular applications for this. Telepsychiatry services are being provided by NIMH, Dhaka at Government level

(Arafat, 2024). Different non-specific, non-specialized telehealth platforms are available like *Maya, Moner Bondhu, Daktarbhai, DocTime* (Arafat, 2024; Muhammad & Arafat, 2024).

4 End of Life Care

Bangladesh is one of the lowest-level countries in Palliative care (Parveen, 2024). Currently, there are around 600,000 people in Bangladesh in need of palliative care. Among them, less than 1% have access to the desired care (Chowdhury et al., 2021). Palliative care in Bangladesh has been formally started in 2007 at *Bangabandhu Sheikh Mujib Medical University (BSMMU)* as the *Centre for Palliative Care*, which was turned to the *Department of Palliative Medicine* (Chowdhury et al., 2023). Currently, there are services providers in Palliative care like *National Institute of Cancer Research and Hospital (NICRH), and Bangladesh Shishu Hospital and Institute, ASHIC, Foundation for Childhood Cancer, Hospice Bangladesh, Bangladesh Palliative & Supportive Care Foundation, Mycare* (palliative and care center of *Bangladesh Cancer Society*). Over the years, there have been several important progress in the sector. However, it is still in an infant state. Importantly, there is an extreme lack of collaboration between mental health professionals and palliative care service providers.

5 Legal and Ethical Aspects of Geriatric Psychiatry

Geriatric psychiatry in Bangladesh encounters considerable legal and ethical issues. The mental health of older adults is often overlooked, resulting in a lack of specialized services and a shortage of trained professionals (Arafat, 2024b). Legal and ethical issues in geriatric psychiatry encompass several critical concerns as follows.

5.1 Ensuring Informed Consent

One fundamental aspect is ensuring informed consent, which requires that older patients fully understand the nature of their treatment, its potential risks and benefits, and alternative options. This process can be complicated by cognitive decline or impairments that may affect a patient's ability to understand information and make decisions.

5.2 Respecting Autonomy

Respecting autonomy is another crucial ethical consideration. Older adults have the right to make their own choices about their care, but this can be challenging in situations where cognitive impairments, such as dementia, hinder their decision-making capacity. Clinicians must navigate these complexities while striving to honor the values and preferences of their patients, which may involve balancing respect for autonomy with the need to protect vulnerable individuals.

5.3 Safeguarding the Rights

On the legal side, safeguarding the rights of elderly patients is paramount, especially in cases where cognitive impairments may compromise their ability to make informed decisions. This includes ensuring that the right legal measures, such as advance directives or guardianship arrangements, are in place to protect their interests. Professionals must be vigilant in advocating for the rights of these individuals and ensuring that their dignity and autonomy are supported, even when their decision-making ability is challenged.

Overall, the intersection of ethical and legal issues in geriatric psychiatry requires a delicate balance between respecting the autonomy of older patients, protecting their rights, and providing the right care that acknowledges the complexities of aging and mental health.

6 Specialist Course and Training Opportunities in Geriatric Psychiatry

As a separate entity, geriatric psychiatry is yet to get adequate attention in Bangladesh. Still, it has been taught as a part of psychiatry in the post-graduate curriculum. There is no specialized geriatrician or geriatric psychiatrist in the country (Alam & Ostler, 2024; Arafat et al., 2024). The *University of Dhaka* runs a Masters course on Gerontology. In addition to that, there is a course on geriatric nursing with 100 marks at graduation level in the Nursing curriculum (Arafat et al., 2024; Nayak, 2018). The country also lacks any specialized training program on geriatric psychiatry. However, the NIMH (Dhaka), could be a potential facility to have experience as it contains a geriatric psychiatry unit.

7 Available Research and Gaps

The evaluation of psychiatric disorders in the elderly population is a relatively neglected field of research in Bangladesh. Notable studies have been mentioned in table 1 the reveals that the majority of the studies conducted on depression (Alam et al., 2021; Alam et al., 2023; Das et al., 2014; Disu et al., 2019; Islam et al., 2021; Rahman et al., 2020; Tabassum et al., 2023; Wahlin et al., 2015), and dementia (Akter et al., 2023; Haq et al., 2015; Naheed et al., 2023; Palmer et al., 2014; Uddin et al., 2019). One study assessed overall psychiatric morbidity among the elderly living in old home facilities (Harun et al., 2022), one study assessed overall distress (Islam, 2019), and one study assessed overall quality of life (Uddin et al., 2017). Barikdar et al. (2016), identifies three categories of vulnerability among elderly people in Bangladesh: Economic, arising from unemployment and low income; Illness, linked to chronic diseases and inadequate healthcare; and Emotional, stemming from stress, anxiety, family conflicts, and trauma (Barikdar et al., 2016). Most of the existing studies focus primarily on depression and anxiety, with minimal consideration given to neurocognitive disorders.

The enduring status indicates an extreme lack of research gaps in other domains of geriatric psychiatry, like longitudinal community-based studies, old age suicide, geriatric sexuality, culture-sensitive interventions in geriatric psychiatry, health economic analysis of geriatric mental disorders, geriatric social services, and geriatric rehabilitations.

8 Programs-Policies-Action Plans for Geriatric Mental Health

Focusing the elder population, there is a policy named *the National Policy for Older Persons 2013* (HelpAge, 2024). It highlights the availability of health care services of for geriatric populations, social facilities, education and training, awareness raising on safe water and sanitation, and nutrition (Dana et al., 2023; HelpAge, 2024). *The Parents Care Act 2013* aimed to ensure social security and responsibilities of child(ren) for their parents at old age. The law suggests that the child(ren) will be responsible for providing food, clothes, treatments, living accommodations and company. It mentions the options of filling cases against the child(ren) by the aggrieved parents. There is a lack of governmental policies by *Older People's Associations (OPAs).* Some non-governmental initiatives are on-going. There is a financial support program for the geriatric population in Bangladesh as "Social Pension" since 1998 (the Old Age Allowance Programme). It provides 500 taka (6 USD) per month to a man with over 65 years of age and to a woman with over 62 years of age (Ahmed, 2023; HelpAge, 2024; Rahman, 2020). However, only one individual from a household is allowed to receive it. Additionally, about two-thirds of the older populations do not get it. The mhGAP (Mental Health Gap Action Programme) began in 2009 to equip health care providers with the skills to recognize and treat mental health issues, including those that impact older adults (World Health Organization, 2020).

9 Current Challenges in Geriatric Mental Health and Ways Out

Geriatric psychiatry in Bangladesh faces some common challenges of mental health services in the country mentioned as high treatment gap and potential underdiagnosis, unregulated help-seeking behavior, malfunctioning referral system, poor budgetary allocation, high out-of-pocket expense, high stigma, low mental health literacy, inadequate and inequitable distribution of manpower, lack of research and inadequate data (Alam & Ostler, 2024; Arafat, 2024; Barikdar et al., 2016; Matthews et al., 2023).

There is no alternative of public mental health interest, augmented research and funding in the geriatric psychiatry field in Bangladesh. Services expansion, proper referral, and awareness raising would help to reduce the treatment gap and underdiagnosis. Increasing the social safety nets, the initiation of mental health insurance will encourage the older adults and their caregivers to seek help from conventional health services (Arafat, 2024). Special training courses, the addition of academic contents would help to ensure better services.

10 Conclusion

Geriatric psychiatry is a neglected entity in Bangladesh and its services are at an inadequate level even though the proportion of geriatric population has been increasing day by day and the psychiatric morbidities are higher than the general population. Among the disorders, depression and dementia has been studied to an extent. Proper attention and policy level implications are warranted to improve the status in the country.

References

Ahmed, N. (2023). Bangladesh needs to do better for its elderly. *The Daily Star*. https://www.thedailystar.net/opinion/views/news/bangladesh-needs-do-better-its-elderly-3470111. (Accessed 09/October/2024).

Akter, N., Banu, B., Chowdhury, S. H., Islam, K. R., Tabassum, T. T., & Hossain, S. M. (2023). Astute exploration of collective mental health events among the residents of elderly care homes. *Heliyon, 9*(7), Article e18117. https://doi.org/10.1016/j.heliyon.2023.e18117

Alam, M. F., Ahmed, H. U., Alam, M. T., Sarkar, M., Khan, N. M., Uddin, M. J., & Sarkar, A. A. (2024). Community prevalence of psychiatric disorders: Findings from a nationwide survey in Bangladesh. *Asian Journal of Psychiatry, 92*, Article 103897. https://doi.org/10.1016/j.ajp.2023.103897

Alam, R. B., & Ostler, T. (2024). Geriatric mental health practice with dementia patients in Bangladesh: Challenges and future directions. *Asian Journal of Psychiatry, 94*, Article 103945. https://doi.org/10.1016/j.ajp.2024.103945

Alam, M. M., Das, R., Clara, A. A., Mohsin, F. M., Rumi, M. A. H., Wahab, A., Hasan, M. A., & Hawlader, M. D. H. (2023). The assessment of geriatric malnutrition, geriatric depression and associated co-morbidities among forcibly displaced Myanmar nationals in Bangladesh. *Public Health Nutrition, 26*(10), 2048–2055. https://doi.org/10.1017/S1368980023001556

Alam, M. R., Karmokar, S., Reza, S., Kabir, M. R., Ghosh, S., & Mamun, M. A. A. (2021). Geriatric malnutrition and depression: Evidence from elderly home care population in Bangladesh. *Preventive Medicine Reports, 23*, Article 101478. https://doi.org/10.1016/j.pmedr.2021.101478

Arafat, S. M. Y. (2024). Mental health services in Bangladesh. In S. M. Y. Arafat (Eds.), *Mental health in Bangladesh.* Springer. https://doi.org/10.1007/978-981-97-0610-5_3

Arafat, S. M. Y., Mazumder, A. H., Maruf, M. M. (2024). Geriatric psychiatry in Bangladesh. In: Arafat, S.M.Y. (Eds.), *Mental health in Bangladesh.* Springer. https://doi.org/10.1007/978-981-97-0610-5_18

Arafat, S. M. Y., Mali, B., & Akter, H. (2020a). Characteristics, methods and precipitating events of suicidal behaviors in Bangladesh: A year-round content analysis of six national newspapers. *Neurology Psychiatry and Brain Research, 36*, 14–17. https://doi.org/10.1016/j.npbr.2020.02.005

Arafat, S. M. Y., Mali, B., & Akter, H. (2020b). Characteristics of suicidal attempts in Bangla online news portals. *Neurology, Psychiatry and Brain Research, 36*, 83–85. https://doi.org/10.1016/j.npbr.2020.03.004

Arafat, S. M. Y., Mali, B., & Akter, H. (2018). Demography and risk factors of suicidal behavior in Bangladesh: A retrospective online news content analysis. *Asian Journal of Psychiatry, 36*, 96–99. https://doi.org/10.1016/j.ajp.2018.07.008

Ates Bulut, E., Soysal, P., & Isik, A. T. (2018). Frequency and coincidence of geriatric syndromes according to age groups: Single-center experience in Turkey between 2013 and 2017. *Clinical Interventions in Aging, 13*, 1899–1905. https://doi.org/10.2147/CIA.S180281

Bangladesh Bureau of Statistics. (2024). Population & Housing Census 2022. https://bbs.gov.bd/site/page/47856ad0-7e1c-4aab-bd78-892733bc06eb/Population-&-Housing. (Accessed 28/September/2024).

Barikdar, A., Ahmed, T., & Lasker, S. P. (2016). The situation of the elderly in Bangladesh. *Bangladesh Journal of Bioethics, 7*(1), 27–36. https://doi.org/10.3329/bioethics.v7i1.29303

Chowdhury, M. K., Saikot, S., Farheen, N., Ahmad, N., Alam, S., & Connor, S. R. (2023). Impact of community palliative care on quality of life among cancer patients in Bangladesh. *International Journal of Environmental Research and Public Health, 20*(15), 6443. https://doi.org/10.3390/ijerph20156443

Chowdhury, M. K., Sarker, M., & Ahmad, N. (2021). A home-based palliative care pilot project for the patients and families with incurable diseases in Bangladesh. *BIRDEM Medical Journal, 11*(3), 202–211. https://doi.org/10.3329/birdem.v11i3.55221

Das, J., Farzana, F. D., Ferdous, F., Ahmed, S, Tegenfeldt, S., Paul, R. C., & Das, S. K. (2014). Factors associated with elderly depression among rural Bangladeshi individuals. *American Journal of Psychiatry and Neuroscience, 2*(1), 1–7. https://doi.org/10.11648/j.ajpn.20140201.11

Dana, G. P. T., Hossain, A. H. M. K., & Hasan, S. (2023). Aging policy of Bangladesh: Issues and challenges for implementation. *Social Science Review, 40*(2), 225–243. https://doi.org/10.3329/ssr.v40i2.72207

Disu, T. R., Anne, N. J., Griffiths, M. D., & Mamun, M. A. (2019). Risk factors of geriatric depression among elderly Bangladeshi people: A pilot interview study. *Asian Journal of Psychiatry, 44*, 163–169. https://doi.org/10.1016/j.ajp.2019.07.050

Ferdous, J., Ali, A., & Ferdousi, A. (2022). Level of satisfaction of geriatric people about services provided by an old home at Gajipur Bangladesh. *Ibrahim Cardiac Medical Journal, 12*(2), 46–52.

Firoz, A. H. M., Karim, M. E., Alam, M. F., Rahman, A. H. M. M., & Zaman, M. M. (2006). Prevalence, medical care, awareness and attitude towards mental illness in Bangladesh. *Bangladesh Journal of Psychiatry, 20*(1), 9–32.

Fischer, C. E., Ismail, Z., & Rapoport, M. J. (2013). Geriatric psychiatry or psychogeriatrics? Partnership at the CAGP/CCSMH 2012 scientific meeting. *Canadian Geriatrics Journal : CGJ, 16*(1), 3–5. https://doi.org/10.5770/cgj.16.66

GBD 2019 Bangladesh Burden of Disease Collaborators. (2023). The burden of diseases and risk factors in Bangladesh, 1990–2019: A systematic analysis for the Global Burden of Disease Study 2019. *The Lancet. Global health, 11*(12), e1931–e1942. https://doi.org/10.1016/S2214-109X(23)00432-1

Government of The People's Republic of Bangladesh. (2022). National Mental Health Strategic Plan, 2020–2030. https://old.dghs.gov.bd/index.php/bd/home/6171-nmu-2020-2030. (Accessed 21/December/2024).

Harun, H. M., Shah, M. A., Mullick, M., Ahmed, A. U., Hasan, M. M., & Solaiman, M. A. (2022). Socio-demographic variation among the elderly people living in old care home. *Bangladesh Journal of Psychiatry, 36*(2), 35–38. https://doi.org/10.3329/bjpsy.v36i2.72751

Haq, A. I., Sarkar, M., Roy, S., & Alam, M. F. (2015). Dementia among older patients attending National Institute of Mental Health (NIMH), Dhaka Bangladesh. *Bangladesh Journal of Psychiatry, 29*(1), 5–9. https://doi.org/10.3329/bjpsy.v29i1.32744

HelpAge. (2024). Ageing population in Bangladesh. https://ageingasia.org/ageing-population-bangladesh/. (Accessed 09/October/2024).

Hossain, Z., Das, J. K., Fahim, N. F., et al. (2023). Prevalence and predictors of cognitive impairment among the elderly in Bangladesh. *J Public Health (Berl.), 31*, 529–537. https://doi.org/10.1007/s10389-021-01569-z

Islam, M. Z., Prue, E., Farjana, S., Al Fidah, M. F., & Efa, S. S. (2024). Cognitive social capital and geriatric depression: A community-based case-control study among the rural elderly people of Bangladesh. *Global Mental Health (Cambridge, England), 11*, Article e89. https://doi.org/10.1017/gmh.2024.72

Islam, F. M. A. (2019). Psychological distress and its association with socio-demographic factors in a rural district in Bangladesh: A cross-sectional study. *PLoS ONE, 14*(3), Article e0212765. https://doi.org/10.1371/journal.pone.0212765

Islam, M. Z., Disu, T. R., Farjana, S., & Rahman, M. M. (2021). Malnutrition and other risk factors of geriatric depression: A community-based comparative cross-sectional study in older adults in rural Bangladesh. *BMC Geriatrics, 21*(1), 572. https://doi.org/10.1186/s12877-021-02535-w

Jesmin, H., Sarkar, A. A., Ahmed, H. U., & Zannat, H. (2022). Psychiatric and physical comorbidity in elderly attending the geriatric clinic of a psychiatric hospital. *Bangladesh Journal of Medicine, 33*(1), 40–43. https://doi.org/10.3329/bjm.v33i1.56788

Kabir, R., Hasan, M. R., Arafat, S. M. Y. (2023). Epidemiology of suicide and data quality in Bangladesh. In S. M. Y. Arafat & M. M. Khan (Eds.), *Suicide in Bangladesh. New perspectives in behavioral & health sciences*. Springer. https://doi.org/10.1007/978-981-99-0289-7_1

Kabir, R., Kabir, M., Uddin, M. S. G., Ferdous, N., & Chowdhury, M. R. K. (2016). Elderly population growth in Bangladesh: Preparedness in public and private sectors. *IOSR Journal of Humanities and Social Science, 21*, 58–73. https://doi.org/10.9790/0837-2108025873

Kahhar, M. A. (2015). Geriatric medicine: Bangladesh perspective. *Journal of Bangladesh College of Physicians and Surgeons, 33*, 63–64.

Macrotrends. (2024). Bangladesh life expectancy 1950–2023. https://www.macrotrends.net/countries/BGD/bangladesh/life-expectancy#:~:text=The%20life%20expectancy%20for%20Bangladesh,a%200.39%25%20increase%20from%202019. (Accessed 29/September/2024).

Mashreky, S. R., Rahman, F., & Rahman, A. (2013). Suicide kills more than 10,000 people every year in Bangladesh. *Archives of Suicide Research, 17*(4), 387–396. https://doi.org/10.1080/13811118.2013.801809

Matthews, N. R., Porter, G. J., Varghese, M., Sapkota, N., Khan, M. M., Lukose, A., Paddick, S. M., Dissanayake, M., Khan, N. Z., & Walker, R. (2023). Health and socioeconomic resource provision for older people in South Asian countries: Bangladesh, India, Nepal, Pakistan and Sri Lanka evidence from NEESAMA. *Global Health Action, 16*(1), 2110198. https://doi.org/10.1080/16549716.2022.2110198

Mistry, S. K., Ali, A. R. M. M., Hossain, M. B., Yadav, U. N., Ghimire, S., Rahman, M. A., Irfan, N. M., & Huque, R. (2021). Exploring depressive symptoms and its associates among Bangladeshi older adults amid COVID-19 pandemic: Findings from a cross-sectional study. *Social Psychiatry and Psychiatric Epidemiology, 56*(8), 1487–1497. https://doi.org/10.1007/s00127-021-02052-6

Muhammad, F., Arafat, S. M. Y. (2024). Technology-Based interventions for mental health support in Bangladesh. In S. M. Y. Arafat (Eds.), *Mental health in Bangladesh*. Springer. https://doi.org/10.1007/978-981-97-0610-5_16

Naheed, A., Hakim, M., Islam, M. S., Islam, M. B., Tang, E. Y. H., Prodhan, A. A., Amin, M. R., Stephan, B. C. M., & Mohammad, Q. D. (2023). Prevalence of dementia among older age people and variation across different sociodemographic characteristics: A cross-sectional study in Bangladesh. *The Lancet Regional Health. Southeast Asia, 17*, Article 100257. https://doi.org/10.1016/j.lansea.2023.100257

Nayak, H. S. (2018). The felt need of home-based geriatric care in Bangladesh. *Journal of Nursing and Health Studies, 3*(2), 7. https://doi.org/10.21767/2574-2825.1000036

Palmer, K., Kabir, Z. N., Ahmed, T., Hamadani, J. D., Cornelius, C., Kivipelto, M., & Wahlin, Å. (2014). Prevalence of dementia and factors associated with dementia in rural Bangladesh: Data from a cross-sectional, population-based study. *International Psychogeriatrics, 26*(11), 1905–1915. https://doi.org/10.1017/S1041610214001392

Parveen, R. (2024). Bangladesh ranked among the worst in palliative care. A decade later, have things gone better? *Bdnews24*. https://bdnews24.com/health/qzszog3lzb. (Accessed 08/October/2024).

Rahman, M. S., Rahman, M. A., Ali, M., Rahman, M. S., Maniruzzaman, M., Yeasmin, M. A., Ahmed, N. A. M. F., Abedin, M. M., & Islam, S. M. S. (2020). Determinants of depressive symptoms among older people in Bangladesh. *Journal of Affective Disorders, 264*, 157–162. https://doi.org/10.1016/j.jad.2019.12.025

Rahman, A. (2020). The increasing 'burden' of the elderly in Bangladesh. The Daily Star. https://www.thedailystar.net/opinion/news/the-increasing-burden-the-elderly-bangladesh-1970349 (accessed on 09 October, 2024).

Reza, A. M. S., Feroz, A. H. M., Islam, S. M. N., Karim, M. N., Rabbani, G. M., Alam, M. S., et al. (2013). Risk factors of suicide and para suicide in rural Bangladesh. *Journal of Medicine, 14*(2), 123–129. https://doi.org/10.3329/jom.v14i2.19653

Shah, M. M. A., Ahmed, S., & Arafat, S. M. Y. (2017). Demography and risk factors of suicide in Bangladesh: A six-month paper content analysis. *Psychiatry Journal, 2017*, 3047025. https://doi.org/10.1155/2017/3047025

Shah, M. M. A., Sajib, M. W. H., & Arafat, S. M. Y. (2018). Demography and risk factor of suicidal behavior in Bangladesh: A cross-sectional observation from patients attending a suicide prevention clinic of Bangladesh. *Asian Journal of Psychiatry, 35*, 4–5. https://doi.org/10.1016/j.ajp.2018.04.035

Salam, S. S., Alonge, O., Islam, M. I., Hoque, D. M. E., Wadhwaniya, S., Baset, M. K. U., Mashreky, S. R., & El Arifeen, S. (2017). The burden of suicide in rural Bangladesh: Magnitude and risk factors. *International Journal of Environmental Research and Public Health, 14*(9), 1–16. https://doi.org/10.3390/ijerph14091032

Statista. (2024). Life expectancy (from birth) in Bangladesh from 1865 to 2020*. https://www.statista.com/statistics/1071009/life-expectancy-bangladesh-historical/. (Accessed 29/September/24).

Tabassum, T., Suzuki, T., Iwata, Y., & Ishiguro, H. (2023). Depression and associated factors among the elderly population in an urban tertiary geriatric hospital in Bangladesh. *Gerontology & Geriatric Medicine, 9*, 23337214231178144. https://doi.org/10.1177/23337214231178145

Tarannum, S., Sultana, B., Algin, S., & Majumder, A. H. (2014). Common behavioral problems among patients with dementia attending in tertiary care hospitals in Dhaka city. *Bangladesh Journal of Psychiatry, 28*(2), 50–52. https://doi.org/10.3329/bjpsy.v28i2.32736

Tithy, S. A., Ara, N. R., Pervej, A. M. A., Afrin, K., & Ara, I. (2022). Depression among the elderly people. *Bangladesh Journal of Psychiatry, 36*(1), 6–10. https://doi.org/10.3329/bjpsy.v36i1.72237

Tohan, M. M., Ahmed, F., Juie, I. J., et al. (2024). Outdoor recreational activities and mental well-being of geriatric people in Bangladesh: Structural equation modelling. *Discov Psychol, 4*, 33. https://doi.org/10.1007/s44202-024-00131-8

Uddin, M. A., Soivong, P., Lasuka, D., & Juntasopeepun, P. (2017). Factors related to quality of life among older adults in Bangladesh: A cross sectional survey. *Nursing & Health Sciences, 19*(4), 518–524. https://doi.org/10.1111/nhs.12385

Uddin, M. S., Mamun, A. A., Takeda, S., Sarwar, M. S., & Begum, M. M. (2019). Analyzing the chance of developing dementia among geriatric people: A cross-sectional pilot study in Bangladesh. *Psychogeriatrics: The Official Journal of the Japanese Psychogeriatric Society, 19*(2), 87–94. https://doi.org/10.1111/psyg.12368

Wahlin, Å., Palmer, K., Sternäng, O., Hamadani, J. D., & Kabir, Z. N. (2015). Prevalence of depressive symptoms and suicidal thoughts among elderly persons in rural Bangladesh. *International Psychogeriatrics, 27*(12), 1999–2008. https://doi.org/10.1017/S104161021500109X

World Health Organization. (2023). Mental health of older adults. Retrieved September 29, 2024, from https://www.who.int/news-room/fact-sheets/detail/mental-health-of-older-adults

World Health Organization. (2020). Bangladesh WHO special initiative for mental health situational assessment. Retrieved October 21, 2024, from, https://www.who.int/news-room/fact-sheets/detail/the-top-10-causes-of-death

Geriatric Psychiatry in India

K. L. Vidya and Prerak Kumar

Abstract India is experiencing a gradual yet steady ageing of its population. It is accompanied by significant changes in its social and familial structures, particularly due to urbanization. These demographic shifts bring forth various challenges, including an increasing dependency ratio, which will impact multiple sectors, especially health care. As a low- and middle-income country, India already faces a considerable treatment gap in addressing psychiatric disorders. Geriatric psychiatry, as a super specialty field, is still in its nascent stages in the country. This chapter underscores the growing need for geriatric mental health services in India, examining the current state of gero-psychiatry, end-of-life care, and related legal and ethical issues. It also explores the training opportunities, government programmes, policies, and action plans, while identifying the key challenges and suggesting strategies for the future development of geriatric mental health care in India.

Keywords Ageing · Geriatric psychiatry · Geriatric mental health · India · Old age psychiatry · Mental health services

1 Introduction

The most recent census in India was conducted in 2011. According to the census, India has 104 million older people aged 60 years and above constituting 8.6% of the total population (International Institute for Population Sciences & United Nations Population Fund, 2023). The proportion of the geriatric population has increased to 10.5% in 2022 and is projected to reach 20.8% by the year 2050, according to the United Nations Population Fund's India Ageing Report 2023 (International Institute for Population Sciences & United Nations Population Fund, 2023). However, this

K. L. Vidya (✉) · P. Kumar
Department of Geriatric Mental Health, King George's Medical University, Lucknow, UP, India
e-mail: vidya.kl@kgmcindia.edu

P. Kumar
e-mail: dr.prerak@kgmcindia.edu

N. Kar et al. (eds.), *Geriatric Psychiatry in South Asia*, South Asian Perspectives in Mental Health and Psychology , https://doi.org/10.1007/978-981-96-7469-5_3

number is relatively less when compared to the global proportion of older people 13.9% in 2022, and projected to be 22% of the global population by 2050 (Gerland et al., 2014). The average life expectancy at birth in India in 2019, just before the COVID-19 pandemic was 70.7 years. The life expectancy is higher for females with 72.4 and for males 69.2, which are projected to increase to 74.5 years and 79.1 years, for males and females respectively, by 2050. India is also witnessing the feminization of ageing. The sex ratio among senior citizens was 1033 females per 1000 males as per census data 2011. There is ruralization of ageing with 70% of the older people living in rural India. Projections indicate that from 2022 to 2050, India's overall population will grow by only 18%, but the number of senior citizens will increase by 134% (International Institute for Population Sciences & United Nations Population Fund, 2023). During this time, the population of people aged 80 years and above is expected to jump by 279%, with a large number of these elderly being widowed and highly dependent women (Sahoo et al., 2023).

India is currently in the late expanding stage of demographic transition, that is where the population growth is starting to level off. This is the result of decreasing birth rate and further decrease in the death rate due to better health and sanitation measures. The population pyramid of India has been an expansive pyramid with tapering at the top for decades since independence in the year 1947. However, this decade has begun witnessing the narrowing of base with a barrel-shaped pyramid, with a maximum number of economically productive age group (Malik et al., 2021). Population projections indicate that in 2021, there were 16 older persons per 100 working-age persons in India (IIPS, 2021). With the demographic shifts, this dependency ratio is expected to increase in the coming years, and the greater the old age dependency, reflecting higher levels of demand for care.

Old age comes with vulnerabilities of an ageing brain, physical morbidities, and declining intrinsic capacities. The burden of mental disorders is increasing among the Indian old age population also due to social factors like changing family structures, loss of spouse, social isolation, decrease in economic independence, neglect, and loneliness.

2 Epidemiology and Burden of Geriatric Mental Disorders and Suicide

2.1 Mental Disorders

The National Mental Health Survey (NMHP), 2016, conducted in 12 states of India with a total number of 34,802 subjects aged 18 years and above, found that weighted lifetime prevalence and the current lifetime prevalence of psychiatric morbidity in the older adults to be 15.1% and 10.9%, respectively which is slightly higher than in the younger adults. This study had 5,590 old age subjects, which is 16.1% of the total subjects. Lifetime and current prevalence of severe mental disorders also were higher when compared to adults, namely 2% and 0.68% respectively (Gautham et al., 2020).

A study reported a higher lifetime (6.93%) and current (3.53%) prevalence of depressive disorders in older adults as compared to younger adults (4.96% and 2.54%) (Sinha et al., 2020). This estimate included a range of mental disorders in the categories of F10–F49 in the International Classification of Diseases 10th revision (ICD-10). Since the categories between F00-F09 were not assessed, a significant chunk of geriatric psychiatric disorders has been missed including delirium and dementia. However, a nationally representative epidemiological study focusing exclusively on geriatric psychiatric disorders is yet to be done.

Longitudinal ageing study in India (LASI) is a national landmark study with a goal to provide valid, reliable and continuous scientific data on the health, social and economic well-being of older adult (aged 45 and above) population of India. The wave 1 of this large survey done between 2017–2018 covered all 30 states and 6 union territories of India with a sample size of 73,396 older adults aged more than 45 years. The self-reported prevalence of diagnosed depression and dementia were 0.8 and 1% respectively in the geriatric population aged 60 years and above (IIPS, 2021). This approach is limited by underreporting arising from the perceived stigma surrounding the mental disorders as well as the lack of awareness and need for treatment, especially in rural India. The overall age-standardized prevalence of depression was 5·7% among adults aged 45 years and older (Perianayagam et al., 2022a, 2022b). The prevalence of probable major depression as assessed using CIDI-SF (Composite International Diagnostic Interview-Short Form) was 8.3% in elderly above 60 years of age. However, health is only one of the four major subject domains under LASI. Only two psychiatric entities, namely depression and dementia, were assessed as part of this study.

After the first wave survey of LASI, the first national study of dementia in India, the Harmonized Diagnostic Assessment of Dementia for the Longitudinal Aging Study in India (LASI-DAD) was conducted with 4,096 geriatric subjects. This study found the estimated dementia prevalence to be 7.4% (Lee et al., 2023). Most of the other prevalence studies are conducted in small regional areas or hospital-based studies, especially with regard to delirium (Grover et al., 2021).

2.2 *Suicidal Behaviour*

Suicide is a relatively less studied entity in India, especially among older adults. In 2021, the suicide death rate among Indian geriatric men was reported to be 15.5 and among geriatric women (Yadav et al., 2023). As per the National Crime Record Bureau (NCRB) around 13,126 older people per 100,000 population committed suicide in India in the year 2020. Contributing factors for elderly suicide in India were abuse, alcohol dependence, physical diseases, family issues, loneliness, financial loss, and psychiatric illnesses (Patel et al., 2022). A recent community-based cross-sectional study found that 62.5% of older adults had a moderate level of suicidal ideation in Kashmir (Shoib et al., 2021). Another recent review stated the prevalence rate of suicide in studies conducted in India, ranging between 11.7 to 189.0 per 100,000 population (Arafat et al., 2021). However, this data is of the general population and not exclusive to older adults. A study conducted on suicide attempters from the Indian geriatric population found that co-morbid physical illness, mental disorders particularly depression, and family history of psychiatric illness to be the important predictors of suicide attempts in older adults (Kumar et al., 2015).

3 Current Status of Services

3.1 Neuropsychiatry

The absence of clinical infrastructure and geriatric mental healthcare professionals in India has resulted in less advanced mental health care for the older adults. There are only a few geriatric specialty departments in the country at Lucknow, Jaipur, and the National Institute of Mental Health and Neurosciences (NIMHANS). The geriatric neuropsychiatry services at NIMHANS, Bengaluru, Karnataka, is known as *Vayo-Manasa* (Ghosh, 2006).

3.2 End-of-Life Care Aspects in Geriatric Psychiatry

Death is inevitable, when terminally ill patients become aware of the imminence of death and dying, it becomes stressful for them. Many older mentally ill patients suffer from terminal conditions. The three national medical associations of neurologists (Indian Academy of Neurology), palliative care physicians (Indian Association of Palliative Care), and intensivists (Indian Society of Critical Care Medicine) formed the End of Life Care in India Taskforce (ELICIT) in 2015 (Salins et al., 2014).

India has approximately 450–500 palliative care centres documented. The Neighborhood Network of Palliative Care and “Palliative Care in Campus Groups” are community-based initiatives focused on providing clinical treatments, pain management, and palliative nursing care. Two of the nation’s centres of excellence as Collaborating Centers in palliation care are the WHO Collaborating Center for Training and Policy on Access to Pain Relief located in Thiruvananthapuram, Kerala, and the WHO Collaborating Center for Community Participation in Palliative Care and Long-Term Care located in Calicut, Kerala.

End-of-Life Care (EOLC) Policy for dying patients in India is still far behind in the race (Salins et al., 2014). Older adults, their caregivers and even the professionals are often not aware of access to palliative care. Essential steps in an end-of-life care plan focus on identifying, assessing, planning, providing, reassessing, and reflecting.

Important goals in EOLC are decision-makers, time for decision, decision communication, transition of care, and advance care planning. Future end-of-life care in India will require policies guiding hospitals, trained staff, education and training for health professionals, well-organized documentation, and a social support team at the social level.

3.3 *Legal and Ethical Aspects of Geriatric Psychiatry*

The physical and cognitive deterioration that occurs with ageing frequently reduces older adults' independence and increases their reliance on others. Chronic illness, a lack of physical strength, and poor decision-making among older adults are all ethical concerns. Important challenges in legal care include informed consent and the nominated representative of the elderly. Elderly people may encounter confidentiality issues related to their abuse due to cognitive decline. When assessing testamentary capacity, alternative relationships and motives of elderly relatives are important. Legal complications arise in elder care for conditions such as delirium, dementia, depression, suicide, and Parkinson's disease. Some legal acts related to elderly mental health in India are the Mental Health Care Act, 2017 (MHCA), the Rights of Persons with Disabilities Act, 2016 (RPWD), the Maintenance and Welfare of Parents and Senior Citizens Act, 2007 (MWPS), the Legal Services Authority Act, 1987, and the Indian Succession Act, 1925 (Dev & Eljo, 2024). The MHCA 2017 discusses people's rights, which are not limited to the older adults but are still not consistently enforced across the country. Important MHCA-2017 features that apply to older people include supported admission, advanced directives, nominated representative (NR), and assessment of treatment capacity. In older persons, testamentary capacity is particularly crucial. It can be difficult for older people suffering from mental illness, dementia, or other psychotropic medications that impair cognition to exercise their right to make a valid will. When handling dementia cases and testamentary capacity, a geriatric psychiatrist should be well-versed in testamentary capacity assessment and its legal consequences. Another important consideration is the older adult's ability to stand trial. To assist with legal matters, the professional should identify the appropriate mental health disorder, severity, and extent of impairment. Some of the old age specific issues in legal services are disability certification, safeguarding the rights of senior citizens, and preventing abuse. Guardianship of the older adults is another important aspect of legal services when they have dementia, severe mental illness, or multiple disabilities. Without a system of guardianship, the older adults may have difficulty making a valid decision. The geriatric psychiatrist's role in providing legal services to the elderly includes determining older people's capacity to make decisions about residential care and advising families on the type of care and support needed for older people with dementia. According to the Legal Services to the elderly NALSA 2016 scheme, court appeals by senior citizens are prioritized. According to Section 125 of the Criminal Procedure Code, the elderly can legally seek maintenance from their children (Gupta et al., 2016).

3.4 Digital Services in Old Age Psychiatry

Digital technology provides several benefits to older people, including improved quality of life and the ability to live more freely. Older adults can stay in touch with their loved ones through texting, social media, and video chats. Furthermore, technology provides access to a wealth of information, entertainment, and mental-exercise options. On April 14, 2021, the Indian government launched the "Mental Health and Normalcy Augmentation System (MANAS)", a national digital platform programme aimed at improving the mental health of Indian citizens, including the elderly. On June 26, 2020, the Karnataka government launched the online platform "e-Manas: Karnataka Mental Healthcare Management System" to provide digital mental health services throughout the state. Other states also have this online e-Manas services e.g. Jammu Kashmir, Assam, Tamil Nadu, Chhattisgarh, Kerala, Odisha, Rajasthan and is expanding. A nationwide survey found that older adults used digital services in the following ways: 95% used mobile calls, 4% browsed the internet, 1% listened to music, and 36% used Google Information (Vaitheswaran et al., 2020). Additionally, the study discovered that 76% of senior citizens were reluctant to use the Internet and digital services; these were attributed to various factors, including age-related barriers (23%), anxiety and fear (8%), cost concerns (8%), lack of relevance (8%), and restricted access to technology use (12%). The severity of symptoms, lack of social support, financial limitations, and mobility issues are some of the reasons why patients choose teleconsultations, according to a follow-up study on older patients with neurocognitive and mental illnesses (Kalaivanan et al., 2021).

Telepsychiatry services for seniors have become more and more popular. In addition to offering telepsychiatry services to the elderly throughout the state, the Karnataka Telemedicine Mentoring and Monitoring Program (KTM) is recognized for its innovative digital solutions. To address the mental health concerns in rural locations, including the elderly section, another digital platform is the "Clinical Decision Support System (CDSS), mainly to assess for making comprehensive diagnosis strategies. An online service called MANSANWAD was created in Rajasthan to handle mental health issues over the phone for all special populations. The Fortis National Mental Health Program's "Fortis Stress Helpline" is a free, round-the-clock helpline that offers psychologists' advice, crisis intervention, and support to the elderly and gives them online solutions (Wadhwa, 2021).

4 Specialist Course and Training Opportunities in Geriatric Psychiatry

Geriatric mental health as super specialty 3 years' DM (Doctorate in Medicine) course was started in 2011 in India, in King George's Medical University, Lucknow. This has been followed by starting of Geriatric Psychiatry DM course in NIMHANS,

Bengaluru in 2016. Both these institutes have also been offering one-year Post-Doctoral fellowship course in geriatric psychiatry. Although, it has been more than a decade since the inception of these courses, till date no other institutes have super specialty or subspecialty training in geriatric psychiatry. Thus, the number of qualified geriatric psychiatrists remains limited, and most of them are concentrated in metropolitan cities. General psychiatrists continue to play a crucial role in providing mental health services to older adults, especially in tier 2 and tier 3 cities of India. Since the introduction of these specialized courses in India, there has been ongoing debate about whether it is premature to establish them before the required number of general psychiatrists is reached (Shamasundar 2014). However, another perspective supports the development of this field, arguing that trained geriatric psychiatrists can contribute significantly by conducting frontier research on Indian geriatric population and training general psychiatrists, thereby reducing the therapeutic nihilism that has traditionally been linked to geriatric psychiatry (Manjunatha et al., 2013).

Although postgraduate training in psychiatry is well established in India both in government as well as private sector, a trainee in psychiatry gets limited exposure to hone their skills in geriatric psychiatry.

MD (Doctor of Medicine) in Geriatric Medicine is a three-year postgraduate broad specialty course that focuses on the health care of older adults. Competency based medical education curriculum of MD geriatric medicine includes few months of training in psychogeriatrics too.

Further, there are short-term courses which help in increasing the manpower specialized in caring for the geriatric psychiatry patients. A one-year fellowship course on geriatric mental health care after the basic medical degree, psychosocial care for the elderly (for social workers and psychologists) and geriatric mental health nursing is being conducted by NIMHANS, Bengaluru. The focus of this training is on preventive care for the geriatric population. These training courses are designed to develop professionals with comprehensive expertise in multidisciplinary care of patients with cognitive decline, dementia and other geriatric psychiatry related issues. These trainees are expected to become leaders in the geriatric psychiatry field to facilitate expansion of services and training in other parts of the country (Sivakumar & Varghese, 2019).

A one-week workshop was being conducted in the super specialty department of geriatric mental health earlier, which was held up during the COVID-19 pandemic and is yet to be restarted. Caregiver workshops are regular by the department of geriatric psychiatry unit of NIMHANS.

Geriatric psychiatry training at the level of medical undergraduate training is limited to the knowledge domain of concepts of dementia, depression, and delirium. Skill-based training to undergraduates regarding geriatric psychiatry is insufficient.

5 Programmes-Policies-Action Plans for Geriatric Mental Health

India is a signatory to the United Nations Principles for Older Persons, which was adopted in 1991 by general assembly resolutions. Inspired by this in 1992, the Integrated Programme for Older Persons (IPOP) came to being in India focusing on the basic amnesties like food, shelter, medical care, and environment of opportunities for older persons. Subsequently, the National policy for older persons NPOP was launched in 1999 (Gupta & Raju, 2018). Apart from the basic amnesties, the policy also covers issues like social security, intergenerational bonding, caregiving, role of Non-Governmental Organizations (NGO), training of manpower, research and training. Subsequently this paved the way for the development of the National Programme for Health Care of Elderly, NPHCE, in 2011 (Vaishnav et al., 2022) and the most recent Atal *Vayo Abhyuday Yojna* (AVYAY), in 2020 (Ahmad & Saxena, 2023). Table 1 provides a summary of programmes, policies, and action plans in relation to geriatric mental health in India.

Although there have been policies, programmes, and action plans targeting the well-being of older persons, mental health has not been taken up as a primary agenda in any. National Mental Health Programme focuses on making basic mental health care affordable and available to all, including the old. However, the geriatric population has not been the primary focus yet. It does not have a separate provision for geriatric mental health as such. Similarly, NPHCE focuses on geriatric health care but not geriatric mental health per se to provide tertiary level care for older adults (Salins et al., 2014). Regional geriatric centres have been established under NPHCE throughout the country. However, the primary focus has been on physical health. Geriatric physicians or general physicians have been delivering clinical services in these centres and they lack geriatric psychiatrists or even the general psychiatrists. Recruitment of geriatric mental health professionals including psychiatrists, clinical psychologists, or neuropsychologists have been overlooked by the policymakers.

So, geriatric mental health care remains a cross-cutting issue in both these prime programmes of the government of India. There is a need for horizontal integration of NMHP and NPHCE. This would enable the concept of 'care under one roof' for the elderly, which otherwise remains an uphill challenge.

6 Available Research and Gaps

The 3 D's of geriatric psychiatry are Depression, Delirium, and Dementia. Although there is some nationally representative epidemiological data on geriatric depression, epidemiological research on dementia and delirium remains limited. Most of the prevalence studies on dementia are regional, state and small cohort based (Das et al., 2014). Available studies have limitations with regard to regional biases, under representation of rural population and lack of longitudinal data. Epidemiological studies

Table 1 Programmes policies and action plans in relation to geriatric mental health in India

Initiatives	Name and year of launch	Schemes and scopes in relation to Geriatric mental health	Remarks
Programmes	National Mental Health Programme, NMHP, 1982	District Mental Health Programme, 1996 Mental healthcare services at district level Mental health promotion, prevention, treatment and rehabilitation of mental disorders	Applicable to all age groups and no exclusive or specialty clinics for geriatric age group per se
	Integrated Programme for Older Persons, IPOP, 1992	Medical care is one of the objectives to improve the quality of life of older persons Respite care homes and continuous care homes for older persons who need assistance to activities of daily living Awareness generation programmes Running day care centres for elderly with Alzheimer's disease/dementia	Although not exclusive to geriatric mental health, it also includes categories of cognitive impairment and dementia
	National Social Assistance Programme, NSAP, 1995	Old age, widow and disability pension schemes	Disability pensions are being given for mental disorders too including dementia
	National Programme for Health Care of the Elderly (NPHCE), 2011	At the subcentre level, health education related to healthy ageing including behavioural changes At PHC, CHC and district hospital level, there are weekly, biweekly and daily geriatric clinics respectively District hospitals have 10 beds reserved for geriatric ward Regional geriatric centres provide tertiary level services High level tertiary care with multidisciplinary clinical services are being provided at 2 National centres for ageing at Delhi and Chennai	Focus has been on geriatric medicine in general Regional geriatric centres have specialists in geriatric medicine with no mental health manpower

(continued)

Table 1 (continued)

Initiatives	Name and year of launch	Schemes and scopes in relation to Geriatric mental health	Remarks
	Integrated Programme for Senior Citizens, 2020	Continuous Care Homes for Senior Citizens with Alzheimer's/Dementia	Focuses on social justice and empowerment
Policies	National Policy for Older Persons, NPOP, 1999	Health care and nutrition is one of the principal areas of intervention and action strategies	Predominantly focuses on the physical health and nutrition. Mental health is still taking back seat
Action plans	The Maintenance and Welfare of Parents and Senior Citizens Act, 2007	Grievance redressal mechanism Penalties for non-compliance	Focuses on providing legal aid and financial security to older persons. This indirectly helps in reducing the social stressors
	National Plan of Action on Senior Citizens (NPASrC) Renamed as Atal Vayo Abhyuday Yojna (AVYAY), 2020	Day Care Centres for Senior Citizens Training programmes for creation of a pool of trained geriatric caregivers	Goal is to improve the quality of life of older persons focusing on the basic amnesties including medical care, geriatric mental health being one of the many focus areas

on other psychiatric disorders in the elderly population in India are scarce. The diverse socio-cultural landscape of India further complicates the generalizability of findings, as factors such as socioeconomic status, family dynamics, and rural–urban divides influence the manifestation and recognition of mental health issues in older people. Most epidemiological studies also fail to account for minimization, underreporting and stigma around the mental illness in older adults, especially in rural India.

Therapeutic interventions for geriatric psychiatric disorders are gaining momentum in India. However, pharmacological research remains limited. Over the past decade, neuromodulation studies have been making significant strides in this field (Rangarajan et al., 2021).

Geriatric psychiatry phenomenological studies in India are relatively rare, but some research has begun to explore the lived experiences of elderly individuals facing mental health challenges. A few studies have investigated the experience of ageing and mental illness, with a particular emphasis on how older adults cope with cognitive decline. Studies have also highlighted the role of family caregivers, particularly the complex dynamics of caregiving and the emotional toll it takes on families (Danivas et al., 2016). Studies on geriatric mental health related to social factors like social isolation, loneliness, abuse, and maltreatment are still in the nascent stage (Mishra et al., 2023).

Preliminary research on the impact of Indian diet and lifestyle on cognitive health in later life has yielded some promising findings. Traditional Indian foods, rich in phytochemicals and nutrients such as turmeric and saffron, are believed to play a significant role in reducing inflammation, protecting the brain from oxidative stress, and offering neuroprotective benefits. A small non-randomized clinical trial has also shown that a combined intervention of Ayurveda Rasayana and Yoga can enhance cognitive functions like learning, attention, processing speed, and working memory in older adults with mild cognitive impairment (Chobe et al., 2022). However, further research using more robust methodologies is needed to better understand these effects.

7 Current Challenges in Geriatric Mental Health and Ways Ahead

With an ageing population, India is undergoing a demographic shift and turning into a grey nation. Given the growing number of elderly people in India, it is alarming that elder mental health is neglected. There are particular management requirements for the elderly population, but India lacks the infrastructure and professional competency to meet these needs. Some of the current challenges are atypical and varied clinical symptom presentations, a thorough comprehension of cognitive issues, dementia care, including rehabilitation services, a dearth of primary health facilities dedicated to geriatric care, national geriatric research centres, and a lack of standardized Indian diagnostic instruments for geriatric disorders. Other prevalent issues in India include stigmas associated with ageing and policymaking for geriatric mental health care. Geriatric mood disorders, especially late-life depression, substance abuse, sexual disorders, senior suicide, and most commonly, delirium emergencies, are not adequately treated in both the acute and follow-up phases due to a lack of specialized treatment (Rajkumar et al., 2009).

With the exception of a few southern states, palliative care facilities are also not very well established nationwide. Elderly abuse because of caregiver stress is another burning issue in our country. Although government policies for social and pension services seem appropriate on paper, they do not adequately cover the elderly. The availability of comprehensive mental health care for senior citizens in India is impacted by the legal framework and insufficient geriatric clinic infrastructure (Lodha & De Souza, 2018).

The Indian Psychiatry Society has also issued guidelines for depression, anxiety, delirium, and rehabilitation treatments pertaining to elderly services (Tiwari & Sonal, 2018).

The *Indian Association of Geriatric Mental Health* (IAGMH) did a study on late-life depression at several centres: 8 centres, 488 older persons in India, and showed the role of socio-demographic factors influence on the clinical presentation in older adults' depression (Grover et al., 2018). Some Journals like *Journal of Geriatric Mental Health, Indian Journal of Gerontology*, dedicated to the research on *Geriatric Mental Health* are also contributing well to older adults. To combat Geriatric challenges in India some NGOs are doing their services like Banyan organization from Chennai, *Vayah Vikas*, Age-Well Foundation, HelpAge India, ManaVlok main is to improve the quality of life, community kitchen services and maintaining independency in older adults. They provide the psychosocial support, financial supports, and take care of basic needs in older adults. Some Welfare Schemes dedicated to older adults in India for their economic and social domain services are: Vayo Mitra, National Council of Senior Citizens, Rashtriya Vayoshri Yojana, Atal Pension Yojana, Senior Care Ageing Growth Engine, Antyodaya Anna Yojana, Ayushman Bharat (Hans, 2023). In India various initiatives like SACRED—Senior Able Citizens for Re-employment in Dignity, AGRASR—Action groups aimed at social construction are mainly focusing on the self-made dignity and skill assurance in older adults (Khai et al., 2024). For the future way ahead, National clinical and research geriatric centres with qualified geriatric mental health professionals are need of the hour in India. Policymakers need to include geriatric psychiatry subject experts for geriatric care services at the central level. There is need to develop geriatric mental health services in compliance with the culture, religion, and spirituality in elder care. There is also need for establishing strong and effective organization bodies for the elderly that encourage their self-determination and the development of a cohesive, powerful voice for their issues. Furthermore, there is need to increase public awareness of geriatric mental health issues and the appropriate cooperation between senior citizens and geriatric professionals through government initiatives, workshops, panel discussions, and the media.

8 Conclusions

In conclusion, Geriatric psychiatry has been gaining momentum in India from past couple of decades. With the establishment of a dedicated national professional association and journal focused on geriatric mental health, the discipline has seen significant growth in recent years. However, the number of qualified geriatric psychiatrists remains limited, and most are concentrated in metropolitan cities. In contrast, general psychiatrists play a crucial role in providing mental health services to older adults, especially in tier 2 and tier 3 cities. Although the majority of India's ageing population resides in rural areas, these regions still face significant challenges in accessing specialized geriatric mental health care due to long travel distances. The Indian government has launched various programmes aimed at improving health care for the elderly; mental health care has not been a primary focus. So, there is an urgent need for greater advocacy as well as policy attention to geriatric mental health care, at the grassroots levels especially in unreached rural regions of India.

References

Ahmad, M., & Saxena, P. (2023). Ageing and age structural transition in major states of India from 1961 to 2011. *Review of Regional Research, 43*(3), 433–465.

Arafat, S. M. Y., Menon, V., Varadharajan, N., & Kar, S. K. (2021). Psychological autopsy studies of suicide in South East Asia. *Indian Journal of Psychological Medicine, 44(*1), 4–9. https://doi.org/10.1177/02537176211033643

Avasthi, A., & Grover, S. (2018). Clinical practice guidelines for management of depression in the elderly. *Indian Journal of Psychiatry, 60*(Suppl 3), S341–S362.

Chobe, S., Patra, S. K., Chobe, M., & Metri, K. (2022). Efficacy of integrated Yoga and Ayurveda Rasayana on cognitive functions in elderly with mild cognitive impairment: Non randomized three-arm clinical trial. *Journal of Ayurveda and Integrative Medicine, 13*(1), Article 100373.

Danivas, V., Bharmal, M., Keenan, P., Jones, S., Karat, S. C., Kalyanaraman, K., Prince, M., Fall, H. D., & Krishna, M. (2016). An interpretative phenomenological analysis (IPA) of coercion towards community dwelling older adults with dementia: Findings from Mysore studies of natal effects on ageing and health (MYNAH). *Social Psychiatry and Psychiatric Epidemiology, 51*, 1659–1664.

Das, P. C., Kumar, P. R. A. K. A. S. H., Amara, A., & Dey, A. B. (2014). Dementia care in India: Issues & prospects. *International Journal of Medicine and Pharmaceutical Sciences, 4*(1), 29–36.

Dev, P. S., & Eljo, J. G. (2024). Addressing the ethical and legal complexities in elderly care: A study from India. *Nusantara Journal of Behavioral and Social Science, 3*(3), 111–118.

Gangadhar, B. N., Kumar, C. N., Sadh, K., Manjunatha, N., Math, S. B., Kalaivanan, R. C., Rao, G. N., Parthasarathy, R., Chand, P. K., Chandra, P. S., Thirthalli, J., Murthy, P., Varghese, M., Mathur, A., Bairy, B. K., Kishore, C., Gowda, G. S., Basvaraju, V., Harihara, S. N., … Chaturvedi, S. K. (2023). Mental Health Programme in India: Has the tide really turned? *Indian Journal of Medical Research, 157*(5), 387–394.

Gautham, M. S., Gururaj, G., Varghese, M., Benegal, V., Rao, G. N., Kokane, A., Chavan, B. S., Dalal, P. K., Ram, D., Pathak, K., Singh, R. K. L., Singh, L. K., Sharma, P., Saha, P. K., Ramasubramanian, C., Mehta, R. Y., & Shibukumar, T. M. (2020). The National Mental Health survey of India (2016): Prevalence, socio-demographic correlates and treatment gap of mental morbidity. *International Journal of Social Psychiatry, 66*(4), 361–372.

Gerland, P., Raftery, A. E., Ševčíková, H., Li, N., Gu, D., Spoorenberg, T., Alkema, L., Fosdick, B. K., Chunn, J., Lalic, N., Bay, G., Buettner, T., Heilig,G. K., & Wilmoth, J. (2014). World population stabilization unlikely this century. *Science, 346*(6206), 234–237.

Ghosh, A. B. (2006). Psychiatry in India: Need to focus on geriatric psychiatry. *Indian Journal of Psychiatry, 48*(1), 4–9.

Grover, S., Avasthi, A., Sahoo, S., Lakdawala, B., Nebhinani, N., Dan, A., & Kedare, J. (2018). Indian Association for Geriatric Mental Health's multicentric study on depression in elderly: Symptom profile and influence of gender, age of onset, age at presentation, and number of episodes on symptom profile. *Journal of Geriatric Mental Health, 5*(1), 35–48.

Grover, S., Kathiravan, S., & Dua, D. (2021). Delirium research in India: A systematic review. *Journal of Neurosciences in Rural Practice, 12*(2), 236.

Gupta, A. (2016). Ethical, legal and forensic issues in geriatric psychiatry. *American Journal of Geriatric Psychiatry, 24*(3), S11. https://doi.org/10.1016/j.jagp.2016.01.015

Gupta, N., & Raju, S. S. (2018). Policies, programs, and schemes for the elderly in India: A critical review. *Handbook of Research on Multicultural Perspectives on Gender and Aging, 1125*, 3.

Hall, S., Petkova, H., Tsouros, A. D., Costantini, M., & Higginson, I. J. (2011). *Palliative care for older people: Better practices*. World Health Organization.

Hans, V. (2023, December 5). *Niti Aayog*.

International institute for population sciences (IIps), I. C. F. (2021). National Family Health Survey (NFHS-5): 2019–21 India. Mumbai: International Institute for Population.

International Institute for Population Sciences & United Nations Population Fund. (2023). *India Ageing Report 2023, Caring for Our Elders: Institutional Responses*. United Nations Population Fund, New Delhi.

Kalaivanan, R. C., Rahul, P., Manjunatha, N., Kumar, C. N., Sivakumar, P. T., & Math, S. B. (2021). Telemedicine in geriatric psychiatry: Relevance in India. *Indian Journal of Psychological Medicine, 43*(5_suppl), S121–S127.

Kar, S. K., Arafat, S. Y., Pandey, N. M., Kabir, R., & Singh, S. (2022). Suicide in the geriatric population of South East Asia-contexts and attributes. *F1000Research, 11*, 1223.

Khai, T. S., Jacob, N. O., Khan, A. W., & Asaduzzaman, M. (2024). *A comparative analysis of the pension schemes for elderly population in developing countries: Policy insights in the context of financial wellbeing and social justice*.

Kumar, P. S., Anish, P. K., & George, B. (2015). Risk factors for suicide in elderly in comparison to younger age groups. *Indian Journal of Psychiatry, 57*(3), 249–254.

Lee, J., Meijer, E., Langa, K. M., Ganguli, M., Varghese, M., Banerjee, J., Khobragade, P., Angrisani, M., Kurup, R., Chakrabarti, S. S., Gambhir, I. S., Koul, P. A., Goswami, D., Talukdar, A., Mohanty, R. R., Yadati, R. S., Padmaja, M., Sankhe, L., Rajguru, C., & Dey, A. B. (2023). Prevalence of dementia in India: National and state estimates from a nationwide study. *Alzheimer's & Dementia, 19*(7), 2898–2912.

Lodha, P., & De Sousa, A. (2018). Geriatric mental health: The challenges for India. *Journal of Geriatric Mental Health, 5*(1), 16–29. https://doi.org/10.4103/jgmh.jgmh_34_17

Macaden, S. C., Salins, N., Muckaden, M., Kulkarni, P., Joad, A., Nirabhawane, V., & Simha, S. (2014). End of life care policy for the dying: Consensus position statement of Indian association of palliative care. *Indian Journal of Palliative Care, 20*(3), 171.

Malik, C., Khanna, S., Jain, Y., & Jain, R. (2021). Geriatric population in India: Demography, vulnerabilities, and healthcare challenges. *Journal of Family Medicine and Primary Care, 10*(1), 72–76.

Mani, R. K., Bhatnagar, S., Butola, S., Gursahani, R., Mehta, D., Simha, S., Divatia, J. V., Kumar, A., Iyer, S. K., Deodhar, J., Bhat, R. S., Salins, N., Thota, R. S., Mathur, R., Iyer, R. K., Gupta, S., Kulkarni, P., Murugan, S., Nasa, P., & Myatra, S. N. (2024). Indian society of critical care medicine and Indian association of palliative care expert consensus and position statements for end-of-life and palliative care in the intensive care unit. *Indian Journal of Critical Care Medicine: Peer-Reviewed, Official Publication of Indian Society of Critical Care Medicine, 28*(3), 20019.

Manjunatha, N., Thyloth, M., & Rao, T. S. (2013). The rise of super (? sub)-specialties courses in psychiatry: Is India ready for it! *Indian Journal of Psychiatry, 55*(4), 401–402.

Mishra, B., Pradhan, J., & Dhaka, S. (2023). Identifying the impact of social isolation and loneliness on psychological well-being among the elderly in old-age homes of India: The mediating role of gender, marital status, and education. *BMC Geriatrics, 23*(1), 684.

Patel, A. B. (2022). Vulnerability as determinant of suicide among older people in Northern Indian states. *Frontiers in Psychology, 13*, Article 971080. https://doi.org/10.3389/fpsyg.2022.971080

Perianayagam, A., Bloom, D., Lee, J., Parasuraman, S., Sekher, T. V., Mohanty, S. K., Chattopadhyay, A., Govil, D., Pedgaonkar, S., Gupta, S., Agarwal, A., Posture, A., Weerman, A., & Pramanik, S. (2022a). Cohort profile: The longitudinal ageing study in India (LASI). *International Journal of Epidemiology, 51*(4), e167–e176.

Perianayagam, A., Prina, M., Selvamani, Y., Gudekar, D., Salvi, S., Varghese, M., & Dandona, R. (2022b). Sub-national patterns and correlates of depression among adults aged 45 years and older: Findings from wave 1 of the longitudinal ageing study in India. *The Lancet Psychiatry, 9*(8), 645–659.

Philip, S., Gajera, G., Nirisha, P. L., Sivakumar, P. T., Barikar, M. C., Panday, P., Patley, R., Chander, R., Sinha, P.,Basavarajappa, C., Manjunatha, N., & Naveen Kumar, C. (2021). Future-proofing geriatric mental health care services in India: training and policy directions. *Indian Journal of Psychological Medicine, 43*(5_suppl), S134–S141.

Rajkumar, A. P., Thangadurai, P., Senthilkumar, P., Gayathri, K., Prince, M., & Jacob, K. S. (2009). Nature, prevalence and factors associated with depression among the elderly in a rural south Indian community. *International Psychogeriatrics, 21*(2), 372–378.

Rangarajan, S. K., Suhas, S., Reddy, M. S. S., Sreeraj, V. S., Sivakumar, P. T., & Venkatasubramanian, G. (2021). Domiciliary tDCS in geriatric psychiatric disorders: Opportunities and challenges. *Indian Journal of Psychological Medicine, 43*(4), 351–356.

Sahoo, P. M., Rout, H. S., & Jakovljevic, M. (2023). Consequences of India's population aging to its healthcare financing and provision. *Journal of Medical Economics, 26*(1), 308–315.

Salins, N., Muckaden, M., Nirabhawane, V., Simha, S., Macaden, S., Kulkarni, P., & Joad, A. (2014). End-of-life care policy for the dying: Consensus position statement of indian association of palliative care. *Indian Journal of Palliative Care, 20*(3), 171. https://doi.org/10.4103/0973-1075.138384

Sathya, T., Selvamani, Y., & Nagarajan, R. (2022). Elder abuse/mistreatment and associated covariates in India: Results from the longitudinal aging study in India wave 1, 2017–2018. *Epidemiology and Health, 44*. https://doi.org/10.4178/epih.e2022017

Shamasundar, C. (2014). Role of super-specialities in psychiatry. *Indian Journal of Psychiatry, 56*(4), 408–409.

Shoib, S., Islam, S. M. S., Arafat, S. Y., & Hakak, S. A. (2021). Depression and suicidal ideation among the geriatric population of Kashmir. *India. International Journal of Social Psychiatry, 67*(6), 651–655.

Sinha, P., Hussain, T., Boora, N. K., et al. (2021). Prevalence of Common mental disorders in older adults: Results from the National Mental Health Survey of India. *Asian J Psychiatry, 2021*(55), Article 102463.

Sivakumar, P. T., & Varghese, M. (2019). P3–489: Training in geriatric psychiatry and related disciplines to promote dementia care in India. *Alzheimer's & Dementia, 15*, P1155–P1156.

Tampi, R. R., Young, J., Balachandran, S., Dasarathy, D., & Tampi, D. (2018). Ethical, legal and forensic issues in geriatric psychiatry. *Current Psychiatry Reports, 20*, 1–7.

Tiwari, S. C., & Sonal, A. (2018). Clinical practice guidelines for addressing the rehabilitation needs of elderly in the Indian context. *Indian Journal of Psychiatry, 60*(Suppl 3), S410–S425.

Vaishnav, L. M., Joshi, S. H., Joshi, A. U., & Mehendale, A. M. (2022). The national programme for health care of the elderly: A review of its achievements and challenges in India. *Annals of Geriatric Medicine and Research, 26*(3), 183.

Vaitheswaran, S., Lakshminarayanan, M., Ramanujam, V., Sargunan, S., & Venkatesan, S. (2020). Experiences and needs of caregivers of persons with dementia in India during the COVID-19 pandemic—A qualitative study. *The American Journal of Geriatric Psychiatry, 28*(11), 1185–1194.

Wadhwa, M. (2021). *Digital mental health initiatives in India* (No. 60) (ICT India Working Paper).

Yadav, S., Aathavan, K. K., Cunningham, S. A., Bhandari, P., Mishra, U. S., Aditi, A., & Yadav, R. (2023). Changing pattern of suicide deaths in India. *The Lancet Regional Health-Southeast Asia, 16*. https://doi.org/10.1016/j.lansea.2023.100265

Geriatric Psychiatry in Nepal

Pawan Sharma, Rika Rijal, and Omkar Dhungel

Abstract The population of Nepal is rapidly ageing and the prevalence of mental health disorders among the ageing population is high. There is limited expertise and access to geriatric mental health services with a huge treatment gap which makes it a rapidly emerging concern. This area remains significantly under-researched as well. When compared to the past there has been some improvement in the mental health care of the elderly population, however, much more needs to be done. By raising awareness, advocating for policy changes, and investing in research and training, we can work towards improving the mental health and well-being of older adults in this rapidly ageing nation. In this chapter, we aim to discuss the epidemiology of mental health disorders, available services, policies, and action plans, challenges, and ways out for geriatric mental health in Nepal.

Keywords Mental health · Geriatric mental health · Old age psychiatry · Older adults · Nepal

1 Introduction

Nepal, a landlocked country, officially known as the Federal Democratic Republic of Nepal, is situated in the lap of the Himalayas and is extended into the Indo-Gangetic Plain. It borders China to the north, and India to the south, east, and west. It has an area of 147,516 km^2 and a population of about thirty million. Traditionally in most nations, the elderly is considered to be that person who is 65 years of age and

P. Sharma (✉)
Department of Psychiatry, School of Medicine, Patan Academy of Health Sciences, Lalitpur, Nepal
e-mail: pawansharma@pahs.edu.np

R. Rijal
Department of Psychiatry, Kathmandu University School of Medical Sciences, Dhulikhel, Nepal

O. Dhungel
Department of Psychiatry, Shree Birendra Hospital, Chhauni, Kathmandu, Nepal

N. Kar et al. (eds.), *Geriatric Psychiatry in South Asia*, South Asian Perspectives in Mental Health and Psychology , https://doi.org/10.1007/978-981-96-7469-5_4

older. However, this definition in Nepal is complex. For the mandatory retirement from civil services, 58 years has been set whereas 63 years has been set for some academic sectors and even 65 years. The social security allowance is given after the age of 68 years. The Senior Citizen Act of Nepal defines individuals aged 60 years and older as the senior citizen or elderly or older adults (Nepal Law Commission, 2006). There are 2.97 million older people above 60 years in Nepal as of the 2021 census which is 38.2% increase as compared to the census of 2011. The 2021 census indicated that the proportion of the older population reached 10.21% of the total population of Nepal. During this decade, Nepal's average population growth rate is 0.92% and the older population growth rate is 3.29% per year (Chalise, 2023). The life expectancy of the Nepalese population was 37 years and 39.9 years in 1961 which has increased to 71 years for men and 73 years for women in 2021 respectively, which indicates the rising trend of the aging population (Bista, 2024). With this increase in the number of elderlies comes a rise in age-related health issues, including mental disorders, making geriatric mental health a growing concern. In this chapter, we aim to discuss the overview of the prevalence of mental disorders, available services, researches, programs, and policies regarding geriatric mental health in Nepal. In addition, it was intended to provide the recommendations regarding effective public health and welfare approaches to prevent, treat and manage the mental health issues among this vulnerable population in Nepal.

2 Epidemiology

Mental disorders in the elderly are a serious public health concern with the aged population having a greater prevalence of mental disorders (Reynolds et al., 2022). Around 14% of adults aged 60 and over live with a mental disorder and these conditions account for 10.6% of the total disability (WHO, 2023). In context of Nepalese elderly population, the common mental health disorders include depression, anxiety, dementia, and substance use disorders. Only a few studies have been conducted among the elderly to estimate their mental state and the results vary considerably. A systematic review of 26 studies on the prevalence of mental disorders in geriatric population in Nepal showed a prevalence of depressive symptom in a range of 25.5% to 60.6% in the community. The prevalence ranged from 17.3 to 89.1% in aged-care facilities and it was in the range of 53.2–57.1% in hospital settings. The prevalence of depressive disorders varied between 4.4% in community sample and 53.2% in hospital sample. The prevalence of cases of anxiety symptoms ranged from 21.7 to 32.3%. The other identified disorders were psychosis and alcohol use disorder (Thapa et al., 2018). Depression among older persons in rural areas is quite common, with findings ranging from 45.7% to 57.4%. In one of the studies done in rural population, 18.8% of sample were severely depressed as measured by the Geriatric Depression Scale (GDS-15) (Shrestha et al., 2020) Manandhar et al., 2019). Similarly, reports from in-patient study also reported the most common diagnosis as depression (23.2%) followed by psychosis (20.3%) and alcohol use disorder (18.1%)

(Aich et al., 2015). In another study done from in-patients admitted in a tertiary hospital in Kathmandu, the most common diagnosis in the elderly was depression (29.6%) followed by delirium and dementia (Dhungana et al., 2014). In another recent hospital-based study among 140 geriatrics in-patients, depression was seen in 19.3% patients (Rijal et al., 2024). While in old age home, the prevalence of geriatric depression ranged from 29.7% to 89.1% (Ranjan et al., 2013; Simkhada et al., 2018; Timalsina et al., 2014). It was found that elderly females, lower-income households and households with migrated adult children were more likely to report depressive symptoms (Joshi & Chalise, 2021). Studies from other Asian countries indicate that lower levels of education, female gender, marital status (being unmarried, divorced, or widowed), low socio-economic status, higher age, family-related issues, loneliness, and perceived lower health status are also linked with elderly depression which is similar in context of Nepal as well (Chen et al., 2012; Grover & Malhotra, 2015).

A study in Kavre, Nepal revealed a high prevalence of geriatric depression (53.1%), which was higher in comparison to the other Asian countries. It was concluded that depression among the Nepalese elderly was significantly associated with rural habitation, illiteracy, less than enough family time, and exposure to verbal/physical abuse. It had an inverse relationship with the quality of life. Another important issue in elderly people, older adults, is suicide. Suicide rates among older adults are linked to factors like chronic illness, social isolation, poverty, bereavement, and depression. In South Asia, in general, suicide is characterized by higher use of organophosphate insecticides, larger numbers of married women, fewer elderly subjects, and role of causative factors such as interpersonal relationship problems and life events (Khan, 2002). In a cross-sectional study done in 100 geriatric patients presenting to outpatient clinics of different departments in a tertiary care hospital based in Kathmandu, the suicidal component of the *Hamilton Depression Rating Scale* (HDRS) was used to screen for suicidality. The study showed suicidal symptoms in 16% of the subjects with female preponderance. The suicidal ideas or gestures were seen in 4% of subjects with a male preponderance, and there was a history of suicidal attempts among three patients (Khattri & Nepal, 2006). In another recent study done among 248 cases from the suicide registry presenting to a tertiary care center in Kathmandu, the prevalence of patients above 60 who had attempted suicide was found to be 0.4%. As per the same registry, most of the patients attempted suicide inside their home and the most common method used was the ingestion of poison (Sharma et al., 2024a, 2024b). Similarly, in one of the recent studies, suicidal ideation and attempts were reported in 14.2% of in-patients (Rijal et al., 2024). Loneliness, which has been deemed a public health emergency by WHO, has been found to be the commonest cause along with past history of suicide and past traumatic events. Hence, there is clear evidence of geriatric mental health issues in Nepal, which is mostly in line with the global and Asian context.

Dementia and cognitive disorders remain largely misunderstood and largely under-recognized by the community and by healthcare professionals in Nepal (Hossain et al., 2020; Kohrt et al., 2018). With increasing life expectancy in Nepal, it has been predicted that dementia will further complicate the lives of older adults. By 2040, it has been predicted that 71% of persons with dementia will reside in low and middle-income countries. In Nepal, there were 78,000 persons with dementia in 2015. This will be 130,000 by 2030 and 285,000 by 2050 (Kamholz et al., 2022). A number of studies have been conducted in various regions and settings of Nepal to determine the quality of life (QoL) in elderly people. Factors affecting the QoL of elderly people were increased age, female gender, living alone, low education, and economic status. There was a negative correlation between the QoL and increasing level of depression (Samadarshi et al., 2021).

However, the findings from the studies done in the past may not fairly represent the entire geriatric community of Nepal due to the country's variable geo-ecological, economic, and sociocultural characteristics and diverse ethnicities, as most of the studies were conducted in a confined geographic area or within a single caste community. Furthermore, not many of the studies had used well-validated, culturally or age-wise adaptation of psychiatric inventories. It has also been found that the estimates in most of the studies are not associated with individual and societal burden.

3 Risk Factors of Mental Disorders Among Geriatric Population

It is known that with increasing age, objectively measured health and functional status decline, physical and cognitive capacities decrease. On the other hand, the number of chronic diseases and the extent of disability in performing daily activities also increases. Similarly, mental illness and poor socialization among the elderly increase the risk of neglect and abuse at the hands of caregivers, which can land them up in old age homes or even end up homeless.

Nepal has undergone several challenging phases in the last few decades. These include a decade-long armed conflict, the 2015 earthquake, the COVID-19 pandemic, and the recent flood and landslide due to climate change that gripped health services throughout the nation. As a result, many young people are migrating abroad in search of good education and employment opportunities. So, an important psychosocial aspect that needs to be taken into account is the migration of children and the mental health impact on the elderly population.

A cross-sectional, house-to-house survey among 260 community-dwelling elderly residents showed that compared to participants without a migrant child, participants with a migrant child had higher odds of self-reported chronic diseases, presence of depressive symptoms, and self-perceived loneliness (Ghimire et al., 2018).

Another study from the elderly home of Nepal also revealed that the migration of their children leads to emotional problems among 78.8% of the respondents (Khanal et al., 2018). There is no evidence regarding whether remittance is of any benefit to the elderly population groups. The increasing rate of the migration of the younger generation and the increased burden of work among the left-behind elderly population group may in turn have psychological consequences (Ghimire et al., 2018; Shrestha et al., 2021). The evidence from the past highlights the migration of children as an important psychosocial stressor for parents who are left behind in Nepal. They are further prone to loneliness, discrimination, and neglect.

The COVID-19 pandemic has brought even more attention to the issues of social isolation and loneliness, particularly among older adults who are the most vulnerable to psychological aspects of this illness (Pant & Subedi, 2020). Elderly women, in particular, are at higher risk due to gender-based discrimination and economic dependency, making them vulnerable to develop serious mental illnesses (Dahal et al., 2022). Nepal's elderly, especially in rural areas, often face financial insecurity due to the lack of social security systems (Acharya et al., 2023). Another risk factor for mental health issues is elderly abuse. A cross-sectional study of 339 older adults aged 60 or above from eastern Nepal showed that 61.7% of elders experienced some form of mistreatment (physical 2.4%, psychological 22.4%, caregiver neglect 57.5%, financial 12.1% and stranger-inflicted 8.3%) (Yadav et al., 2018).

4 Current Status of Services, Neuropsychiatry, End-of-Life Care

The specialized services for geriatric mental health are lacking in Nepal. However, the services are provided by general psychiatrists and other health workers trained in mental health. Dementia is included in mhGAP-IG (WHO *Mental Health Gap Action Program* Intervention guide) module, the training of which is provided to health workers (Luitel et al., 2023). All the universities and academies running postgraduate psychiatry programs have some provision of geriatric mental health in the curriculum, however, separate posting is not done in any of them, as specialized geriatric mental health units are not available. Also, there are no neuropsychiatry units throughout the country and the cases are seen by either a psychiatrist and/or neurologist. With the information available in 2024, there are only five geriatricians and one geriatric psychiatrist and most of them are providing services in the urban areas (Thapa et al., 2024).

Nepal is classified as "Category 3a" with isolated palliative care provision based on various dimensions of palliative care (Clark et al., 2017). The end-of-life and palliative care services are not well supported, dependent on donor funding, limited availability of morphine, and the services are not proportionate to the population size of the country (Gautam & Adhikari, 2021). For the case of euthanasia, the Nepal Medical Council Code of Ethics and Professional Conduct-2017 states Euthanasia as the act of painless killing of a patient suffering from an incurable and painful disease. This is not legalized in Nepal and hence no medical practitioner should practise it. However, administration of narcotics and sedatives titrated to alleviate pain and distress in a dying patient is palliative care which should be provided and clearly documented in the medical record (Nepal Medical Council, 2017).

5 Available Research and Gaps

Most of the research available from Nepal in geriatric mental health is cross-sectional in nature and mainly focused on the epidemiology of depression, dementia, and quality of life. The studies on the prevalence and risk factors are already discussed in the respective section. Most of the available studies are from urban areas, hospitals, and old age homes which may not represent the entire geriatric population of Nepal. Most of the studies didn't use well-validated or culturally adapted tools of assessment (Risal et al., 2024) There are a limited number of scales validated in the Nepali language used in the geriatric population. The GDS, a 15-item questionnaire to screen depression in the older adults has been validated and is considered a reliable tool for assessing depression in the elderly population in Nepal (Risal et al., 2020a, 2020b). Another scale *Rowland Universal Dementia Assessment Scale* (RUDAS) which is an assessment tool for screening cognitive impairment among the elderly has been translated and culturally adapted into Nepali language. (Nepal et al., 2019).

6 Programs-Policies-Action Plans for Geriatric Mental Health

Right to health is one of the fundamental constitutional rights in Nepal. Nepal has a single, over-arching health policy, with sub-sections related to different health conditions. Mental health is mentioned in Section 6.17.5. Geriatric mental health is addressed through the existing health policy of Nepal (National Health Policy, 2019). The National Mental Health Strategy and Action Plan of 2020 has also identified the elderly population as a vulnerable group and has discussed on capacity building, proper services, and assurance of their rights (Department of Health Services Nepal, 2020). Regarding programs, the Social Security Section, Nursing and Social Security Division, Department of Health Services, Ministry of Health and Population of Nepal, oversees the "*Bipanna Nagarik Ausadhi Upachar* Programme". Under this program, the impoverished senior citizens receive free treatment up to NPR 100,000 (approx. 735$) per patient via the listed hospitals for severe diseases including Alzheimer's disease. The age criterion for the Senior Citizen's Social Security Allowance (SSA) is 68 years and above where the monthly allowance is NPR 4000 (approx. 30$) is provided. In addition, the Ministry of Health and Population has postulated the Geriatric Health Service Strategy from 2021 to 2030 in which the strategy 1.4 focuses on promoting the psychological and spiritual health of senior citizens for enhancing their psychosocial well-being and creating an enabling health-related environment (NHSSP: Nepal Health Sector Support Programme, 2022). Senior Citizens Act provides details about respect, maintenance, and care of senior citizens. There is mention of facilities and concessions. It has also played a vital role in the formation of Central Senior Citizen Welfare Committee, formation of the District Senior

Table 1 Important programs for geriatric population in Nepal (NHSSP: Nepal Health Sector Support Programme, 2022)

Year	Program	Description
2004	Government of Nepal-state-funded senior citizen healthcare service programme	Free medical services for senior citizens and the "Senior Citizens Health Facilities Fund"
2006	Senior citizens act of 2006	Provisions for the protection and social security of senior citizens including health services
2010	*Aarogya Ashram* for senior citizens	Achieved limited coverage, constrained financial resources, weak institutional and service delivery capacity has left the health needs of senior citizens largely unmet
2021–2030	Ministry of health and population—Geriatric health service strategy 2021–2030	Purpose: To protect the health rights of older persons by means of their health promotion and protection, effective delivery of health services and an improved system of social health insurance and to enable them to lead active and quality lives on the basis of optimum health protection and effective health service delivery
2021	The Geriatric care centre implementation guidelines	Established updated, broad, highly informed standards for any organization treating or caring for older persons

Citizen Welfare Committee. It also emphasizes the care of senior citizens through local levels.

As a member state of the UN and as a signature country of the Universal Declaration of Human Rights (UDHR) and various other important international conventions, Nepal has expressed international commitment to develop social security services in line with the constitutional provisions of the country. In response to tackling ageing issues and addressing their needs and challenges, the government of Nepal has formulated national policies and security programs for senior citizens and has committed itself to various regional and international conventions to promote healthy ageing (Bhandari, 2019). Some of the important programs regarding the elderly population and their description are provided in Table 1

Currently, no specialty or fellowship courses in geriatric psychiatry are offered by any medical college or institution in Nepal.

7 Current Challenges in Geriatric Mental Health

The challenges and ways out for geriatric psychiatry are similar to the general mental health issues (Sharma, et al., 2024a, 2024b). Apart from that there are a few important challenges unique to the geriatric population that shall be discussed.

7.1 *Stigma Against Mental Illness*

Like with all mental illnesses, there is a stigma against mental illness among the geriatric population. There is a reluctance to seek help and attribution of mental illness and psychological trauma to bad "*karma*", which stipulates one's past actions (Kudva et al., 2020). There is also a lack of awareness and limited understanding of mental health problems like depression, anxiety, and dementia, which has led to underreporting and neglect (Jeyakumar et al., 2024).

7.2 *Poor Healthcare Infrastructure*

Nepal has a shortage of specialized manpower like geriatric psychiatrists, psychologists, and mental health professionals trained to address the unique needs of the elderly. Very few hospitals or clinics offer geriatric-specific mental healthcare services, particularly in rural areas, and there is an urban–rural disparity in health services (Thapa et al., 2024).

7.3 *Social Isolation and Changing Family Dynamics with Economic Barriers*

A significant proportion of the elderly population in Nepal lives in poverty (Poudel, 2022) limiting their ability to afford healthcare services. Many elderly individuals are economically dependent on their families, who may prioritize other financial needs over mental health care. A study among 88 older people aged 65 years in the central part of Nepal showed that functional dependency, comorbidity, financial dependence, and lower education were significantly associated with psychosocial problems among older people (Poudyal et al., 2024).

7.4 *Policy and Implementation Gaps*

The National Mental Health Strategy and Action Plan 2020 details actions for mental health in the country for the next five years, and the elderly population has been identified as a vulnerable group and has been discussed on capacity building, proper services and assurance of their rights. It emphasizes the integration of mental health services within primary healthcare settings. However, there is inadequate implementation due to resource constraints and a lack of coordination (Acharya et al., 2023; Sharma, et al., 2024a, 2024b).

7.5 Comorbidities and Diagnostic Challenges

The elderly have various chronic physical health conditions like hypertension, diabetes, and arthritis, and they co-exist with mental health issues, which complicate diagnosis and treatment (Yadav et al., 2020). General practitioners often lack the training to identify and manage mental health issues in geriatric patients, which further poses a challenge.

7.6 Research and Data Limitations

There is a scarcity of research and data on geriatric mental health in Nepal, making it difficult to plan and implement effective interventions.

8 Ways Out to the Challenges of Geriatric Mental Health

8.1 Human Resource Development

There is an urgent need for developing human resources, especially geriatric psychiatrists, geriatric psychiatric nurses, and trained paramedics to handle the cases of geriatric psychiatry, including clinical psychologists, and social workers.

8.2 Geriatric Mental Health Service Development

The development of manpower alone is not sufficient to counter this huge challenge. There is a need for proper geriatric, old age-friendly services not only in specialized care but in all domains of care involving the elderly. One way of providing service would be to integrate geriatric mental health in the primary care setting. Also, there should be the provision of mental health screening for mood disorders, cognitive functioning at the point of health contact either a general practice consultation, medicine consultation, or geriatric medicine consultation.

8.3 Research

There is a need for conducting research with robust methodology in order to know the exact mental health status and its associated factors among the older adults. It is imperative to develop culturally validated tools for screening and interventions that suit our local context. Given the lack of adequate expertise and funding, it may be further helpful if more collaboration with international organizations, universities, and funding agencies is made.

8.4 Policy Implementation

There have been multiple pieces of evidence of poor implementation of laws and policies regarding elderly (Tausig & Subedi, 2022), hence it is of utmost importance that the mental health professionals implement the documented programs and policies relating to geriatric health and elderly. This would ultimately help in better mental health services and outcomes.

8.5 Improved Social Security of Older Generation

There is a need to ensure proper nutrition, medication, and safety of the elderly. The establishment of senior citizen centers for socialization, and programs for home visits at a local level may be helpful to counter loneliness.

8.6 Use of Tele-Mental Health Services

Older individuals with mobility, transportation, or other physical limitations would have difficulty attending in-person interventions. In addition, the landscape of Nepal, centralization of services, and limited transportation facilities make in-person visits difficult. The digital interventions in the form of tele-consultation might increase the accessibility and convenience to geriatric population.

9 Conclusion

Geriatric mental health in Nepal is an emerging field that requires more attention and resources. With the increase in the ageing population, the prevalence of mental health issues among the elderly is also increasing. Recent developments in Nepal do present a promising approach to elderly care. The importance of a collaborative approach integrating physical therapy, long-term care, sensory impairment and assistive devices, rehabilitation, nutrition, and community-based care, has been realized. Despite the growing need for geriatric mental health services, there is still lack of specialized services and trained professionals in the field. In the recent years, policies have been made with special regards to geriatric health, they are yet to be implemented. To improve the situation, there is a need for implication and supervision of government policies and programs to prioritize geriatric mental health care, including increasing funding for research and training programs for healthcare providers.

References

Acharya, T., Dhungana, G. K., Traille, K., & Dhakal, H. (2023). *Gerontology and Geriatric Medicine, 9*. https://doi.org/10.1177/23337214231179902

Aich, T. K., Shah, S., & Subedi, S. (2015). Pattern of neuropsychiatric illnesses in geriatric population: An outpatient study report. *Journal of Psychiatrists' Association of Nepal*, *4*(1), https://doi.org/10.3126/jpan.v4i1.16737

Bhandari, K. (2019). Social security system of elderly population in Nepal. *NUTA Journal, 6*(1–2), 1–2. https://doi.org/10.3126/nutaj.v6i1-2.23223

Bista, S. (2024). Trends of aged population in Nepal. *Patan Prospective Journal*, *4*(01), https://doi.org/10.3126/ppj.v4i01.70218

Chalise, H. N. (2023). Aging trend and situation in Nepal. *Advances in Aging Research*, *12*(3), https://doi.org/10.4236/aar.2023.123003

Chen, Y., Hicks, A., & While, A. E. (2012). Depression and related factors in older people in China: A systematic review. *Reviews in Clinical Gerontology, 22*(1), 52–67. https://doi.org/10.1017/S0959259811000219

Clark, D., Baur, N., Clelland, D., et al. (2020). Mapping levels of palliative care development in 198 countries: The situation in 2017. *Journal of Pain and Symptom Management, 59*, 794–807.

Dahal, P., Joshi, S. K., & Swahnberg, K. (2022). A qualitative study on gender inequality and gender-based violence in Nepal. *BMC Public Health, 22*(1), 2005. https://doi.org/10.1186/s12889-022-14389-x

Dhungana, S., Chapagai, M., Tulachan, P., & Ojha, S. P. (2014). A retrospective review of elderly patients admitted in psychiatry department of a tertiary care center over 3 years. *Journal of Institute of Medicine Nepal*, *36*(3), https://doi.org/10.59779/jiomnepal.571

Gautam, D., & Adhikari, S. (2021). Palliative care services for cancer patients in Nepal, a lower-middle-income country. *Palliative Care and Social Practice, 15*, 26323524211021104. https://doi.org/10.1177/26323524211021105

Ghimire, S., Baral, B. K., Pokhrel, B. R., Pokhrel, A., Acharya, A., Amatya, D., Amatya, P., & Mishra, S. R. (2018). Depression, malnutrition, and health-related quality of life among Nepali older patients. *BMC Geriatrics, 18*(1), 191. https://doi.org/10.1186/s12877-018-0881-5

Grover, S., & Malhotra, N. (2015). Depression in elderly: A review of Indian research. *Journal of Geriatric Mental Health, 2*(1), 4. https://doi.org/10.4103/2348-9995.161376

Hossain, M., Crossland, J., Stores, R., Dewey, A., & Hakak, Y. (2020). Awareness and understanding of dementia in South Asians: A synthesis of qualitative evidence. *Dementia (London, England), 19*(5), 1441–1473. https://doi.org/10.1177/1471301218800641

Jeyakumar, S., Nealon, M., Shrestha, A., Koirala, R., Kamholz, B., & Grossberg, G. (2024). Implementing culturally-informed solutions for addressing geriatric mental health in Nepal. *The American Journal of Geriatric Psychiatry*, *32*(4, Supplement), S118–S119. https://doi.org/10.1016/j.jagp.2024.01.204

Joshi, M. R., & Chalise, H. N. (2021). Elderly abuse and quality of life: A study of community living older people of Nepal. *Journal of Medical Evidence, 2*(2), 113. https://doi.org/10.4103/JME.JME_140_20

Kamholz, B., Marahatta, K., & Magar, S. T. (2022). The Implications of accelerated aging in Nepal. *The American Journal of Geriatric Psychiatry, 30*(8), 854–858. https://doi.org/10.1016/j.jagp.2022.01.003

Khan, M. M. (2002). Suicide on the Indian subcontinent. *Crisis: The Journal of Crisis Intervention and Suicide Prevention, 23*(3), 104–107. https://doi.org/10.1027/0227-5910.23.3.104

Khanal, P., Rai, S., & Chalise, H. N. (2018). Children's migration and its effect on elderly people: A study at old age homes in Kathmandu. *American Journal of Gerontology and Geriatrics, 1*(1). https://www.remedypublications.com/american-journal-of-gerontology-and-geriatrics-abstract.php?aid=2031

Khattri, J. B. K., & Nepal, M. K. (2006). Suicidal symptoms among elderly patients attending outpatient department of Tribhuvan University Teaching Hospital. *Journal of Institute of Medicine Nepal, 28*(2), Article 2. https://nepjol.info/index.php/JIOM/article/view/598

Kohrt, B. A., Jordans, M. J. D., Turner, E. L., Sikkema, K. J., Luitel, N. P., Rai, S., Singla, D. R., Lamichhane, J., Lund, C., & Patel, V. (2018). Reducing stigma among healthcare providers to improve mental health services (RESHAPE): Protocol for a pilot cluster randomized controlled trial of a stigma reduction intervention for training primary healthcare workers in Nepal. *Pilot and Feasibility Studies, 4*, 36. https://doi.org/10.1186/s40814-018-0234-3

Kudva, K. G., El Hayek, S., Gupta, A. K., Kurokawa, S., Bangshan, L., Armas-Villavicencio, M. V. C., Oishi, K., Mishra, S., Tiensuntisook, S., & Sartorius, N. (2020). Stigma in mental illness: Perspective from eight Asian nations. *Asia-Pacific Psychiatry, 12*(2), Article e12380. https://doi.org/10.1111/appy.12380

Luitel, N. P., Neupane, V., Lamichhane, B., Koirala, G. P., Gautam, K., Karki, E., Adhikari, S., Votruba, N., Jordans, M. J. D., Kohrt, B. A., Carswell, K., Thornicroft, G., & Lempp, H. (2023). Experience of primary healthcare workers in using the mobile app-based WHO mhGAP intervention guide in detection and treatment of people with mental disorders: A qualitative study in Nepal. *SSM - Mental Health, 4*, Article 100278. https://doi.org/10.1016/j.ssmmh.2023.100278

Manandhar, K., Risal, A., Shrestha, O., Manandhar, N., Kunwar, D., Koju, R., & Holen, A. (2019). Prevalence of geriatric depression in the Kavre district, Nepal: Findings from a cross sectional community survey. *BMC Psychiatry, 19*(1), 271. https://doi.org/10.1186/s12888-019-2258-5

National Health Policy 2074. (2019, January 27). https://dohs.gov.np/national-health-policy-2074/

NCD and Mental Health Section. (n.d.). Retrieved February 14, 2023, from https://dohs.gov.np/ncd-and-mental-health-section/

Nepal Medical Council. (2017). *Code of ethics and professional conduct*. Retrieved December 8, 2024, from https://nmc.org.np/code-of-ethics-and-professional-conducts-2017

Nepal, G. M., Shrestha, A., & Acharya, R. (2019). Translation and cross-cultural adaptation of the Nepali version of the Rowland universal dementia assessment scale (RUDAS). *Journal of Patient-Reported Outcomes, 3*(1), 38. https://doi.org/10.1186/s41687-019-0132-3

NHSSP: Nepal Health Sector Support Programme. (2022). Retrieved February 8, 2023, from https://www.nhssp.org.np/GESI-Report.html

Pant, S., & Subedi, M. (2020). Impact of COVID-19 on the elderly. *Journal of Patan Academy of Health Sciences, 7*(2), Article 2. https://doi.org/10.3126/jpahs.v7i2.31104

Paudel, B. B. (2022). Socio-economic and health status of elderly people in Nepal. *Journal of Development and Social Engineering, 8*(01), 1–8.

Poudyal, S., Sharma, K., Subba, H. K., & Subba, R. (2024). Psycho-social problems among older people residing in community of Chitwan, Nepal—A cross-sectional study. *PLoS ONE, 19*(9), Article e0310849. https://doi.org/10.1371/journal.pone.0310849

Ranjan, S., Bhattarai, A., & Dutta, M. (2013). Prevalence of depression among elderly people living in old age home in the capital city Kathmandu. *Health Renaissance, 11*(3), Article 3. https://doi.org/10.3126/hren.v11i3.9634

Reynolds, C. F., 3rd., Jeste, D. V., Sachdev, P. S., & Blazer, D. G. (2022). Mental health care for older adults: Recent advances and new directions in clinical practice and research. *World Psychiatry, 21*(3), 336–363.

Rijal, R., Pokhrel, P., Adhikari, A., & Shrestha, P. (2024). Sociodemographic, clinical and treatment profile in geriatrics patients: A retrospective hospital based study in a psychiatric hospital in Nepal. *Journal of Psychiatrists' Association of Nepal (JPAN), 13*(2), 13–19.

Risal, A., Giri, E., Shrestha, O., Manandhar, S., Kunwar, D., Amatya, R., Manandhar, N., Manandhar, K., & Holen, A. (2020). Nepali version of geriatric depression scale-15—A reliability and validation study. *Journal of Nepal Health Research Council, 17*(4), 506–511. https://doi.org/10.33314/jnhrc.v17i4.1984

Risal, A., Kunwar, D., & Shrestha, B. (2024). Mental health among the elderly in Nepal: Special emphasis on depression. *OBM Geriatrics, 8*(1), Article 1. https://doi.org/10.21926/obm.geriatr.2401268

Risal, A., Manandhar, S., Manandhar, K., Manandhar, N., Kunwar, D., & Holen, A. (2020b). Quality of life and its predictors among aging people in urban and rural Nepal. *Quality of Life Research: An International Journal of Quality of Life Aspects of Treatment, Care and Rehabilitation, 29*(12), 3201–3212. https://doi.org/10.1007/s11136-020-02593-4

Samadarshi, S. C. A., Taechaboonsermsak, P., Tipayamongkholgul, M., & Yodmai, K. (2021). Quality of life and associated factors amongst older adults in a remote community, Nepal. *Journal of Health Research, 36*(1), 56–67. https://doi.org/10.1108/JHR-01-2020-0023

Senior Citizens Act, 2063 (2006)—Nepal Law Commission. (n.d.). Retrieved February 4, 2023, from https://lawcommission.gov.np/en/?cat=575

Sharma, P., Bhandari, A. R., Shakya, R., Sapkota, N., Joshi, S., Bhattarai, G., Shah, B., & Marahatta, K. (2024). Development and use of suicide registry for recording patient profile with self-harm visiting tertiary hospital of Nepal: A descriptive cross-sectional study. *JNMA; Journal of the Nepal Medical Association, 62*(276), 526–531. https://doi.org/10.31729/jnma.8733

Sharma, P., Gautam, K., & Marahatta, K. (2024). Access to mental health care in Nepal: Current status, potential challenges, and ways out. In S. M. Y. Arafat & S. K. Kar (Eds.), *Access to mental health care in South Asia: Current status, potential challenges, and ways out* (pp. 91–111). Springer Nature. https://doi.org/10.1007/978-981-99-9153-2_6

Shrestha, R., Shrestha, A. P., Shrestha, A., & Kamholz, B. (2020). Unrecognized geriatric depression in the emergency Department of a Teaching Hospital in Nepal: Prevalence, contributing factors, and metric properties of 5 item geriatric depression scale in this population. *BMC Psychiatry, 20*(1), 533. https://doi.org/10.1186/s12888-020-02910-8

Shrestha, S., Aro, A. R., Shrestha, B., & Thapa, S. (2021). Elderly care in Nepal: Are existing health and community support systems enough. *SAGE Open Medicine, 9*, 20503121211066380. https://doi.org/10.1177/20503121211066381

Simkhada, R., Wasti, S. P., Gc, V. S., & Lee, A. C. K. (2018). Prevalence of depressive symptoms and its associated factors in older adults: A cross-sectional study in Kathmandu, Nepal. *Aging & Mental Health, 22*(6), 802–807. https://doi.org/10.1080/13607863.2017.1310803

Tausig, M., & Subedi, J. (2022). Aging in Nepal. *The Gerontologist, 62*(6), 803–808. https://doi.org/10.1093/geront/gnac047

Thapa, D. K., Visentin, D., Kornhaber, R., & Cleary, M. (2018). Prevalence of mental disorders among older people in Nepal: A systematic review. *Kathmandu University Medical Journal (KUMJ), 16*(62), 181–190.

Thapa, P., Marahatta, K., Upadhyay Raj, S., Sapkota, N., Baral, P., Lama, S., Kamholz, B., Paudel, S., & Basnet, M. (2024). Dementia care landscape in Nepal: Understanding the context, barriers, and opportunities for the development of a national dementia care plan. *International Journal of Geriatric Psychiatry, 39*(6), Article e6111. https://doi.org/10.1002/gps.6111

Timalsina, R., Sherpa, P. D., & Dhakal, D. K. (2014). Factors associated with depression among elderly living in old age homes in Kathmandu Valley. *Journal of Institute of Medicine Nepal, 36*(1), Article 1. https://doi.org/10.59779/jiomnepal.616

WHO. (2023). *Mental health of older adults*. Retrieved December 4, 2024, from https://www.who.int/news-room/fact-sheets/detail/mental-health-of-older-adults

Yadav, U. N., Tamang, M. K., Paudel, G., Kafle, B., Mehta, S., Chandra Sekaran, V., & Gruiskens, J. R. J. H. (2018). The time has come to eliminate the gaps in the under-recognized burden of elder mistreatment: A community-based, cross-sectional study from rural eastern Nepal. *PLoS ONE, 13*(6), Article e0198410. https://doi.org/10.1371/journal.pone.0198410

Yadav, U. N., Thapa, T. B., Mistry, S. K., Pokhrel, R., & Harris, M. F. (2020). Socio-demographic characteristics, lifestyle factors, multi-morbid conditions and depressive symptoms among Nepalese older adults. *BMC Psychiatry, 20*(1), 261. https://doi.org/10.1186/s12888-020-02680-3

Geriatric Psychiatry in Pakistan

Osamah Khan, Saima Sheikh, and Saeed Farooq

Abstract Pakistan is currently confronted with the significant challenge of an increasingly ageing population that experiences a heightened prevalence of psychiatric and neurocognitive disorders. However, the field of geriatric psychiatry remains critically underdeveloped. The existing challenges are intensified by the limitations in psychiatric infrastructure, shortages in the workforce, and insufficient investment in healthcare. Furthermore, cultural stigma and a predominant reliance on family caregiving serve to obstruct timely interventions. Addressing these deficiencies necessitates expanding specialised training programs, strengthening community-based services, and incorporating telemedicine to enhance accessibility. In addition, legal and ethical reforms are crucial to protecting older adults against neglect and exploitation. A multidisciplinary, policy-driven framework is essential for the establishment of a sustainable geriatric mental healthcare system in Pakistan, guaranteeing equitable and evidence-based care for its ageing population. This chapter thoroughly examines the systemic barriers present and highlights the imperative need for an integrated approach to care.

Keywords Geriatric psychiatry · Dementia care · Caregiver burden · Societal stigma · Mental health · Healthcare infrastructure · Community-based care · Neurocognitive disorders · Public health interventions · Integrated mental healthcare

---

The original version of the chapter has been revised. A correction to this chapter can be found at https://doi.org/10.1007/978-981-96-7469-5_13

O. Khan (✉)
NHS Education for Scotland, Edinburgh, Scotland, UK
e-mail: osamah.khan@nhs.scot

S. Sheikh · S. Farooq
School of Medicine, Keele University, Staffordshire, UK

S. Farooq
National Institute of Health and Care Research, London, UK

N. Kar et al. (eds.), *Geriatric Psychiatry in South Asia*, South Asian Perspectives in Mental Health and Psychology , https://doi.org/10.1007/978-981-96-7469-5_5

1 Introduction

The world is experiencing an unprecedented demographic transition, with the proportion of older adults growing at an accelerated rate.According to the World Health Organization, by 2050, the global population aged 60 years and older is projected to surpass 2.1 billion, with nearly 80% of these individuals residing in low- and middle-income countries (LMICs) (World Health Organization, 2024). This transition places substantial pressure on healthcare systems, particularly in geriatric psychiatry, a field that remains underdeveloped in many LMICs, including Pakistan. While high-income countries have progressively integrated geriatric mental health services into their primary care and psychiatric systems, Pakistan lacks the specialised workforce, policies, and infrastructure required to support the growing mental health needs of its ageing population (Ahmad et al., 2013).

Pakistan, the fifth-most populous country in the world, is experiencing a rapid rise in its older adult population. As of 2024, 7% of its 240 million residents are aged 60 and above, a figure projected to triple by 2050, reaching 43.3 million (Asian Development Bank, 2024). Despite this demographic surge, Pakistan's geriatric healthcare infrastructure remains ill-equipped, particularly in addressing psychiatric and neurocognitive disorders (Karim et al., 2017). With a life expectancy of 67 years and a high burden of non-communicable diseases (NCDs) such as hypertension, diabetes, and cardiovascular illnesses, older adults are at an increased risk of developing psychiatric conditions, including depression, anxiety, dementia, and post-traumatic stress disorder (PTSD) (Khan et al., 2018; Sabzwari et al., 2019).

Studies suggest that geriatric depression rates in Pakistan range from 40% to 60%, significantly exceeding the global median prevalence of 11.7% observed in international community-based samples (Barua et al., 2011; Bhamani et al., 2013; Minallah et al., 2019; WHO, 2017). Similarly, dementia cases are expected to rise sharply, with an estimated 875,000 individuals projected to be affected by 2050 (Leroi et al, 2019; Zaidi et al., 2018). Despite this increasing disease burden, mental health services remain severely under-resourced, with only 0.19 psychiatrists per 100,000 people, one of the lowest ratios in the Eastern Mediterranean region (Javed et al., 2020; WHO, 2023).

The barriers to establishing geriatric psychiatric services in Pakistan are complex and multifaceted. Structural deficiencies; including a lack of specialised geriatric mental health units and an acute shortage of trained professionals, and limit access to care (Karim et al., 2017). Financial constraints further exacerbate the issue, as mental health services receive only 0.4% of Pakistan's total healthcare budget, significantly lower than India (1.3%) and Brazil (2.2%) (Malik & Khan, 2016; WHO, 2023). Additionally, the deep-seated cultural stigma surrounding mental health leads to widespread misconceptions, where psychiatric conditions in older adults are often attributed to supernatural causes or dismissed as natural ageing (Ali et al., 2023). Consequently, many older adults turn to traditional healers rather than seeking clinical interventions, resulting in delayed diagnoses and inadequate treatment (Javed et al., 2020; Minallah et al., 2019).

2 Mental Health Burden

The burden of mental health disorders among older adults in Pakistan is substantial, with conditions such as depression, anxiety, and PTSD being particularly prevalent. The rise in mental health issues is strongly linked to societal violence, disrupted social structures, and economic struggles (Minallah et al., 2019; Rashid, 2015; Saleem et al., 2021).

Several socio-economic and health-related factors have been identified as key contributors to geriatric depression in Pakistan. Financial insecurity, social isolation, and a lack of family support further compound mental health challenges for older adults (Saleem et al., 2021; Minallah et al., 2019). Moreover, chronic illnesses often exacerbate psychological distress, leading to a cycle of deteriorating physical and mental health. NCDs, including cardiovascular disease and diabetes, are among the leading causes of morbidity, and they often coexist with mental health disorders such as depression and anxiety. The bidirectional relationship between chronic illnesses and psychiatric conditions further complicates disease management and highlights the need for integrated care approaches (Leroi et al., 2019).

2.1 Psychiatric Disorders

Psychiatric disorders, including depression, anxiety, and posttraumatic stress disorder (PTSD,) represent significant challenges for the older adult population of Pakistan.

2.1.1 Depression

Depression among Pakistan's older adult population in Pakistan represents a significant public health challenge, as evidenced by numerous studies that have consistently reported elevated prevalence rates. A study from Karachi in 2008 reported a prevalence of 22.9% among older adults, identifying polypharmacy, urinary incontinence, financial stress, and unmet spiritual needs as key factors, with women (27.8) more affected than men (20.7) (Ganatra et al., 2008). Subsequent research has revealed even higher rates. For example, a notable study conducted in Karachi in 2013 revealed that approximately 40.6% of older adults were afflicted by depression, with prevalence rates notably higher in women (50%) compared to their male counterparts (32%) (Bhamani et al., 2013). Furthermore, familial dynamics emerged as a critical factor; older adults without spouses exhibited a 60% increased likelihood of experiencing depression, while those lacking financial support from offspring faced a twofold increase in their risk of depression (Bhamani et al., 2013).

A 2014 study conducted in Rawalpindi examined depression among older adults in care homes and community settings, revealing notable disparities. The findings reveal that the prevalence of depression is significantly higher in care home residents (60.6% on the Geriatric Depression Scale) compared to community residents (31.5%), with notable associations to factors such as gender, marital status, education, and perceived social support (Qadir et al., 2014).

By 2019, an outpatient study found that 51.6% of older adults were depressed, with women (58%) and those aged 61–70 years (57%) being the most affected (Minallah et al., 2019). Depression was more common in urban areas (56%) than in rural areas (45.5%). The study also showed higher depression rates among divorced (100%), unmarried (83%), and widowed (72%) older adults. Additionally, 72% of older adults without children had depression, compared to 46.6% of those with children, with having more male children reducing the risk by 10% (Minallah et al., 2019). More recently, a 2022 hospital-based study in Karachi found that 80.2% of older adults screened positive for depression using the Geriatric Depression Scale −15, with retirement status, financial difficulties, and absence of peer support emerging as significant independent predictors (Ali et al., 2022).

The mental health burden of depression among older adults in conflict-affected regions of Pakistan, particularly in Khyber Pakhtunkhwa, is severe but underreported. According to Rashid (2015), older individuals who have lost family members, faced displacement, or experienced violence are particularly vulnerable to major depressive disorders. However, due to cultural stigma and lack of mental health services, many do not seek professional help. A clinic-based study in Khyber Pakhtunkhwa reported significantly high depression rates, with female patients being disproportionately affected. Despite depression being a leading cause of morbidity among the elderly, mental health support systems remain inadequate, especially in rural and conflict-stricken areas (Rashid, 2015).

Globally, Pakistan's older adult depression rates, ranging from 40 to 60% in earlier community and outpatient studies, and reaching over 80% in more recent hospital-based research. This exceeds the global median of 11.7%, aligning more closely with India's range of 6%–50% (Ali et al., 2022; Bhamani et al., 2013; Minallah et al., 2019). Initial studies significantly underestimated the burden, while later research has revealed widespread underdiagnosis, unmet psychosocial needs and persistent treatment gaps (Ali et al., 2022; Bhamani et al., 2013; Minallah et al., 2019).

2.1.2 Post-Stroke Depression and Multi-Morbidity in Older Adults

Post-stroke depression (PSD) is a major public-health concern in Pakistan. A cross-sectional study at Abbasi Shaheed Hospital, Karachi, reported that 46.4% of ischemic-stroke patients experienced depression, with smoking, marital status, and lower education identified as significant risk factors (Jabeen et al., 2023). Similarly, studies from Khyber Pakhtunkhwa found that 63.3% of stroke patients experienced depression and 83.5% anxiety, with women more frequently affected and hemorrhagic stroke slightly predominating (Hussain et al., 2023; Ullah et al., 2023), further highlighting the urgent need for comprehensive post-stroke rehabilitation and mental health interventions.

2.1.3 Anxiety Disorders

Anxiety disorders represent a significant but under-researched mental health concern among older adults in Pakistan. Globally, anxiety disorders affect 16% to 27% of the geriatric population, with significantly higher rates observed in regions such as Asia and Africa due to socioeconomic challenges and healthcare barriers (Bano et al., 2021; Jalali et al., 2024). However, empirical data specific to Pakistan's ageng population remains sparse, and much of the literature draws from small, cross sectional studies or samples not exclusively focused on older adults.

Despite this limitation, available evidence suggests a high burden of anxiety disorders among Pakistan's older adults, often coexisting with depression and other chronic health conditions. For instance, elderly residents of old age homes in Lahore exhibited substantially higher anxiety and depression scores compared to those living with families, alongside poorer coping strategies and reduced quality of life (Parshad & Tufail, 2014).

Additionally, multimorbidity has been strongly associated with increased psychological distress, as older adults managing multiple chronic conditions face even higher rates of depression and anxiety, leading to functional decline (Farooq et al., 2019; Sharif et al., 2024).

2.1.4 Post-Traumatic Stress Disorder

PTSD manifests following exposure to or witnessing traumatic events. Notably, PTSD represents a significant mental health concern in Pakistan, primarily due to the pervasive issues of torture, violence, deprivation, and conflict within Pakistani society. Furthermore, the ongoing war on terrorism has subjected the Pakistani populace to a continuous series of traumatic experiences (Khan, 2023; Rashid, 2015).

In addition, a study conducted 30 months after the 2005 earthquake found high PTSD prevalence among survivors, particularly older adults, women, unmarried individuals, and those with low incomes being the most vulnerable. Moreover, living in temporary housing further increased the risk; however, social support and religious faith served as protective factors (Ali et al., 2012). Similarly, a study on flood survivors in Sindh reported elevated PTSD rates, especially among older women and individuals with lower education levels (Shah et al., 2014).

In Khyber Pakhtunkhwa, prolonged periods of violence, military operations, drone strikes, and insurgency have imposed a significant psychological burden on the population. A clinic-based study conducted in the region revealed that 36% of elderly women experienced adjustment disorders, whereas 21% of elderly men were diagnosed with PTSD (Rashid, 2015).

2.1.5 Impact of Chronic Illness and Social Determinants

Biopsychosocial factors significantly influence the quality of life (QoL) among older adults, emphasising the interconnectedness of biological, psychological, and social elements in their overall well-being (Batool et al., 2024). Chronic illnesses, such as hypertension, diabetes, and arthritis, not only lead to physical impairments but are also strongly correlated with adverse mental health outcomes (Ganatra et al., 2008). Moreover, social determinants, including family dynamics, poor spousal relationships, widowhood, lack of children, financial stress, and social isolation, intensify the mental health challenges encountered by older adults (Batool et al., 2024; Minallah et al., 2019). Notably, elderly women experience disproportionately lower QoL, frequently due to caregiving responsibilities and economic dependency, which underscores the pressing necessity for gender-sensitive interventions (Batool et al., 2024). Additionally, research indicates that older Pakistani adults experience an enhancement in QoL when they receive care from caregivers within their own homes (Qidwai & Ashfaq, 2011).

2.1.6 Late-Life Schizophrenia

Late-life schizophrenia presents distictive challenges within geriatric psychiatry, often manifesting with symptoms such as paranoia, delusions, and hallucinations and in some cases, aggression. According to the WHO, schizophrenia affects approximately 0.32% of the global population and about 0.45% of adults (WHO, 2022). Among individuals aged 65 and older, the prevalence ranges from 0.1% to 0.5% based on epidemiological studies (Howard et al., 2000). These variations can be attributed to differences in diagnostic criteria, healthcare access, and reporting practices across regions.

However, in Pakistan, the epidemiology of late-life schizophrenia remains unknown, mainly due to the absence of epidemiological studies. Despite this gap, a retrospective observational study found that 90% of hospitalised older adult schizophrenia patients were between 60 and 65 years old, with males comprising 74% of the study population. Over half of these patients (52%) lacked insight into their illness, making long-term management more complex. Additionally, medical comorbidities were present in 56%, with hypertension and diabetes among the most common, which further complicated treatment approaches (Fatima et al., 2011).

From a pharmacological perspective, atypical antipsychotics were the most frequently prescribed medications for older adult schizophrenia patients, either alone (50%) or in combination with typical agents (22%). However, polypharmacy was prevalent with many patients recieving five or more medications, increasing the risk of drug-related complications such as cognitive impairment, falls, and metabolic disturbances. Unfortunately, non-pharmacological interventions including psychotherapy and counselling were notably underutilised despite their potential benefits in improving long-term outcomes. Additionally, the absence of clinical pharmacy services in psychiatric institutions further exacerbates these challenges.

Evidence suggests that enhancing pharmaceutical care and education can significantly improve rational drug use and reduce medication-related complications among the older adult psychiatric patients (Fatima et al., 2011).

2.2 Neurocognitive Disorders

2.2.1 Dementia: A Growing Public Health Concern

Dementia is an increasing global concern, impacting over 55 million individuals as of 2020. Projections indicate that this figure may nearly double every 20 years, potentially reaching 139 million by 2050 (Alzheimer's Disease International, 2020). Alarmingly, at least 60% of these cases are expected to arise in low- and middle-income countries (LMICs), including Pakistan, where systemic healthcare constraints exacerbate the burden of this condition (Thaver & Ahmad, 2018).

In Pakistan, dementia has been recognised as one of the leading contributors to disease burden among older adults, with a standardised prevalence of 5–7% in individuals aged 60 and above (Karim et al., 2017; WHO, 2017). By 2050, approximately 1.42 million by 2050, people in Pakistan are projected to be living with dementia highlighting the urgent need for targeted interventions and healthcare reforms (Alzheimer's Disease International, 2014). Currently, estimates suggest that between 150,000 and 200,000 individuals in Pakistan are living with dementia, a number expected to rise significantly as the population ages (Khan et al., 2019). Among those aged 65 years and older, prevalence rates are projected to increase over the next three decades (Thaver & Ahmad, 2018).

The economic impact of dementia is also substantial, with annual costs exceeding $1.3 trillion and projected to rise to $2.8 trillion by 2030 (Alzheimer's Disease International, 2020). Alarmingly, a significant number of dementia cases remain undiagnosed; estimates suggest that approximately 25% individuals in low- and middle-income countries receive a formal diagnosis, leaving approximately 75% of individuals without access to appropriate treatment and support (Alzheimer's Disease International, 2014). In Pakistan, where mental illness accounted for an estimated economic burden of £2.97 billion in 2020 (Alvi et al., 2023), dementia-related care is further constrained by limited public mental health infrastructure, underfunding, and inadequate service coverage.

In Pakistan, dementia is accompanied by considerable stigma, which profoundly affects help-seeking behavi*ou*rs and caregiving experiences. A low level of public awareness leads to misinterpretation of symptoms and results in delayed diagnoses (Ali et al., 2023; Willis et al., 2020). Many families perceive dementia as a natural consequence of ag*e*ing or attribute its symptoms to spiritual issues, including black magic, often postponing necessary medical intervention (Ali et al., 2023; Khan et al., 2019; Willis et al., 2020; Zaidi et al., 2019; Zaman et al., 2019). Qualitative studies highlight widespread misconceptions, compounded by poor public awareness, inadequate diagnostic services, and weak referral systems (Ali et al., 2023; Zaman et al.,

2019). Caregivers, particularly women, face emotional distress, isolation, and lack of formal support while managing numerous responsibilities (Zaidi et al., 2019). Religious decline due to cognitive impairment, such as difficulty performing daily prayers, adds to the emotional burden for both patients and caregivers in a culturally devout society (Willis et al., 2020).

2.2.2 Addressing Dementia Through National Guidelines and Community-Based Care

Acknowledging the critical need for dementia care, the Pakistan Society of Neurologists has developed National Guidelines for Clinicians to enhance diagnosis and management. These guidelines emphasise early detection via public awareness and thorough assessments, integrating medical, cognitive, functional, and psychosocial evaluations. Recommended treatments include pharmacological options like acetylcholinesterase inhibitors and non-pharmacological methods like cognitive stimulation therapy. Caregiver education and support are vital, acknowledging families' key role in dementia care (Ahmad et al., 2013).

While the National Guidelines for Dementia were mainly developed by neurologists (Ahmad et al., 2013), psychiatric involvement remains minimal. This is concerning, as dementia is a neuropsychiatric disorder, the management of which requires a multidisciplinary approach, involving neurologists, geriatricians, and psychiatrists to ensure accurate diagnosis and comprehensive care (Berrios & Markovά, 2002). This is important because multidisciplinary team improves diagnostic accuracy, with each speciality offering complementary expertise for tailored evaluations (Leroi et al., 2019). The interplay between psychiatric and neurological conditions highlights the need for integrated care. Psychiatric symptoms may serve as early indicators underlying neurodegenerative disorders, while such conditions can also modify the course of pre-existing psychiatric illnesses, leading to atypical presentations (Berrios & Markovά, 2002). Recent evidence demonstrates that psychiatrists are actively involved in diagnosing and managing mild cognitive impairment and Alzheimer's disease, frequently conducting mental status examinations and neurological assessments (Gopalakrishna et al., 2023).

The shortage of specialised geriatric mental health services in Pakistan worsens the treatment gap, leaving many older adults without proper psychiatric care (Karim et al., 2017). Research shows that developing countries face a high burden of dementia, with rates reaching 60% of older adults in some areas (WHO, 2017). In Pakistan, the number of dementia cases is expected to exceed 1.4 million by 2050, which emphasises the urgent need for the development of dementia-specific services. Community-based care models can effectively bridge this gap. Memory clinics and outreach programs in urban areas have shown promise in delivering specialised dementia services (Khan, 2014). These initiatives improve early diagnosis and treatment, addressing significant deficits in awareness and resources within Pakistan's healthcare system (Balouch et al., 2021). However, rural populations still face severe disparities in dementia care due to cultural stigmas, inadequate infrastructure, and a lack of trained professionals (Zaidi et al., 2018).

Pakistan's mental health system remains vastly unequipped to meet the growing psychosocial needs of its ageing population (Karim et al., 2017). The Pakistan Psychiatric Society (PPS) and other stakeholders must take an active role in shaping dementia care policies, advocating for specialist geriatric mental health services, and training healthcare professionals to manage the complex interplay between dementia, psychiatric comorbidities, and social determinants of health. Collaboration between neurologists, psychiatrists, and geriatricians is essential to establish a holistic and effective dementia care framework in Pakistan (Karim et al., 2017).

2.2.3 The Socioeconomic Burden of Dementia in Pakistan

Beyond its clinical implications, dementia has profound socioeconomic consequences. Findings from the *Cognitive Impairment and Dementia in Afghanistan, Pakistan, and South Africa (CIDAPSA)* study reveal that older adults diagnosed with dementia face disproportionate levels of multidimensional poverty, further complicating their care. Families often shoulder the financial, social, and emotional burdens associated with the diseases, particularly as affected individuals lose their ability to contribute to household responsibilities. In countries like Pakistan, where social security systems are weak or underdeveloped, caregiving responsibilities frequently fall on family members—especially women—who may experience disruptions in employment or education due to their caregiving roles (CIDAPSA, 2024).

2.2.4 Challenges in Dementia Care and the Need for Systemic Reforms

Dementia care in Pakistan is hampered by deep-rooted socio-cultural factors and a fragile healthcare infrastructure. A major barrier is the social stigma surrounding mental health as the sense of *shame* or *disgrace* often prevents families from acknowledging dementia symptoms, which are frequently misinterpreted as a normal part of ageing or a 'shortcoming of character' rather than a medical condition (Khan et al., 2019).

Furthermore, Pakistan is deficient in specialised training in geriatric psychiatry, which leaves healthcare professionals inadequately prepared to address dementia-related symptoms. There is a pressing need for structured training for physicians and public awareness campaigns to address dementia and mental health conditions in older adults adequately (Karim et al., 2017). To remedy these deficiencies, a strategic roadmap for dementia research has been proposed, advocating for dedicated inpatient facilities, national screening programs, and enhanced training for healthcare professionals (Ali et al., 2023; Leroi et al., 2019).

Moreover, caregiver burnout remains a critical concern, as family members, particularly women, bear most caregiving responsibilities (Khan et al., 2019; Zaidi et al., 2019). The absence of structured training programs and professional support further exacerbates stress and fatigue among caregivers (Vahia & Kirwin, 2019). While memory clinics in urban centres provide some relief, their limited accessibility underscores the need for expanded caregiver support programs, increased access to training, and large-scale public health campaigns to promote early diagnosis and intervention (Balouch et al., 2021).

2.2.5 Traumatic Brain Injury and Its Role in Dementia Progression

Another emerging concern in dementia research is the connection between traumatic brain injuries (TBIs) and neurodegenerative disorders. In Pakistan, high rates of TBIs are exacerbated by sociopolitical instability, road traffic accidents, and terrorism, leading to long-term cognitive impairments (Razzak et al., 2015). Chronic traumatic encephalopathy (CTE), a progressive taupathy associated with repeated mild TBIs, has been linked to gradual emergence of dementia-like symptoms, including memory loss, executive dysfunction and behavioral changes, particularly in advanced stages of the disease. Emerging evidence highlights underlying mechanisms such as axonal injury, neuroinflammation and vascular dysfunction, reinforcing the need for greater awareness and preventive measures (McKee et al., 2013; Wu et al., 2020).

To address these challenges, initiatives such as the Pakistan Brain Injury Consortium (PBIC) have been established to enhance clinician training, develop dementia registries, and improve diagnostic facilities for neurodegenerative conditions. However, significant obstacles persist, including a shortage of dementia specialists, limited access to neuroimaging services, and economic barriers that hinder many older adults from receiving adequate care (Adamson et. al, 2020).

2.2.6 The Future of Dementia Care in Pakistan

Despite these challenges, some promising developments have emerged in dementia care. Memory clinics, particularly those affiliated with institutions such as Aga Khan University in Karachi, have initiated dementia screening programs aimed at early detection and intervention (Khan, 2014). However, these efforts remain insufficient, given the rapid ageing of Pakistan's population, which is projected to increase the number of individuals affected by dementia significantly (Ahmad et al., 2013). Moving forward, scaling up these programs and integrating dementia care into Pakistan's broader healthcare system will be essential in meeting the growing needs of older adults (Thaver & Ahmad, 2018).

3 Status of Geriatric Mental Health Services in Pakistan

Efforts to enhance geriatric mental healthcare in Pakistan have been diverse, focusing on raising awareness, training healthcare professionals, and developing specialised programs tailored to the needs of older adults. In urban areas, the establishment of memory clinics has provided diagnostic and therapeutic services for neurocognitive disorders such as dementia, offering much-needed support for conditions like Alzheimer's disease (Zaidi et al., 2019).

Despite the escalating demand for specialised geriatric care, the availability of dedicated facilities remains insufficient, resulting in a significant shortfall of professionals specifically trained in geriatric psychiatry. The limited accessibility of psychiatric services further exacerbates healthcare disparities, particularly affecting marginalised communities that remain underserved (Ahmad et al., 2013; Zaman et al., 2019; Ali et al., 2023). Both Zaman et al. (2019) and Ali et al. (2023) emphasise that specialist care is mostly concentrated in urban centres, leaving rural populations underserved. Addionally, primary care providers are often ill-equipped to identify or manage dementia due to lack of training, resulting in missed or delayed diagnoses (Zaman et al., 2019)

It is noteworthy that psychiatric services in Pakistan, as a whole, are severely under-resourced. According to data, Pakistan has merely 0.19 psychiatrists per 100,000 inhabitants, one of the lowest ratios in the World Health Organization (WHO) Eastern Mediterranean Region and globally (WHO Eastern Mediterranean Regional Health Observatory, 2023).This situation is worsened by inadequate dementia education amongst medical and allied healthcare disciplines (Ali et al., 2023; Zaman et al., 2019), thereby pointing out the necessity for structured training programs. Recent research has demonstrated that initiatives such as the Dementia Detectives workshop significantly enhanced knowledge and attitudes among medical and pharmacy students. Initially, only 27% of participants were able to identify symptoms and risk factors associated with dementia accurately. However, this percentage rose to 51% following the workshop, accompanied by a notable shift in their perceptions of individuals living with dementia (Ahsan et al., 2022).

In addition, Pakistan lacks specialised training programs in geriatric psychiatry, leaving many healthcare professionals ill-equipped to manage dementia-related neuropsychiatric symptoms. It has been stressed that the country needs structured training programs for physicians, alongside public awareness campaigns, to address misconceptions surrounding dementia and mental health in older adults (Karim et al., 2017).

4 Barriers to Geriatric Mental Healthcare

Pakistan faces numerous obstacles to providing effective geriatric mental healthcare, including cultural, economic, systemic, and workforce-related challenges (Murad & Siraj, 2024; Noreen et al., 2022). Collectively, these impediments obstruct access to high-quality psychiatric services for older adults, especially within marginalised and rural communities (Riaz et al., 2024). Tackling these concerns necessitates a comprehensive strategy that includes policy reforms, workforce enhancement, and improvements in healthcare infrastructure.

4.1 Cultural Stigma and Misconceptions

The lack of awareness and understanding about dementia among the general public hinders early diagnosis and proper management of the condition. Mental health conditions such as dementia and depression are frequently dismissed as natural consequences of ageing, leading to significant delays in diagnosis and care (Zaidi et al., 2019). The lack of awareness and understanding about dementia among the general public hinders early diagnosis and proper management of the condition. Furthermore, cultural beliefs often attribute dementia to supernatural causes, such as black magic, which further discourages timely medical intervention (Ali et al., 2023). Additionally, societal norms strongly emphasise family caregiving, discouraging institutionalisation, even in cases where professional support is essential (Ahmad et al., 2013).

4.2 Economic Constraints and High Out-Of-Pocket Costs

Financial burden disproportionately impacts older adults, especially those in rural areas with scarce healthcare services (Riaz et al., 2024). Moreover, socio-economic factors such as unemployment and poverty contribute to poor mental health outcomes, particularly in peri-urban and slum populations, as demonstrated in a Karachi-based study (Sharif et al., 2024).

4.3 Lack of Specialised Training & Research Provision

Pakistan lacks specialised training programs in geriatric psychiatry, leaving many healthcare professionals ill-equipped to manage dementia-related neuropsychiatric symptoms (Ali et al., 2023; Karim et al., 2017). Furthermore, there exists only one research centre dedicated to dementia care (Adamson et al., 2020).

4.4 Gaps in Healthcare Infrastructure and Service Availability

Despite the rising burden of dementia and other geriatric psychiatric disorders, mental health services remain underfunded and fragmented. Moreover, clinical assessments for dementia in Pakistan are inadequately informed by localised research, leading to a "diversity crisis" in brain health studies, as clinical current evaluations are primarily based on data collected from Caucasian populations from relatively wealthy backgrounds (Ahmad et al., 2013; Khan, 2014). Notably, healthcare services, encompassing psychiatric and dementia care, continue to exhibit a disproportionate concentration in urban areas (Ahmad et al, 2013). Conversely, rural regions are afflicted by inadequate infrastructure, a significant shortage of trained healthcare providers, and cultural barriers that impede older adults from seeking professional mental health support (Minallah et al., 2019; Riaz et al., 2024).

This disparity may be mitigated by the engagement of community health workers and general practitioners, who play a crucial role in delivering mental health services (Leroi et al., 2019). Nevertheless, these professionals frequently lack adequate training and resources, which are insufficiently developed (Hussain et al., 2018), thereby obstructing their capacity to manage geriatric patients' conditions effectively.

Research findings indicate that consistent mental health screenings and integrated care models significantly enhance patient outcomes. This is evidenced by the incorporation of mental health services into primary healthcare, which has resulted in improved identification and management of anxiety and depression within urban populations (Sharif et al., 2024). Moreover, available evidence suggests that general practitioners who provide psychiatric care can attain results comparable to those of specialists for mild to moderate cases (Pervez et al., 2024).

4.5 Caregiver Burdens and Lack of Support Services

Caregiver burnout remains a critical concern, as family members—particularly women—bear most caregiving responsibilities (Zaidi et al., 2019). They often experience immense physical, emotional, and financial strain (Vahia & Kirwin, 2019). Misconceptions about dementia and a lack of structured institutional support further exacerbate these challenges, leaving caregivers overwhelmed and unprepared for long-term care responsibilities. The absence of respite care services and structured caregiver training programs significantly adds to the burden (Vahia & Kirwin, 2019). The absence of structured training programs and professional support further exacerbates stress and fatigue among caregivers (Vahia & Kirwin, 2019). While memory clinics in urban centres provide some relief, their limited accessibility underscores the need for expanded caregiver support programs, increased access to training, and large-scale public health campaigns to promote early diagnosis and intervention (Balouch et al., 2021).

4.6 *Limited Adoption of Telemedicine and Digital Health Solutions*

Telemedicine has the potential to bridge rural–urban disparities in healthcare access. However, its adoption remains limited in Pakistan due to challenges such as poor internet penetration, low digital literacy among older adults, and insufficient investment in telehealth infrastructure (Asian Development Policy Report, 2024).

4.7 *Lack of Neuroimaging Techniques*

Pakistan's high rates of TBI resulting from sociopolitical instability, road traffic accidents, and terrorism pose a significant risk for dementia development. The lack of neuroimaging and rehabilitation services further complicates outcomes for patients with TBI-related cognitive decline (Adamson et.al, 2020).

5 Legal Aspects of Geriatric Care

Following the 18th Constitutional Amendment in 2010, mental health legislation in Pakistan was devolved to the provinces, rendering the Pakistan Mental Health Ordinance of 2001 largely obsolete at the federal level (Government of Pakistan, 2001; Tareen & Tareen, 2016). While provinces such as Sindh, Punjab, and Khyber Pakhtunkhwa enacted their own mental health acts, these laws remain largely silent on the specific needs of older adults care particularly capacity assessments, long-term care and financial protections. In contrast, the UK's Deprivation of Liberty Safeguards (DoLS) under the Mental Capacity Act 2005 provide structured legal mechanisms to protect individuals lacking capacity, including patient advocacy, and access to judicial review (Age UK, 2025). The Cheshire West judgement further clarified that continuous supervision and a lack of freedom to leave constitute a deprivation of liberty under human rights law, even in community-based care (Supreme Court of the United Kingdom, 2014). This comparison highlights critical legislative gaps in Pakistan's evolving mental health framework.

Beyond legal shortcomings, financial exploitation is a growing issue among older adults, including coerced property transfers, pension misuse, and financial neglect, which remain primarily unregulated under existing frameworks (Peterson et al., 2014). Additionally, cultural barriers further complicate legal and ethical dilemmas. At the same time, family involvement is crucial; it sometimes conflicts with individual autonomy, leading to undue influence or decision-making based on familial rather than patient interests (Minallah et al., 2019). Implementing advance directives, caregiver education programs, and culturally sensitive policies could help balance legal protections with traditional caregiving norms (Ali et al., 2023). Finally, Comprehensive Geriatric Assessments (CGA) that incorporate medical, legal, and social evaluations to ensure holistic, patient-centred care planning for older adults with neurocognitive disorders and psychiatric conditions (Ellis et al., 2017), are a crucial requirement for Pakistan.

6 Recommendations

The challenges facing geriatric mental healthcare in Pakistan highlight the need for a holistic and sustainable strategy. To address the critical gaps in geriatric mental health services in Pakistan, a comprehensive and multidisciplinary approach is required. Currently, Pakistan lacks formal training programmes or specialised degrees in geriatric psychiatry, limiting the availability of professionals to address the growing mental health needs of older adults. Unlike high-income countries with structured pathways, no dedicated fellowships or diplomas exist in Pakistan's postgraduate training bodies, such as the College of Physicians and Surgeons, Pakistan (Karim et al., 2017). While some institutes integrate some elements into general psychiatry training, this remains inadequate given the rising prevalence of geriatric psychiatric disorders (Zaidi et al., 2019). The absence of specialised training has contributed to a severe treatment gap, leading to delayed diagnoses and suboptimal management (Ali et al., 2023). Therefore, developing structured training frameworks through the Pakistan Psychiatric Society and partnerships with international institutions could bridge this gap and improve mental health services for older adults (Karim et al., 2017). Additionally, interdisciplinary collaboration between psychiatrists, neurologists (Gopalakrishna et al., 2023) and primary care physicians must be strengthened to provide more comprehensive and continuous care for older adult patients.

From a policy and infrastructure perspective, studies such as those by the Asian Development Bank (2024), WHO (2023), and Malik and Khan (2016) highlight the need for more significant financial investment in geriatric healthcare. Pakistan allocates only a fraction of its health budget to mental health services, which is insufficient given the growing burden of dementia, depression, and anxiety among older adults. A reallocation of resources is required to establish structured screening programs for early dementia detection and psychiatric disorders in older adults. Furthermore, expanding mental health infrastructure, particularly in rural and underserved regions, will ensure equitable access to essential services. Creating dedicated geriatric psychiatric units in tertiary hospitals and community health centres will significantly enhance service delivery.

Beyond institutional settings, community-based mental health models have shown promising outcomes in countries with similar socioeconomic constraints. Zaidi et al. (2019), Balouch et al. (2021), and Pervez et al. (2024) advocate for integrating geriatric psychiatric care into primary healthcare. This approach involves training general practitioners to diagnose and manage common psychiatric disorders in older adults, reducing the burden on specialised services. Community outreach programs are equally important, as they help educate families and caregivers on dementia management, encourage early intervention, and promote social inclusion. Expanding home-based interventions and support services will allow ageing individuals to maintain independence and avoid unnecessary institutionalisation.

One of the most significant barriers to accessing mental healthcare in Pakistan is the widespread cultural stigma surrounding psychiatric illnesses in older adults. Ali et al. (2023), Minallah et al. (2019), and Rashid (2015) identify societal misconceptions as key contributors to delayed diagnosis and treatment. Many individuals and families attribute symptoms of dementia and depression to supernatural causes, leading them to seek treatment from traditional healers rather than medical professionals. Nationwide awareness campaigns are necessary to change these perceptions, and the involvement of religious and community leaders can help challenge these deeply ingrained beliefs. Public education on mental health, mainly through media and community-based programs, will be crucial in normalising psychiatric care for older adults.

In parallel with improving clinical services, support for caregivers remains a crucial but neglected area in Pakistan's geriatric psychiatry landscape. Research by Vahia and Kirwin (2019), Zaidi et al. (2019), and Karim et al. (2011) point out the immense psychological and financial strain faced by family caregivers, particularly women, who bear the primary responsibility for caring for older relatives. Structured training programs should be implemented to equip caregivers with the knowledge and skills to manage dementia and psychiatric conditions effectively. Additionally, financial and psychosocial support systems must be developed to alleviate the caregiving burden. Introducing respite care services would provide much-needed relief for caregivers, allowing them temporary breaks while ensuring continued patient support.

Integrating digital health solutions presents another avenue for improving access to geriatric mental healthcare. The Asian Development Policy Report (2024), Noorullah et al. (2024) and Adamson et al. (2020) emphasise the role of telemedicine in bridging rural–urban healthcare disparities. Expanding telepsychiatry services would enable older adults in remote regions to receive consultations from mental health professionals without travelling long distances. However, this requires investment in digital literacy programs for older adults and their caregivers, as well as the development of affordable and user-friendly telehealth platforms. Furthermore, advances in artificial intelligence and cognitive assessment tools should be explored to facilitate the early diagnosis of dementia and other neuropsychiatric disorders.

Legal and ethical protections for older adults with mental illnesses remain insufficient under Pakistan's current mental health laws. The Pakistan Mental Health Ordinance (2001), as noted, lacks specific provisions addressing the rights and protections of older adults with cognitive and psychiatric disorders. Legal frameworks must be revised to introduce stronger safeguards against elder abuse, financial exploitation, and inadequate psychiatric care. Establishing independent advocacy roles and ensuring comprehensive assessments of mental capacity would help protect vulnerable older adults from coercion and neglect. Additionally, integrating ethical considerations into psychiatric treatment plans will help uphold patient autonomy and dignity.

7 Conclusion

Addressing the mental health needs of Pakistan's ageing population requires a proactive, multidisciplinary approach. With rising rates of dementia, depression, and anxiety among older adults, the country must invest in specialised training, infrastructure, and community-based interventions. Overcoming cultural stigma, expanding caregiver support, and integrating digital solutions will ensure accessible and sustainable mental health services. Legal reforms are also necessary to safeguard vulnerable elderly individuals. By implementing these measures, Pakistan can create a more inclusive and effective geriatric mental healthcare system, improving the quality of life for its ageing population.

References

Adamson, M. M., Shakil, S., Sultana, T., Hasan, M. A., Mubarak, F., Enam, S. A., & Razi, A. (2020). Brain injury and dementia in Pakistan: Current perspectives. *Frontiers in Neurology, 11*, 299. https://doi.org/10.3389/fneur.2020.00299

Age UK. (2025). *Factsheet 62: Deprivation of Liberty Safeguards*. Retrieved from https://www.ageuk.org.uk/globalassets/age-uk/documents/factsheets/fs62_deprivation_of_liberty_safeguards_fcs.pdf

Ahmad, A., Owais, K., Siddiqui, M., Mamun, K., Rao, F., & Yousufzai, A. W. (2013). Dementia in Pakistan: national guidelines for clinicians. *Pakistan Journal of Neurological Sciences (PJNS), 8*(3), 17–27. http://ecommons.aku.edu/pjns

Ahmed, S., Chase, L. E., Wagnild, J., Akhter, N., Sturridge, S., Clarke, A., & Hampshire, K. (2022). Community health workers and health equity in low-and middle-income countries: Systematic review and recommendations for policy and practice. *International Journal for Equity in Health, 21*(1), 49. https://doi.org/10.1186/s12939-021-01615-y

Ali, M., Farooq, N., Bhatti, M. A., & Kuroiwa, C. (2012). Assessment of prevalence and determinants of posttraumatic stress disorder in survivors of earthquake in Pakistan using Davidson Trauma Scale. *Journal of Affective Disorders, 136*(3), 238–243. https://doi.org/10.1016/j.jad.2011.12.023

Ali, S., Zehra, M., Fatima, T., & Nadeem, A. (2023). Advancing dementia care in Pakistan: Challenges and the way forward. *Frontiers in Dementia, 2*, 1241927. https://doi.org/10.3389/frdem.2023.1241927

Ali, Z., Amin, F., Saeed, R., Durrani, N., Pasha, M. S., & Ahmed, I. (2022). Frequency and predictors of depression among the elderly population of Karachi. *Journal of Family Medicine and Primary Care, 11*(11), 6920–6928. https://doi.org/10.4103/jfmpc.jfmpc_947_22

Alvi, M. H., Ashraf, T., Kiran, T., Iqbal, N., Gumber, A., Patel, A., & Husain, N. (2023). Economic burden of mental illness in Pakistan: An estimation for the year 2020 from existing evidence. *Bjpsych International, 20*(3), 54–56. https://doi.org/10.1192/bji.2023.4

Alzheimer's Disease International. (2020). *World Alzheimer Report 2020*. Retrieved from https://www.alzint.org/

Alzheimer's Disease International. (2014). *Dementia in the Asia Pacific region*. Alzheimer's Australia. https://www.alzint.org/u/dementia-in-the-asia-pacific-region.pdf

Ahsan, M., Anwer, K., Raza, H., Ali, S., Ali, M., & Akhter, P. (2022). Knowledge, perceptions, and attitudes towards dementia among medical students in Pakistan. *Indonesian Journal of Community and Special Needs Education, 2*(1), 29–38. https://doi.org/10.17509/ijcsne.v2i1.38408

Asian Development Bank. (2024). *Ageing well in Asia: Asian development policy report*. https://doi.org/10.22617/SGP240253-3

Bano, Z., Ejaz, M., & Ahmad, I. (2021). Assessment of prevalence of anxiety in adult population and development of anxiety scale: A study of 819 patients with anxiety disorder. *Pakistan Journal of Medical Sciences, 37*(2), 472–476. https://doi.org/10.12669/pjms.37.2.2158

Balouch, S., Zaidi, A., Farina, N., & Willis, R. (2021). Dementia awareness, beliefs and barriers among family caregivers in Pakistan. *Dementia, 20*, 899–918. https://doi.org/10.1177/1471301220915066

Barua, A., Ghosh, M. K., Kar, N., & Basilio, M. A. (2011). Prevalence of depressive disorders in the elderly. *Annals of Saudi Medicine, 31*(6), 620–624. https://doi.org/10.4103/0256-4947.87100

Batool, S. S., Tanveer, S., Chatrath, S. K., & Batool, S. A. (2024). Biopsychosocial determinant of quality of life of older adults in Pakistan and Canada. *Front. Psychiatry, 15*, 1364443. https://doi.org/10.3389/fpsyt.2024.1364443

Berrios, G. E., & Marková, I. S. (2002). The concept of neuropsychiatry: a historical overview. *Journal of psychosomatic research, 53*(2), 629–638. https://doi.org/10.1016/s0022-3999(02)00427-0

Bhamani, M. A., Karim, M. S., & Khan, M. M. (2013). Depression in the elderly in Karachi, Pakistan: a cross sectional study. *BMC Psychiatry, 13*, 181. https://doi.org/10.1186/1471-244X-13-181

CIDAPSA Study. (2024). *Cognitive impairment and Dementia in Afghanistan, Pakistan, and South Africa*. https://sites.wustl.edu/globaldisability/items/dementia-and-aging-projectdementia-and-aging/

Ellis, G., Gardner, M., Tsiachristas, A., Langhorne, P., Burke, O., Harwood, R. H., Conroy, S. P., Kircher, T., Somme, D., Saltvedt, I., Wald, H., O'Neill, D., Robinson, D., & Shepperd, S. (2017). Comprehensive geriatric assessment for older adults admitted to hospital. *The Cochrane Database of Systematic Reviews, 9*(9), CD006211. https://doi.org/10.1002/14651858.CD006211.pub3

Fatima, A., Barkat, U., Mahmood, K. T., & Zaka, M. (2011). Schizophrenia in elderly patients. *Journal of Pharmaceutical Sciences and Research, 3*(1), 952–960.

Farooq, R., Jawad, U., Khan, I., Rehman, M., Irfan, M. S., & Ullah, S. (2022). A cross-sectional study on behavioral manifestation in Alzheimer's disease patients and their association with cognitive impairment. *Pakistan Journal of Medical & Health Sciences, 16*(02), 952. https://doi.org/10.53350/pjmhs22162952

Farooq, S., Khan, T., Zaheer, S., & Shafique, K. (2019). Prevalence of anxiety and depressive symptoms and their association with multimorbidity and demographic factors: A community-based, cross-sectional survey in Karachi. *Pakistan. BMJ Open, 9*(11), Article e029315. https://doi.org/10.1136/bmjopen-2019-029315

Ganatra, H. A., Zafar, S. N., Qidwai, W., & Rozi, S. (2008). Prevalence and predictors of depression among an older adult population of Pakistan. *Aging & Mental Health, 12*(3), 349–356. https://doi.org/10.1080/13607860802121068

Gopalakrishna, G., Brunton, S., Pruzin, J., Alford, S., Hamersky, C., & Sabharwal, A. (2023). Understanding the role of psychiatrists in the diagnosis and management of mild cognitive impairment and mild Alzheimer's disease dementia: a cross-sectional survey. *BMC psychiatry, 23*(1), 716. https://doi.org/10.1186/s12888-023-05129-5

Government of Pakistan. (2001). The Mental Health Ordinance, 2001. *Islamabad: Ministry of Law and Justice.* Retrieved from https://health.punjab.gov.pk/system/files/Mental%20Health%20Ordinance%202001.pdf

Jabeen, S. J. S., Sadia, M., Begum, S., & Khan, M. N. A. (2023). The frequency of depression in post stroke patients presenting at outpatient department of Abbasi Shaheed hospital, Karachi: Depression in post stroke patients. *Pakistan Journal of Health Sciences*, 231–235. https://doi.org/10.54393/pjhs.v4i06.866.

Jalali, A., Ziapour, A., Karimi, Z., Rezaei, M., Emami, B., Kalhori, R. P., & Kazeminia, M. (2024). Global prevalence of depression, anxiety, and stress in the elderly population: A systematic review and meta-analysis. *BMC Geriatrics, 24*(1), 809. https://doi.org/10.1186/s12877-024-05311-8

Javed, A., Khan, M. N. S., Nasar, A., & Rasheed, A. (2020). Mental healthcare in Pakistan. *Taiwanese Journal of Psychiatry, 34*(1), 6–14. https://doi.org/10.4103/TPSY.TPSY_8_20

Howard, R., Rabins, P. V., Seeman, M. V., Jeste, D. V., & The International Late-Onset Schizophrenia Group. (2000). Late-onset schizophrenia and very-late-onset schizophrenia-like psychosis: An international consensus. *American Journal of Psychiatry, 157*(2), 172–178. https://doi.org/10.1176/appi.ajp.157.2.172

Hussain, S. S., Khan, M., Gul, R., & Asad, N. (2018). Integration of mental health into primary healthcare: Perceptions of stakeholders in Pakistan. *Eastern Mediterranean Health Journal, 24*(2), 146–153.

Hussain, S. S., Ullah, Z., Bacha, M., & Khalil, S. U. (2023, April 17). Prevalence of post-stroke depression and anxiety among patients admitted in Khyber Teaching Hospital Peshawar [Preprint]. *medRxiv*. https://doi.org/10.1101/2023.04.10.23288355

Karim, S., Minhas, H. M., Bhattacharya, S., Sein, K., Nayar, B., Morris, J., Nizami, A., Minhas, F., & Burns, A. (2011). The symptomatology of Alzheimer's disease: A cross-cultural study. *International Journal of Geriatric Psychiatry, 26*(4), 415–422. https://doi.org/10.1002/gps.2544

Karim, S., Rana, M. H., & Rana, R. Z. (2017). The need for developing specialist mental health services for the elderly in Pakistan. *Journal of Pakistan Psychiatric Society*, *14*(4), 6–7. https://www.jpps.pk/index.php/journal/article/view/520

Khan, Q. (2014). Dementia: Challenges of practice in Pakistan. *Neurology, 83*(22), 2091–2092. https://doi.org/10.1212/WNL.0000000000001018

Khan, A. (2023). Cognitive behavioral therapy for posttraumatic stress disorder in Pakistan. In *Handbook of cognitive behavioral therapy by disorder* (pp. 365–375). Academic Press. https://doi.org/10.1016/B978-0-323-85726-0.00010-7

Khan, A. T., Toor, R. H., & Amjad, Q. (2018). Assessment and management of geriatric care in Pakistan. *Journal of Gerontology & Geriatric Research, 7*(5). https://doi.org/10.4172/2167-7182.1000488

Khan, M. N. S., Afridi. M. I,, & Javed, A. (2019). Pakistan. In A. Burns, P. Robert, & Ideal steering group. (2019, March). Dementia care: International perspectives. *Current Opinion in Psychiatry*, *32*(4), 361–365. https://doi.org/10.1097/YCO.0000000000000511

Khan, Q. (2014). Dementia: Challenges of practice in Pakistan. *Neurology, 83*(24), 2091–2092. https://doi.org/10.1212/WNL.0000000000001018

Leroi, I., Chaudhry, N., Daniel, A., Dunne, R., Eman, S., Farina, N., & Wasay, M. (2019). A roadmap to develop dementia research capacity and capability in Pakistan: A model for low-and middle-income countries. *Alzheimer's & Dementia: Translational Research & Clinical Interventions, 5*, 939–952. https://doi.org/10.1016/j.trci.2019.11.005

Malik, A. M., & Khan, M. M. (2016). Economic burden of mental illnesses in Pakistan. *Journal of Mental Health Policy and Economics, 19*(3), 155–166.

McKee, A. C., Stern, R. A., Nowinski, C. J., Stein, T. D., Alvarez, V. E., & Daneshvar, D. H. (2013). The spectrum of disease in chronic traumatic encephalopathy. *Brain, 136*(1), 43–64. https://doi.org/10.1093/brain/aws307

Minallah, A., Azam, N., & Merani, I. (2019). Frequency of depression with associated risk factors among elderly in two tertiary care hospitals in Rawalpindi. *Pakistan Armed Forces Medical Journal, 2*, S317.

Murad, S., & Siraj, S. (2024). Bridging the void: Unravelling mental health policies for the older adults in Pakistan's tapestry—A literature review. *Journal of Clinical Psychology and Neurology, 2*(17), 1–4. https://doi.org/10.61440/JCPN.2024.v2.17

Noreen, N., Abdullah, M., & Lalani, N. (2022). Geriatric care in Pakistan: Current realities and way forward. *Pakistan Journal of Public Health, 11*(4), 214–219. Available from: https://pjph.org/pjph/article/view/872

Noorullah, A., Asad, N., Pirani, S., Iqbal, S., & Khan, M. M. (2024). Mental health care in Pakistan. In S. M. Y. Arafat & S. K. Kar (Eds.), *Access to mental health care in South Asia* (pp. 123–144). Springer. https://doi.org/10.1007/978-981-99-9153-2_7.

Parshad, N., & Tufail, A. (2014). Depression, anxiety, coping and quality of life among elderly living in old age homes and in family setup. *Pakistan Journal of Professional Psychology: Research and Practice, 5*(1). https://doi.org/10.62663/pjpprp.v5i1.93

Pervez, A., Bukhari, M. M., Chhapra, R., Baig, M. I., Martins, R. S., Pirzada, S., Rizvi, N. A., Aamdani, S. S., Ayub, B., Rehman, A. A., Mustafa, M. A., Nadeem, S., Asad, N., Haider, A. H., & Nadeem, T. (2024). Adolopment of clinical practice guidelines and creation of referral pathways for psychiatric conditions in Pakistan. *The Lancet Regional Health. Southeast Asia, 23*, Article 100387. https://doi.org/10.1016/j.lansea.2024.100387

Peterson, J. C., Burnes, D. P., Caccamise, P. L., Mason, A., Wells, M. T., Berman, J., Cook, A. M., Shukoff, D., Brownell, P., Powell, M., Salamone, A., Pillemer, K. A., & Lachs, M. S. (2014). Financial exploitation of older adults: A population-based prevalence study. *Journal of General Internal Medicine, 29*(12), 1615. https://doi.org/10.1007/s11606-014-2946-2

Qadir, F., Haqqani, S., Khalid, A., Huma, Z., & Medhin, G. (2014). A pilot study of depression among older people in Rawalpindi, Pakistan. *BMC Research Notes, 7*, 1–9. https://doi.org/10.1186/1756-0500-7-409

Qidwai, W., Ashfaq, T. (2011). Elderly patients and their health in Pakistan: current status, issues, challenges and opportunities. *Journal of Liaquat University of Medical and Health Sciences, 10*(3). Available at: http://ecommons.aku.edu/pakistan_fhs_mc_fam_med/68

Rashid, A. (2015). Elderly mental health in Northwest Pakistan: An overview in the context of violence and trauma. *Journal of Geriatric Care and Research, 2*(1), 14–15.

Razzak, J. A., Baqir, S. M., Khan, U. R., Heller, D., Bhatti, J., & Hyder, A. A. (2015). Emergency and trauma care in Pakistan: A cross-sectional study of healthcare levels. *Emergency Medicine Journal, 32*(3), 207–213. https://doi.org/10.1136/emermed-2013-202590

Riaz, K., Sajid, M., Ishtiaq, M., & Amin, H. (2024). Barriers and access to mental health care in rural areas of Pakistan: An inferential statistical analysis. *Journal of Population Therapeutics and Clinical Pharmacology, 31*(9), 2892–2902. https://doi.org/10.53555/mhznzr83

Sabzwari, S. R., Iqbal, R., Fatmi, Z., & Azam, I. (2019). Factors associated with geriatric morbidity and impairment in a megacity of Pakistan. *PLoS ONE, 14*(6), Article e0218872. https://doi.org/10.1371/journal.pone.0218872

Shah, S., Van den Bergh, R., Van Bellinghen, B., Severy, N., Sadiq, S., Afridi, S. A., & Zachariah, R. (2014). Offering mental health services in a conflict affected region of Pakistan: Who comes, and why? *PLoS ONE, 9*(6), Article e97939. https://doi.org/10.1371/journal.pone.0097939

Sharif, H., Sheikh, S. S., Thompson, A. M., Hashim, M., Seemi, T., Zaidi, K., & Saleem, S. M. (2024). Prevalence of mental disorders among patients with multimorbidity visiting primary care settings in Slums of Karachi, Pakistan. *Journal of Primary Care & Community Health, 15*, 21501319241258656. https://doi.org/10.1177/21501319241258658

Saleem, S., Baig, A., Sajun, S., Bird, V., Priebe, S., & Pasha, A. (2021). A mixed methods exploration of the role of multi-family groups in community treatment of patients with depression and anxiety in Pakistan. *International Journal of Mental Health Systems, 15*(1), 78. https://doi.org/10.1186/s13033-021-00500-z

Supreme Court of the United Kingdom. (2014). *P v Cheshire West and Chester Council and another; P and Q v Surrey County Council [UKSC 19]*. Retrieved from https://www.supremecourt.uk/cases/uksc-2012-0068.html
Tareen, A., & Tareen, K. I. (2016). Mental health law in Pakistan. *BJPsych international, 13*(3), 67–69. https://doi.org/10.1192/s2056474000001276
Thaver, A., & Ahmad, A. (2018). Economic perspective of dementia care in Pakistan. *Neurology, 90*(5), e993–e994. https://doi.org/10.1212/WNL.0000000000005108
Ullah, I., Khan, A., Tariq, M., Akhtar, N., Kousar, & Rabnawaz. (2023). The burden of post-stroke depression and anxiety among stroke patients admitted to tertiary care teaching hospitals of Khyber Pakhtunkhwa. *Journal of Health and Rehabilitation Research, 3*(2), 1047–1051. https://doi.org/10.61919/jhrr.v3i2.292
UNDP. (2019). *Human development report*. United Nations Development Programme.
Vahia, I. V., & Kirwin, P. D. (2019). Education in geriatric psychiatry. In M. Hermans, T. Chay-Hoon, & E. Pi (Eds.), *Education about mental health and illness* (pp. 198–217). Springer. https://doi.org/10.1007/978-981-10-2350-7_15
World Bank. (2024). *World development indicators*. Retrieved from https://www.worldbank.org.
WHO Eastern Mediterranean Reginal Health Observatory Pakistan > News > press release 2023. https://www.emro.who.int/pak/pakistan-news/who-pakistan-celebrates-world-mental-health-day.html
World Health Organization. (2017). *Pakistan: WHO statistical profile*. Retrieved from https://www.who.int/docs/default-source/mental-health/dementia/gdo-country-profiles/gdo-pakistan.pdf
World Health Organization. (2023). *Mental health atlas 2023*. WHO. https://www.who.int/publications/i/item/mental-health-atlas-2023
World Health Organization. (2022, January 10). *Schizophrenia*. https://www.who.int/news-room/fact-sheets/detail/schizophrenia
World Health Organization. (2024, October 1). Ageing and health. https://www.who.int/news-room/fact-sheets/detail/ageing-and-health
Willis, R., Zaidi, A., Balouch, S., & Farina, N. (2020). Experiences of people with dementia in Pakistan: Help-seeking, understanding, stigma, and religion. *The Gerontologist, 60*(1), 145–154. https://doi.org/10.1093/geront/gny143
Wu, Z., Wang, Z. H., Liu, X., Zhang, Z., Gu, X., Yu, S. P., Keene, C. D., Cheng, L., & Ye, K. (2020). Traumatic brain injury triggers APP and Tau cleavage by delta-secretase, mediating Alzheimer's disease pathology. *Progress in Neurobiology, 185*, Article 101730. https://doi.org/10.1016/j.pneurobio.2019.101730
Zaidi, A., Willis, R., Farina, N., & Balouch, S. (2018). Understanding, beliefs, and treatment of dementia in Pakistan: Final report. *Age International*. https://www.ageinternational.org.uk/globalassets/documents/final_report_dementia_in_pakistan_september209.pdf
Zaidi, A., Willis, R., Farina, N., Balouch, S., Jafri, H., Ahmed, I., Khan, Q., & Jaffri, R. (2019). *Understanding, beliefs and treatment of dementia in Pakistan: Final report. University of Southampton*. https://www.southampton.ac.uk/assets/imported/transforms/content-block/UsefulDownloads_Download/B179D58B112C4B79BCAFBE9D774D649C/Dementia%20in%20Pakistan%20Final%20Report%2031%20January%202019.pdf
Zaman, Q., Siddiqui, M., & Malik, Z. I. (2019). Dementia in Pakistan: An unprecedented challenge and local cultural beliefs, problems and actions required. *Pakistan Journal of Neurological Sciences, 14*(1), Article 4, https://ecommons.aku.edu/pjns/vol14/iss1/4

Geriatric Psychiatry in Sri Lanka

Anuprabha Wickramasinghe and Malsha Gunathilake

Abstract Sri Lanka is the fastest-ageing country in South Asia, probably due to its long-standing commitment towards the health and literacy of the people. This expansion of the elderly population is happening before the country's economy is ready for such a transformation, posing many challenges. With certain key policies and action plans that came into place across the globe, Sri Lanka is gearing up for the challenge of catering for the varied demands of the ageing population. Still, there is a lot of uncertainty and apprehension whether we are doing enough in preparation for the avalanche ahead. Recent economic troubles and the massive out bound migration of young workforce have made the country weaker and more vulnerable. Inadequate understanding of the problem, the lack of coordination between stakeholders and the lack of vision for the future are concerning. Country needs stronger political and financial commitment and changes to the existing policies and practices such as increasing the retirement age, and more active participation of the young old in the country's development journey. Efficient top-down as well as bottom-up approaches are needed in order to face the challenges with more confidence.

Keywords Older adults · Sri Lanka · Population ageing · Services · Dementia

1 Introduction

Sri Lanka, an island located in the Indian Ocean, has a total land area of 62,710 square kilometres. The total population of Sri Lanka at mid-year 2024 stood at 23 104 000, out of which 3 966 000 (17.2% of the population) were above 60 years and 2 796 000 (12.1%) were above 65 years (ESCAP, 2024).

A. Wickramasinghe (✉)
Department of Psychiatry, Faculty of Medicine, University of Colombo, Colombo, Sri Lanka
e-mail: anuprabha@psych.cmb.ac.lk

M. Gunathilake
Colombo South Teaching Hospital, Kalubowila, Sri Lanka

N. Kar et al. (eds.), *Geriatric Psychiatry in South Asia*, South Asian Perspectives in Mental Health and Psychology , https://doi.org/10.1007/978-981-96-7469-5_6

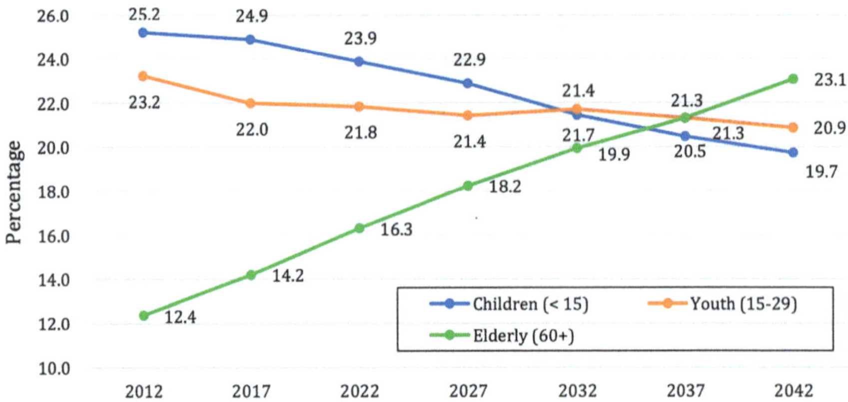

Fig. 1 Relative size of children (< 15 years), youth (15–29 years) and older adults (60 + years) populations in Sri Lanka, 2012–2042 (*Source* de Silva and De Silva, 2023)

Sri Lanka is currently experiencing a notable demographic transformation, characterised by a rapidly ageing population that represents the fastest-growing older adult demographic in South Asia (Solano, 2021). It has been projected that by year 2050, above 60 years age category will represent 25.9% of the population and above 65 years 20.3% (ESCAP, 2024).

Figure 1 illustrates the current and projected population percentages across different age groups (Silva and de Silva, 2023). While children currently outnumber the older adult population, this trend is expected to reverse by 2037, when the older adult population will surpass the number of children and youth.

Improvements in healthcare services and infrastructure over the past decades have led to a significant increase in life expectancy for both males and females in Sri Lanka. As of the latest data, the life expectancy for females is 80.7 years, while for males, it is 74.4 years (WHO, 2024). Female life expectancy is forecasted to increase to 84.3 years and male life expectancy to 78.7 years by 2050 (www.healthdata.org, 2025).

This trend presents both challenges and opportunities, particularly in the domain of mental health. As the older adult population grows, addressing their mental health needs becomes crucial to ensuring their quality of life and reducing the societal and economic burdens of untreated mental health conditions.

2 Epidemiology

Sri Lanka recognises 60 years as the beginning of old age, for administrative purposes. Currently, the country has nearly four million older adults, out of which nearly three out of four belong to the above 65 years age group (ESCAP, 2024).

A shrinking working age population to support an expanding older adult population will result in a rapid rise in the dependency ratio. Moreover, an ageing workforce will be less efficient, and an ageing population will have increased expenditure on pensions, health and long-term care provisions. For Sri Lanka, this transformation is happening ahead of an expected economic development and at a lower level of per capita income (Asian Development Bank, 2019).

2.1 Determinants of Health of Older Adults

Both environmental and personal characteristics determine the health of an older person, and a lower socio-economic position makes a person vulnerable to lower health (WHO, 2024).

Income and Social Status

Income of citizens in Sri Lanka declines with age, especially between 55 and 64 years. As most of the elders live in multigenerational households with their children and their families, their poverty levels correlate with the poverty rates of the population. Rural and estate sector elders are more vulnerable to poverty, and about 1 in 10 elders above 70 years in these sections may be getting senior citizens' allowance. In 2006, Sri Lanka Ageing Survey showed that about half of the older adults receive cash assistance from their adult children as a primary source of income (World Bank, 2008). About 75% of elders receive food and other material goods from adult children, especially when they do not have a pension. More than half of EPF members in Sri Lankan spend their EPF money without saving for the future. Very old citizens have a higher risk of poverty than young old citizens (Asian Development Bank, 2019).

It is also not uncommon to see elders begging for food or money in the streets, revealing a segment of the older adults suffering from hunger, extreme poverty and homelessness (HelpAge International, 2022). They are also seen gathering around religious sites where they might receive free food and other donations. People are de-sensitised to such sights partly because it may be difficult to differentiate a true sufferer from an impersonator by an untrained eye. Older adults suffering from extreme poverty are not able to represent themselves for a number of reasons including negative emotions such as shame and embarrassment, and this is an area that needs due attention (World Bank Blogs, 2013).

Education

Higher level of education and literacy bring better health, social, economic and living standards for people. In the 2012 census, the overall language literacy rate among Sri Lankans was reported as 95.7%. The older cohorts of people had relatively lower levels of literacy and education than the younger cohorts. About 10% of the older population had not attended school, while only about one-third completed primary education. Females have a lower literacy rate than males. The introduction of free education in 1947 drove higher literacy rates among the younger-old groups, which put Sri Lanka ahead in the demographic transformation.

Physical Environment

The country has nine provinces and 25 districts. The Western province accommodates approximately one-third of older adults above 60 years of age. The western province is home to administrative capital as well as the commercial capital of Sri Lanka, and high level of migration to the capital as well as lower fertility rate may have caused this skewed distribution of older adults in the Western province.

Despite the urbanisation of the population, three out of four older adults in Sri Lanka still live in rural areas (Asian Development Bank, 2019). Many of the rural elders are left behind by their younger families due to out migration for education and employment.

The country provides safe water, clean air and a thriving ground for fauna and flora. Natural disasters are not common, although climate change is posing a threat to the equilibrium. Road networks are somewhat underdeveloped overall, especially in the rural settings. Most of the older adults depend on public transport for commuting, which is in a poor state. The use of three-wheelers is common, but they have a poor safety record.

Housing and Living Arrangements

In 2012, 70% of older adults lived in permanent houses, most of the rest lived in semi-permanent houses, while a very small percentage lived in improvised houses (United Nations Population Fund, Sri Lanka, 2016).

Overall, about 60% of older adults live in multigenerational households with their extended families. This is a phenomenon common among the oldest old, showing the important role played by younger family members towards the wellbeing of older members. The number of older adults living independently however is steadily increasing in Sri Lanka (United Nations Population Fund, Sri Lanka, 2016).

Loneliness and Social Networks

Many factors contribute to the loneliness in old age such as children leaving family homes, migration, retirement, bereavement, sensory impairment and disability with restricted mobility. Old age is packed with negative life events such as losses of loved ones demanding constant adjustment from this vulnerable group.

Ageing migrant populations, mainly in cities, face loneliness, lack of access to social networks, and lack of aged friendly living arrangements, and therefore need opportunities to social activities and participation (United Nations Population Fund, Sri Lanka, 2016).

A study conducted in care homes in Colombo district showed significant level of loneliness among the residents which they related to feeling abandoned by their families. Many had moved to residential institutions due to the inadequate care by the families in the first place. They understood loneliness as a feeling of inner suffering that they try to cope with various ways such as acceptance, religious practices, staying in touch with family, and by engaging in social activities (Anna-Karin Edberg, 2019).

Older adults living in the community are also vulnerable to loneliness which has both psychological and physical consequences. One study looking at social and emotional loneliness in older adults living in a coastal suburb in Sri Lanka found an overall prevalence of social and emotional loneliness to be 47.8% (Subathevan et al., 2022).

2.2 *Burden of Health Issues Among the Older Adults in Sri Lanka*

The ageing population of Sri Lanka is posing many challenges in providing for the extra demands of the needs of the older citizens. The needs arise from several areas such as deterioration of their physical health, increased vulnerability to neurocognitive and mental disorders as well as social factors such as loss of job, grief, loneliness, isolation and poverty (Mendonc, 2013; Pandey et al., 2022). Further to this, they are vulnerable to violations of human rights and stigma.

2.2.1 Physical Health

Non-communicable Disease

Cardiovascular diseases were the most common cause of death, while sense organ disease was responsible for the most number of years of healthy life lost due to disability in the above 60 years of age group in Sri Lanka.

Sri Lanka Health and Aging Survey 2018/19 found the crude prevalence of diabetes among adults to be 23% and age standardised prevalence to be 21.8%. Prevalence of pre-diabetes was 30.5%. Diabetes prevalence was shown to be increasing up until > 70 years of age (Rannan-Eliya et al., 2023). Diabetes was the second most common cause of years of healthy life lost due to disability among above 60 years in Sri Lanka.

Prevalence of hypertension among adults was 28.2% in Sri Lanka, and this increased almost linearly with increasing age between 30 and 69 years, with the prevalence peaking at 68.5% among the age group 70–79 years (Rannan-Eliya et al., 2022).

Musculoskeletal conditions are the third most common cause of healthy years lost due to disability among the older people in Sri Lanka. With a rapidly ageing female population, osteoarthritis is predicted to increase. A study of a sample of females above 50 years of age, an estimated age standardised prevalence of clinical knee osteoarthritis for Sri Lanka was reported as 21.8%, out of which 59% of them had radiological evidence of OA and 30% of them had evidence of moderate to severe osteoarthritis of the knee (Hettihewa et al., 2018). Malignant neoplasms are a common cause of death in the above-60-years age group in Sri Lanka. Cancer is on the rise due to population ageing and increased exposure to risk factors such as tobacco, alcohol and obesity. A 77% increase in the new cancers has been predicted by 2050 globally, which will mainly affect the low and middle-income countries (LMIC) (Weerakoon., 2024).

The incidence of home accidents among the older adults was reported as 10.9%, while the above-75-years age group showed a higher incidence of 16.4%, and the 60–74 years age group showed a lower incidence of 8.9% (Jayasekera & Abeysena, 2018).

Nutrition

Old age is susceptible to poor nutritional status due to physiological and psychosocial changes in this population. One study looking at 396 elders above 60 years showed about 31% of the sample were at risk of malnutrition, which was somewhat lower than such rates in the region. Increasing age, poverty and living in rural areas were associated with poor nutritional state (De Silva et al., 2017). Older adults living in residential homes are especially vulnerable with 59% showing to be at risk of malnourishment (Fernando & Wijesinghe, 2011).

Infectious Diseases

The highest number of deaths due to infectious diseases is due to tuberculosis, which is about 500–600 deaths annually. The incidence of tuberculosis is 65 per 100,000. Sri Lanka is only detecting slightly more than 50% of the cases it should be detected, and therefore, several thousand cases go undetected and untreated. It has a target to bring down tuberculosis incidence to 13 per 100,000 by 2035 as per Sustainable Development Goals by the United Nations.

Disability

According to the census and statistics report 2012, out of 2 520 573 older persons, 548, 776 (21.8%) experienced difficulty in seeing, 284 285 (11.3%) experienced difficulty in hearing, 488,209 (19.4%) experienced difficulty in walking, and 208 657 (8.3%) had experienced difficulty related to cognition. Sense organ disease, diabetes, musculoskeletal diseases, cardiovascular diseases, mental health conditions and substance use disorders, neurological diseases, respiratory conditions and injuries were among the top 10 causes of disability among the above 60 years age group in Sri Lanka.

3 Geriatric Mental Disorders and Suicide in Sri Lanka

3.1 Depression

Depression is an important mental health issue among the older adult population in Sri Lanka, especially in the urban areas (Rajapakshe et al., 2019). A study was done on 1283 young elders living in the urban Colombo district using the Geriatric Depression Scale (cut off 8) which revealed a prevalence of depression to be

13.9% (mild depression 11.2%, moderate to severe 2.7%) (Rajapakshe et al., 2019). The same study found that socio-demographic factors; female sex, being unmarried, separated, divorced or widowed, and having a lower income, were significantly associated with depression. Smoking, alcohol, the presence of chronic disease, limitation to Instrumental Activities of Daily Living (IADL), poor partner relationship, perceived inadequate social support and experiencing abuse and life events were significantly related to depression among young elders (Rajapakshe et al., 2019).

An island-wide study; Sri Lanka Ageing Survey done by the world bank in 2006 looked into 14 dimensions of health in older adult citizens. In that study men were more likely to be free of stress and worry and not depressed than women (Østbye et al., 2009). Another publication from the same survey reported that clinically significant depressive symptoms that were taken as a score of more than 6 in the 15-item GDS were present in 27.8% of the community-dwelling older adult population. For men, the figure was 24% whereas for women this was 30.8% (Malhotra et al., 2010).

A study of 100 older adults systematically recruited from care homes in Colombo district showed that 52% of males and 60% of females were depressed with an overall prevalence of 56% which is much higher than the community prevalence (Wijeratne et al., 2008).

3.2 *Suicide*

Globally, suicide rate among all ages has come down, but the rate remains the highest in the oldest population groups (De Leo, 2022). The overall age-standardised suicide rate in Sri Lanka dropped from 38 per 100,000 in 1997 to 15 per 100,000 in 2022 (Bandara et al., 2024). The reduction in the suicide rate was mainly seen in the youth, whereas the suicide rate in the older adults has remained constant in the last two decades (Fig. 1). In 2022, the highest suicide rate in the country, 65 per 100,000, was reported in males above 55 years of age (Bandara et al., 2024). Among the older adults, the oldest old has the highest suicide rate. At present, hanging is the most common method used to commit suicide in the island.

Depression and debilitating physical illness have been identified as significant contributors to suicide risk in the older adults (Obuobi-Donkor et al., 2021). A qualitative study from Sri Lanka that looked at 30 psychological autopsies of older adult suicide victims reported that almost all subjects had mood or behavioural symptoms during the time leading up to the suicide, and these warning signs were identified as anger outbursts, sleep disturbances, isolating behaviour, reduced speaking, and contemplation on meaninglessness of life (Rasnayake & Navratil, 2023). Directly expressing suicidal ideas was not commonly reported. Factors such as having a weak social network, poor understanding of depression and suicide warning signs by the family, negative attitude towards the old age and a crisis of personal perspectives in help-seeking adversely influenced help-seeking behaviour (Rasnayake & Navratil, 2023).

Improving the understanding of depression symptoms and encouraging help-seeking among the older adults is a primary prerequisite in bringing down older adult suicides. Combating ageism and stigma of the communities, including self-stigma, is important in order to remove barriers to help-seeking. In order to facilitate the detection of at-risk older adults, improving overall health literacy of the community, and of the health care staff will be helpful, with special focus on the gatekeepers of the community. Addressing social isolation, ensuring active participation with mainstream socio-economic and cultural activities, and improving determinants of health among the older adults will also be a priority in making an impact on reducing suicides among this age group.

3.3 Cognitive Functions and Dementia

Alzheimer's and other dementias are within the top 10 causes of mortality, and they are also showing an upward trend in mortality statistics among older adults in Sri Lanka. Diagnosis of cognitive impairment is often missed in general health care settings attended by the older adults which represents a missed opportunity (Samaraweera, 2015). Sri Lankan health care system is not geared up to face the rapidly increasing numbers of patients with dementia projected. A negligible percentage of patients are thought to be on memory enhancers and are accessing specialised memory services in the country.

Both men and women showed a decline in cognition with increasing age, although women showed lower cognition than men (Østbye et al., 2009). A semi-urban regional survey found the prevalence of dementia to be around 4% in Sri Lanka (De Silva et al., 2003). The number of dementia patients in Sri Lanka was estimated to be around 147,000 in 2015 and 267,000 in 2030, and 463,000 in 2050 (*Data Collection Survey on Ageing Sector in Sri Lanka Final Report*, 2021).

Patients with dementia are mostly cared for by their own families, often living in the same household as the patient. Carer burden was reported in 26% in a hospital out-patient study (Abeywickrema et al., 2015). Adequate household income and access to external help were associated with less carer burden, and 3.9% of the carers had major depression (Abeywickrema et al., 2015).

Institutional care for dementia patients is still minimal. Care homes in the government sector do not specialise in dementia care at present and have not expanded in recent times although the private care homes are starting to be established in the country.

Ensuring a good quality of life is one of the important arms of dementia care, especially considering the lack of a cure and limited options to improve symptoms. In an unmatched case–control study that compared different QoL groups, identified using Dementia Specific Quality of Life tool (DEMQOL), characteristics such as education up to ordinary level and above, ever been employed, good social functioning, mild functional impairment, little or no caregiver burden, absence of apathy and absence of irritability were found to be associated with good Quality of Life

(Jayakody and Arambepola, 2022). Authors suggested that 60% of the variance of good QoL was explained by these factors. Therefore, programs to improve QoL among patients with dementia should focus on strategies to improve ADL's (activities of daily living), reducing and managing neuropsychiatric symptoms effectively, promoting activities to enhance social functioning and addressing caregiver burden (Jayakody and Arambepola, 2022).

3.4 Anxiety, Somatoform and Other Psychiatric Disorders

Anxiety and somatoform symptoms are common among the older adult patients. Lack of epidemiological data precludes quantifying of the psychological problems in this population. Research is mainly based on patients presenting to various institutions than representative community samples.

3.5 Substance Use Disorders

Substance use disorders cause a significant disability among older adults. The depth of the problem is not studied among older adults in Sri Lanka. More and more older adults are seeking treatment for alcohol-related problems, which indicates alcohol use disorders are prevalent in this age group. A high index of suspicion is needed to recognise alcohol and other substance misuse among older adults in Sri Lanka (Health Care for Older People, Sri Lankan Association of Geriatric Medicine 2021).

3.6 Other Psychosocial Aspects

Elder Abuse

A study that focused on older adult out-patient attendees of a tertiary care hospital reported physical abuse, verbal abuse, psychological abuse or neglect among 45% of the participants. Loneliness was reported in 26% of the participants. Psychological abuse was the most common type reported, and physical abuse was the least common (Edirisinghe et al., 2014). It is important that the service providers and caregivers have a sound knowledge about how to identify elder abuse early and what steps to be taken to prevent or address such situations.

Stigma and Ageism

The societal norm for older adults in Sri Lanka is to enjoy retirement, to live a peaceful and dignified life at home in harmony with their extended families and also to observe religious practices in most cases. They are also expected to transfer their worldly possessions to the younger members of the family without undue delay. Spending their savings on leisure activities or re-marrying after death of the spouse is uncommon. Adult children become the informal guardians when they are as young as mid-50 s or early 60 s. Older adults may feel that their financial freedom and independence in decision-making are restricted but, these issues are rarely brought up in any informal or formal discussions by either party. Stigma against the aged is subtle but prevalent and under-explored.

Quality of Life

One cross-sectional study looking at the quality of life among 3573 community-dwelling older adults between the ages of 60 and 74 years in rural Sri Lanka reported a moderate quality of life among the participants. Social support, absence of chronic disease and good education level were positively associated with better quality of life.

Overall quality of life score among older persons living in Jaffna was 11.5 ± 2.2 out of 20 as per WHOQOL, with low scores recording for all four individual domains compared to global reference scores. QoL of the older persons studied was found to be negatively associated with the presence of a health condition, limitations to ADL's, and the exposure to addictive substances.

4 Current Status of Services

4.1 Mental Health Services in Sri Lanka

Mental health services in Sri Lanka are primarily delivered by the government through the Mental Health Directorate under the Ministry of Health (mentalhealth.health.gov.lk, n.d.). These services are provided free of charge and have a wide reach across the country, ensuring accessibility for the majority of the population. The private sector is gradually expanding and offers both inpatient and outpatient psychiatric care. However, it represents a smaller proportion of mental health service providers, and access remains limited to those who can afford it.

4.2 Mental Health Services for Older Adults

Until 2022, mental health care for older adults in Sri Lanka was primarily provided by general adult psychiatrists. Across the country, inpatient and outpatient services were typically shared between young and older adult patients, with few dedicated resources for the older adults. Only a limited number of teaching hospitals conducted specialised clinics for older adults, which were also managed by general adult psychiatrists with an interest or additional training in Old Age Psychiatry.

The National Institute of Mental Health (NIMH) in Angoda, the primary governmental institution for mental health treatment and training, established the country's first and only inpatient unit dedicated to older adult patients in 2000. Recently, NIMH expanded its services with the opening of a day centre exclusively for older individuals, making it the only facility of its kind in Sri Lanka.

With the introduction of subspecialty training in Old Age Psychiatry by the Postgraduate Institute of Medicine in 2017, there are now three board-certified consultants in Old Age Psychiatry practising in Sri Lanka while two are in the training pathway. At present these consultants are based at NIMH, Colombo South Teaching Hospital (CSTH), and Colombo North Teaching Hospital (CNTH). They provide inpatient, outpatient, and liaison psychiatry services for older adult patients. However, among these institutions, still only NIMH has a dedicated inpatient unit for older individuals; other facilities continue to share wards between young and older patients. At present, specialised Community Mental Health Teams or Home Treatment Teams focused on older adult care are not available. The same team which manages both inpatient and outpatient units, conducts domiciliary visits when necessary.

4.3 Day Centres and Activities for Older Adults

In addition to the dedicated day centre at NIMH, a few other day centres, including CSTH and the National Hospital of Sri Lanka (NHSL), provide day centre services and therapeutic activities for older individuals with mental health conditions.

A significant development in non-pharmacological treatment is the adaptation of Cognitive Stimulation Therapy (CST) for dementia to the Sri Lankan context. CST, an evidence-based intervention for individuals with mild to moderate dementia, became available in 2023 (UCL, 2024). Currently, CST groups operate at NIMH, CSTH, NHSL, Thalangama Hospital, and the Teaching Hospital in Anuradhapura. Several non-governmental organisations (NGOs) contribute to dementia care in Sri Lanka. The Lanka Alzheimer's Foundation provides services such as caregiver training, public awareness programs, cognitive screening, and day centre activities. HelpAge International has been running HelpAge Sri Lanka for over 30 years, contributing with advocacy, day centres, and services such as active case finding of visually impaired and organising cataract surgeries and other provisions (HelpAge International, 2016).

4.4 Specialised Services

While there are no dedicated neuropsychiatry services currently established in Sri Lanka, the needs of patients with neuropsychiatric conditions are generally met through existing general or Old Age Psychiatry services mainly through liaison psychiatry services based on hospital settings.

4.5 End-Of-Life Care

Palliative care for older adult patients is still in its developmental stages in Sri Lanka. Some general hospitals have formed specialised palliative care teams to support both inpatients and community-dwelling individuals nearing the end of life. A significant advancement in this area is the introduction of End-of-Life Care Guidelines by the Sri Lanka Medical Association. These guidelines provide healthcare professionals with a framework for delivering care to terminally ill patients, including those with advanced dementia.

4.6 Legal and Ethical Aspects of Geriatric Psychiatry

The legal provisions for mentally ill patients in Sri Lanka are governed by the Mental Health Ordinance, which was originally enacted in 1873 and amended in 1956 (Policy Repository—Ministry of Health—Sri Lanka, n.d.). Efforts are currently underway by the Sri Lanka College of Psychiatrists and the Ministry of Health to draft a new Mental Health Act to better address contemporary needs. While the current ordinance covers involuntary admissions and treatments, there is no Capacity Act in Sri Lanka to address issues related to decision-making capacity in older individuals.

4.7 Digital Services

The use of digital health services in Old Age Psychiatry remains limited in Sri Lanka. Some private sector services provide remote assessments and treatments, but their availability is restricted by several barriers, including resource constraints and the lack of familiarity with digital devices among the older adult population.

5 Specialist Course and Training Opportunities in Old Age Psychiatry

5.1 Sub-Specialty Training in Old Age Psychiatry

The development of specialist training in Old Age Psychiatry in Sri Lanka represents a significant step forward in addressing the mental health needs of the ageing population. Recognising the importance of this subspecialty, the Postgraduate Institute of Medicine (PGIM) at the University of Colombo introduced Old Age Psychiatry as a formal subspecialty in 2017.

Eligible candidates for this subspecialty are trainees in psychiatry who have completed the MD Part 2 examination. The training program spans three years and is structured to provide comprehensive expertise in psychogeriatrics.

- Local Training:

The initial 2 years of training are completed in Sri Lanka. Trainees spend one year working in an Old Age Psychiatry service within a tertiary care setting at a general hospital, gaining exposure to clinical and multidisciplinary management of older adult patients with mental health disorders. The second year is based at the psychogeriatric unit at the National Institute of Mental Health (NIMH), Sri Lanka.

- Overseas Training:

Trainees are required to complete a minimum of 1 year of overseas training in a recognised Old Age Psychiatry unit. This international exposure ensures that trainees gain advanced skills, knowledge of diverse care models, and experience with cutting-edge interventions.

5.2 Integration of Old Age Psychiatry in General Psychiatry Training

In addition to the subspecialty training, general adult psychiatry training programmes in Sri Lanka incorporate training in Old Age Psychiatry during the pre-MD period. This ensures that all psychiatrists, regardless of their chosen subspecialty, develop foundational knowledge and skills in managing mental health conditions in the older adult population.

5.3 Workshops and Continuous Professional Development (CPD)

The Sri Lanka College of Psychiatrists actively promotes professional development in Old Age Psychiatry through regular workshops and conference sessions:

- An annual workshop on psychogeriatrics or neuropsychiatry is organised to provide updates on recent advancements and evidence-based practices.
- Topics related to Old Age Psychiatry are routinely included in the scientific programmes of the Sri Lanka College of Psychiatrists annual conferences, fostering academic discussions and collaboration.

5.4 *Cognitive Stimulation Therapy (CST) Training Initiatives*

The Old Age Psychiatry Subcommittee of the Sri Lanka College of Psychiatrists is in the process of promoting cognitive stimulation therapy (CST) as a non-pharmacological intervention for dementia. Regular workshops are conducted to train facilitators, including doctors, occupational therapists, psychologists, and volunteers, to effectively conduct CST groups. These workshops aim to enhance the quality of care and improve the cognitive and social well-being of patients with dementia (UCL, 2024).

5.5 *Specialised Training for Nurses*

The Faculty of Allied Sciences at the University of Ruhuna is planning to offer a specialised training course focusing on neurodegenerative disorders, including dementia care. This initiative is designed to equip nurses with advanced skills in managing older adult patients with neurodegenerative conditions.

5.6 *Residential Care Homes and Long-Term Care for Older Adults*

Elder care homes provide housing for elders who lack shelter and these amount to approximately 255 care homes accommodating about 7000 residents. Out of these, 2 were owned by the central government, 3 by provincial councils, 20 by the private sector and others by not-for-profit organisations.

Charitable organisations such as the Welcome Village at Makandura, and the Little sisters of the poor Home for the Elderly in Colombo are some of such organisations that provide residential care for older adults on a large scale. Sri Lankan organisations such as Sarvodaya, and YMBA also show dedication towards residential care for the older adults.

6 Research Gap

Research on the large community samples such as true epidemiological studies that focus on the older adults are severely lacking in Sri Lanka. Studies on mental health conditions were mostly conducted in hospital-based small samples or on samples of people attending a health care facility. Population projections and estimates are often used in several internationally funded project reports as the next best option to quantify the disease prevalence in the absence of original research.

Community figures for determinants of health were mostly provided by the census and statistics department surveys, which were found to be very helpful but the last available population census was in 2012. The next census is planned to start immediately, which is expected to provide very useful information.

Dementia research conducted in the country also showed a deficit in the island-wide prevalence studies. Most studies were about translation and validation of screening tools, and this is still useful as a lack of screening tools was a significant barrier to conducting research in the past. Clinical trials were almost non-existent in this field. Challenges faced by family members who are caregiving were understudied (Kalpani et al., 2020). There were only a very few genetic or family studies and studies exploring pathophysiology, which is very likely to be due to additional investigations involving extra costs. A severe lack of local funding for research or lack of understanding about how to obtain international research funding could explain these deficits.

Certain areas are clearly understudying, such as the status of substance abuse in older adults and ageism and stigma related to old age.

Treatment protocols for the older adults were not available thus far, and currently, the College of Geriatric Medicine has shown interest by releasing delirium and dementia care pathways tailor made for Sri Lankan setup. Physicians often use foreign guidelines such as NICE, Maudsley and RANZCP in the absence of equivalent guidelines in the country.

A situational analysis of elderly women in institutionalised care showed the older women felt isolated from family and community, and there is a wide scope to strengthening the ties between the residents and the community. The use of a variety of study methods such as situational analysis, feasibility studies, technical evaluations, cohort studies and clinical trials need to be promoted.

Genetic and laboratory-based studies are seriously lagging behind when compared to epidemiological studies in Sri Lanka reflecting the resource limitations and lack of expertise in these fields.

Sri Lanka should invest in research and development more liberally to understand the needs of the older adults, to advance the care of the older adults and to benefit from a healthy older adult population.

7 National Legislations, Policies and Programmes to Enhance the Lives of Older Citizens

Respecting and looking after the older adults are engraved in the country's culture which is still preserved especially in the more rural settings. However, when the country enters a faster phase of industrialisation and development, it is going to need a robust supportive framework to ensure the rights of the older citizens, as the goodwill of the fellow citizens alone becomes inadequate and unreliable.

Madrid International Plan of Action on Ageing (MIPAA) presented during the World Assembly on Ageing in April 2002 provided the guiding framework to prepare for the needs of the ageing population in three main areas; older persons and development, advancing health and well-being in old age, and enabling a supportive environment. Sri Lanka also welcomed United Nations General Assembly Resolution "Towards a comprehensive and integral international legal instrument to promote and protect the rights and dignity of older persons" as a timely initiative that will guide the development agenda of the country. In keeping with the international initiatives, Sri Lanka has levelled up its commitment to enhance the lives of older citizens by bringing in several new legislations, policies, programmes and action plans.

7.1 Protection of the Rights of the Elders Act, no 9 of 2000 and Its Amendment Act, no. 5 of 2011

Parliament of the democratic Socialist Republic of Sri Lanka introduced the protection of the rights of the Elders Act, no. 9 of 2000, to operate under the Ministry of Social Empowerment and Welfare. This enabled the establishment of National Council for the Elders for the promotion and protection of the welfare and the rights of elders. National Secretariat for the Elders was established to assist the council to achieve its tasks. The act also directs registration of services, handling of funds, staff, appointment of the board, adoption and compliance with international conventions, education, training and research, and other provisions for the older citizens such as health, welfare and legal facilities. This also provides directions to issue identity cards to the senior citizens and creation of older adult committees local to the members.

7.2 National Secretariat for the Elders

The National Secretariat for Elders aims to encourage participation of older persons on social development, and to ensure their independence, care, participation, self-fulfilment, and dignity and to protect the rights of the elders. Making policies, launching programmes, providing welfare assistance to the older adults and maintaining a database relating to the older adults are some of the key functions. The director of the National Secretariat is helped by 95 elders' Rights Protection Assistants attached to the divisional secretaries across the country who implement the programme.

One currently ongoing project, JAICA project for capacity enhancement of older adult services in the community, is working in collaboration with the National Secretariat for the Elders to introduce an integrated older adult service care model inspired by the Japanese way.

Senior citizens' allowance is given by the National Secretariat for the Elders to the elders over 70 years of age, and centenary allowance is given to the elders over 100 years of age.

National Secretariat for the Elders also collaborates with other organisations to raise awareness such as Pre-retirement seminars and caregiver training. They closely collaborated with the Legal Aids Foundation in order to bring about legal empowerment of elders.

7.3 National Charter for Senior Citizens

National charter for senior citizens was adopted by the cabinet ministers in March 2006. It sets out the rights and responsibilities of senior citizens of Sri Lanka in order to reinforce the values of independence, dignity, participation, self-fulfilment and good quality of life in old age. It also provides the norms against which the quality of care, health and welfare programmes for senior citizens will be judged.

7.4 National Policy for Senior Citizens, Sri Lanka

National policy for senior citizens was formulated as per the Madrid Plan of Action and strategies mainly follow themes; elders and development, advancing health and well-being and ensuring supportive environment.

7.5 National Plan of Action on Ageing 2012–2021

The National Secretariat in collaboration with the WHO formulated the above in 2010 to reflect priority areas identified in the National Policy.

7.6 The National Fund for Elders

The National Fund for Elders was established to address poverty among the elders and the fund receives contribution from both public and private donors.

7.7 Maintenance Board

An elder who is unable to look after his/her needs can apply to the maintenance board for an order that one or more of his/her children pay a monthly allowance or a lump sum for his/her maintenance.

7.8 Older Adult Committees

Currently, there are around 10,000 older adult committees functioning at different levels in the community such as village level, divisional level, district level and provincial level. These committees encourage the participation of the elders in decision-making processes on issues affecting the older citizens as well as economic, social and cultural activities. Members have opportunities continuous learning programmes.

7.9 Protection of the Rights of Persons with Disabilities Act no 28 of 1996 and Its Amendment Act, no 33 of 2003

This enabled the establishment of the National Council for Persons with Disabilities and the protection of the rights of the people with disabilities such as ensuring disabled people can access any premises safely.

7.10 Caregiver

In a Sri Lankan study, both elders and adult children saw in-home caregiving as ideal and as a moral obligation. Here, the family was seen as a reciprocal unit where parents make sacrifices when raising children and children look after the parents when the parents are old. Elders often felt useful when they could contribute to the household chores and when they took responsibilities for caring for grandchildren. With shifts in the modern society such as females starting to work, and multi-generational households becoming nuclear families, and migration, availability of adult children for caregiving is becoming less and less.

Due to parents living to very old ages, and due to other reasons mentioned, the need for outside carers' input is steadily going up. There is a huge demand for caregivers outside the family, but this group is rapidly shrinking due to high demands for them abroad.

8 Current Challenges in Geriatric Mental Health and Way Forward

8.1 Poor Public Awareness of Mental Illnesses Among Elders and Stigma

One of the critical challenges in addressing geriatric mental health in Sri Lanka is the lack of awareness and understanding of mental health conditions among the older adult population and their caregivers. Mental health issues in older adults, such as depression, dementia, and anxiety, are often dismissed as part of ageing, leading to underdiagnosis and untreated cases. Additionally, the stigma associated with mental health disorders discourages elders from seeking help, further exacerbating their conditions.

To tackle this issue, it is imperative to initiate an island-wide program aimed at mental health promotion and increasing awareness about mental illnesses among elders. This program should leverage community engagement, media campaigns and local leaders to educate the public, reduce stigma and encourage timely interventions. Collaborative efforts between governmental and non-governmental organisations can significantly amplify the impact of such initiatives.

8.2 Lack of Human Resources and Infrastructure

Sri Lanka currently has few trained Old Age Psychiatrists and other mental health professionals specialising in geriatric care. This disparity in human resources limits the availability of services in many parts of the country, particularly in rural and underserved areas. Additionally, financial constraints hinder the development of adequate infrastructure and the establishment of specialised geriatric mental health services.

A long-term solution involves increasing funding allocations for the training of specialists and the establishment of dedicated geriatric mental health units in major hospitals. Policymakers must prioritise these investments to ensure equitable access to care for all older citizens, irrespective of their geographic location.

8.3 Lack of Collaboration Between Agencies

The fragmentation of mental health services due to limited collaboration between different organisations and agencies presents another significant challenge. This lack of coordination leads to duplication of efforts, inefficiencies and gaps in service delivery. The Ministry of Health should take the lead in conducting comprehensive service mapping to identify existing resources and areas of overlap. Developing a centralised system for planning and coordination will streamline efforts and foster better collaboration between governmental bodies, NGOs and private healthcare providers.

8.4 Lack of Training and Learning Opportunities for Other Staff Categories

Doctors, nurses and other allied healthcare staff often lack adequate training in geriatric mental health, making it difficult for them to identify and manage mental health conditions among elders.

Regular updates and continuing medical education (CME) activities focused on Old Age Psychiatry are essential to bridge this gap. Structured training programs, workshops and mentorship opportunities should be provided to healthcare staff across the country to enhance their skills and confidence in managing geriatric mental health issues.

8.5 Lack of Local Study Data on Epidemiology and Intervention Effectiveness

The absence of local research data on the prevalence of geriatric mental health disorders and the effectiveness of various interventions hinders evidence-based policymaking and program development.

There is a need to conduct comprehensive epidemiological studies and clinical trials tailored to the Sri Lankan context. Collaborative research efforts involving universities, healthcare institutions, and international organisations can generate valuable insights to guide policy and practice.

8.6 Limited Legal Framework, Including Lack of a Mental Capacity Act

Sri Lanka's current legal framework for mental health, including the outdated Mental Health Act, does not adequately address the unique needs of the older adult population, such as issues related to decision-making capacity and guardianship.

Enacting a new Mental Health Act that incorporates provisions for a Mental Capacity Act is essential to safeguard the rights and autonomy of older individuals with mental health conditions. This updated legislation should be aligned with international human rights standards and developed through a consultative process involving stakeholders from diverse sectors.

9 Conclusion

It is imperative that a clear vision to provide holistic care for the older adults is present, and a master plan is formulated incorporating all organisations involved in the care of the older adults. Strong political commitment and financial backing are mandatory in order to implement such an action plan. Ways to improve coordination between the organisations should be sought. Sri Lanka should also work with regional and global partners to identify correct policies and innovations that can bring a positive impact.

References

Abeywickrema, S., Weerasundera, R., & Ranasinghe, K. (2015). Assessment of the level of care-burden in informal caregivers of patients with dementia. *Sri Lanka Journal of Psychiatry, 6*(1), 4. https://doi.org/10.4038/sljpsyc.v6i1.8053

Ageing Population of Sri Lanka. Thematic report based on census of population and housing 2012. United Nations Population Fund. 2016. Available at: http://srilanka.unfpa.org

Asian Development Bank (2019). *Growing Old Before Becoming Rich: Challenges of an aging population in Sri lanka.* S.L.: Asian Development Bank.

Bandara, P., et al. (2024). Reflections on the trends of suicide in Sri Lanka, 1997–2022: The need for continued vigilance. *PLOS Global Public Health, 4*(4), 1–11. https://doi.org/10.1371/journal.pgph.0003054

De Leo, D. (2022). Late-life suicide in an aging world. *Nature Aging, 2*(1), 7–12. https://doi.org/10.1038/s43587-021-00160-1

De Silva, H. A., Gunatilake, S. B., & Smith, A. D. (2003). Prevalence of dementia in a semi-urban population in Sri Lanka: Report from a regional survey. *International Journal of Geriatric Psychiatry, 18*(8), 711–715. https://doi.org/10.1002/gps.909

De Silva, K., et al. (2017). Nutritional status of elders in Galle district, Sri Lanka. *Galle Medical Journal, 22*(1), 1. https://doi.org/10.4038/gmj.v22i1.7958

Edberg, A.-K. (2019). Loneliness among older people living in care homes in Sri Lanka. *International Journal of Older People Nursing*, (February), 1–11. https://doi.org/10.1111/opn.12253

Edirisinghe, P. A. S., et al. (2014). Elder abuse among outpatient department attendees in a tertiary care hospital in Sri Lanka. *The Ceylon Medical Journal, 59*(3), 84–89. https://doi.org/10.4038/cmj.v59i3.6527

ESCAP. (2024). *ESCAP population data sheet 2024.* [online] Available at: https://www.unescap.org/kp/2024/escap-population-data-sheet-2024

Fernando, W., & Wijesinghe, D. (2011). Assessment of nutritional status and disease prevalence among elderly population in Elderly Homes in Kandy. *Tropical Agricultural Research, 21*(3), 229. https://doi.org/10.4038/tar.v21i3.3296

Policy Repository -Ministry of Health -Sri Lanka. (n.d.). Available at: https://www.health.gov.lk/wp-content/uploads/2022/10/7_Mental-Health-1.pdf

Health Care for Older People Holistic Approach Mental Health Problems in Old Age, Sri Lankan Association of Geriatric Medicine 2021

HelpAge International. (2016). *HelpAge Sri Lanka is proud of what it has achieved over 30 years.* [online] Available at: https://www.helpage.org/blog/helpage-sri-lanka-is-proud-of-what-it-has-achieved-over-30-years

HelpAge International. (2022). *The struggle for survival faced by Sri Lanka's senior citizens.* [online] Available at: https://www.helpage.org/news/the-struggle-for-survival-faced-by-sri-lankas-senior-citizens

Home (2024) *Alz Lanka.* Available at: https://alzlanka.org

Jayakody, S., & Arambepola, C. (2022). Determinants of quality of life among people with dementia: evidence from a South Asian population. *BMC Geriatrics, 22*(1), 1–7. https://doi.org/10.1186/s12877-022-03443-3

Jayasekera, R., & Abeysena, C. (2018). Incidence, pattern and factors associated with home accidents among the elderly in Wattala Medical Officer of Health area. *Sri Lanka Journal of the College of Community Physicians of Sri Lanka 2018, 24*(4). http://repository.kln.ac.lk/handle/123456789/20475

Kalpani, A. et al. (2020). Dementia research activity in Sri Lanka: A review. *Journal of Neurodegenerative Disorders, 3*(1), 89–100. https://doi.org/10.36959/459/603

Malhotra, R., Chan, A., & Østbye, T. (2010). Prevalence and correlates of clinically significant depressive symptoms among elderly people in Sri Lanka: Findings from a national survey. *International Psychogeriatrics, 22*(2), 227–236. https://doi.org/10.1017/S1041610209990871

Mendonc, C. A. De (2013). Mental health and wellbeing of older people: Opportunities and challenges, 125–128.

mentalhealth.health.gov.lk. (n.d.). *Home - Directorate of Mental Health.* [online] Available at: https://www.mentalhealth.health.gov.lk/index.php?lang=en

Obuobi-Donkor, G., Nkire, N., & Agyapong, V. I. O. (2021). 'Prevalence of major depressive disorder and correlates of thoughts of death, suicidal behaviour, and death by suicide in the geriatric population—a general review of literature. *Behavioral Sciences, 11*(11). https://doi.org/10.3390/bs11110142

Østbye, T., Malhotra, R., & Chan, A. (2009). Thirteen dimensions of health in elderly Sri Lankans: Results from a national Sri Lanka aging survey. *Journal of the American Geriatrics Society, 57*(8), 1376–1387. https://doi.org/10.1111/j.1532-5415.2009.02350.x

Pandey, N. M. et al. (2022). Organization South-East Asia region: Needs and resource gaps, *12*(1), 117–127. https://doi.org/10.5498/wjp.v12.i1.117

Practice guidelines in the end-of-life care Palliative and End-of-life Care Task Force Sri Lanka Medical Association. (n.d.). Available at: https://slma.lk/wp-content/uploads/2021/12/Practice-guidelines-in-EoL-care.pdf

Prashansanie Hettihewa, A., Gunawardena, N. S., Atukorala, I., Hassan, F., Lekamge, I. N., & Hunter, D. J. (2018). Prevalence of knee osteoarthritis in a suburban, Srilankan, adult female population: A population-based study. *International Journal of Rheumatic Diseases, 21*, 394–401. https://doi.org/10.1111/1756-185X.13225

Rajapakshe, O. B. W., Sivayogan, S., & Kulatunga, P. M. (2019). Prevalence and correlates of depression among older urban community-dwelling adults in Sri Lanka. *Psychogeriatrics, 19*(3), 202–211. https://doi.org/10.1111/psyg.12389

Rannan-Eliya, R. P., et al. (2023). Prevalence of diabetes and pre-diabetes in Sri Lanka: A new global hotspot-estimates from the Sri Lanka Health and Ageing Survey 2018/2019. *BMJ Open Diabetes Research and Care, 11*(1), 1–11. https://doi.org/10.1136/bmjdrc-2022-003160

Rannan-Eliya, R. P. et al. (2022). Prevalence and associations of hypertension in Sri Lankan adults: Estimates from the SLHAS 2018–19 Survey Using JNC7 and ACC/AHA 2017 guidelines. *Global Heart, 17*(1). https://doi.org/10.5334/gh.1135

Rasnayake, S., & Navratil, P. (2023). Warning signs of elderly suicide and factors affecting professional help-seeking: Case of Sri Lanka. *Journal of Population and Social Studies, 31*, 1–19. https://doi.org/10.25133/JPSSv312023.001

Samaraweera, D. N. (2015). Care of the elderly: A multidisciplinary approach. *Journal of the Ceylon College of Physicians, 45*(1–2), 45. https://doi.org/10.4038/jccp.v45i1-2.7728

Silva, W. I. D., & de Silva, R. (2023). n Galle district, Sri Lanka', of dementia in a semi-urban population in Sri Lanka: Report from a regional survey.

Solano, L., R., (2021). *Sri Lanka must increase its efforts to protect and promote the human capital of the elderly. World Bank Blogs.* Available at: https://blogs.worldbank.org/en/endpovertyinsouthasia/sri-lanka-must-increase-its-efforts-protect-and-promote-human-capital-elderly

Sri Lanka Population (2024) - Worldometer, Available at: https://www.worldometers.info/world-population/sri-lanka-population/

Sri Lanka Development Update: Demographic changes in Sri Lanka. Available at: https://www.dailymirror.lk/print/news-features/Sri-Lanka-Development-Update:--Demographic-changes-in-Sri-Lanka/131-163033

Subathevan, S., et al. (2022). Aging and Health Research Social and emotional loneliness among older adults in a coastal suburb in Sri Lanka. *Aging and Health Research, 2*(2), Article 100075. https://doi.org/10.1016/j.ahr.2022.100075

Data Collection Survey on Aging Sector in Sri Lanka Final Report Data Collection Survey on Aging Sector in Sri Lanka Final Report Sri Lanka Democratic Socialist Republic Aging Sector Information Gathering and Confirmation Survey CONTENTS (2021).

UCL. (2024). *Sri Lanka, International Cognitive Stimulation Therapy (CST) Centre.* Available at: https://www.ucl.ac.uk/international-cognitive-stimulation-therapy/international-cst-training/sri-lanka

Weerakoon, K. (2024). Weekly Epidemiological Report A publication of the Epidemiology Unit Ministry of Health, March 2024.*Welcome to NIMH - Sri Lanka.* Available at: https://nimh.health.gov.lk/

WHO. (2024). *Determinants of health.* [online] World Health Organization. Available at: https://www.who.int/news-room/questions-and-answers/item/determinants-of-health

Wijeratne, M. D. M., Wijerathne, S. A. W. S. G., & Wijesingha, I. (2008). Prevalence of depression among institutionalized elders in the Colombo district. *Student Medical Journal, 1*(1), 27–32.

World Bank Blogs. (2013). *Ending the shame and stigma of poverty.* [online] Available at: https://blogs.worldbank.org/en/endpovertyinsouthasia/ending-shame-and-stigma-poverty

Worldbank.org. (2022). *Sri Lanka - Aging survey 2006 | Data catalog.* [online] Available at: https://datacatalog.worldbank.org/search/dataset/0050033/Sri-Lanka---Aging-Survey-2006

www.healthdata.org. (n.d.). *Sri Lanka | The Institute for Health Metrics and Evaluation.* [online] Available at: https://www.healthdata.org/research-analysis/health-by-location/profiles/sri-lanka

Geriatric Psychiatry in Other South Asian Countries: Afghanistan, Bhutan, the Maldives

Sujita Kumar Kar and S. M. Yasir Arafat

Abstract Geriatric psychiatry is underdeveloped in South Asian countries such as Afghanistan, Bhutan, and the Maldives. This is not surprising, as overall mental health services in these regions face several challenges, including pervasive stigma, low literacy rates, a lack of mental health professionals, a significant treatment gap, and limited research. Among the eight countries in South Asia, research on mental health is particularly lacking in these three nations.

In this chapter, we aim to examine the burden of geriatric mental health, the current status of available services, end-of-life care, research, and training in geriatric psychiatry, as well as the legal and ethical issues surrounding geriatric mental health. We will also discuss existing policies and programs, along with the current challenges in geriatric mental health, based on the available evidence.

Keywords Geriatric psychiatry · Old age psychiatry · Afghanistan · Bhutan · Maldives · Mental health · Psychiatric services

1 Introduction

South Asia consists of eight low-middle-income countries and caters to 25% of the world population (Arafat & Kar, 2024). Approximately 2 billion people live in this region, with 95% residing in Bangladesh, India, and Pakistan. Among these countries, India is recognized for having a stronger output in mental health research, followed by Pakistan and Sri Lanka. Mental health has also received increased attention in Bangladesh recently. However, there is a noticeable lack of evidence on mental health

S. K. Kar
Department of Psychiatry, King George's Medical University, Lucknow, Uttar Pradesh, India

S. M. Y. Arafat (✉)
Department of Psychiatry, Bangladesh Specialized Hospital, Dhaka, Bangladesh
e-mail: arafatdmc62@gmail.com

Biomedical Research Foundation, Dhaka, Bangladesh

N. Kar et al. (eds.), *Geriatric Psychiatry in South Asia*, South Asian Perspectives in Mental Health and Psychology , https://doi.org/10.1007/978-981-96-7469-5_7

from Afghanistan, Bhutan, and the Maldives, as well as a shortage of consistent mental health researchers in these countries.

The region has made progress in mental health services in recent decades. However, there are enduring challenges like high stigma, low mental health literacy, inadequate mental services and providers, inequitable availability of mental health professionals, and low budget (Arafat & Kar, 2024; Sayed, 2011; Trivedi et al., 2007). Branches of psychiatry, particularly geriatric psychiatry, remain largely undeveloped in countries such as Afghanistan, Bhutan, and the Maldives. In this chapter, we will explore the landscape of geriatric psychiatry in these regions, drawing on existing evidence and the expertise of professionals in the field. We will discuss the unique challenges these countries face in addressing the mental health needs of their aging populations and highlight the importance of establishing specialized services to support older adult individuals struggling with psychiatric disorders.

2 Country-Wise Geriatric Mental Health

2.1 Afghanistan

2.1.1 Country Profile

Afghanistan is a low-income country in South Asia with a population of about 42 million, troubled with war and political conflict (ESCAP, 2024; World Health Organization, 2024). It is an Islamic Republic where more than 99% of the population are Muslims (Arafat & Kar, 2024; Arafat et al., 2022). Along with war and political turmoil, the country faces natural disasters. The median age of the population is 17 years, and the life expectancy at birth in Afghanistan is 64.2 years. Among them, 1.6 million (about 4%) had an age above 60 years, and 56.3% of them are females (ESCAP, 2024; World Health Organization, 2024). The proportion of the population with an age above 60 years will be more than 11% in 2050.

2.1.2 Epidemiology and Burden of Geriatric Psychiatry

The prevalence of dementia among persons with an age of more than 65 years was 5.8% (Kovess Masfety et al., 2018). The rate is higher among females than among males (Trani et al., 2023). Dementia in Afghanistan is affected by multiple domains of poverty, especially among females (Trani et al., 2023), indicating the importance of social determinants of mental disorders.

2.1.3 Mental Health Services

The first mental health service was noted in 1985 in Afghanistan. Psychiatric services have been officially extended to primary, secondary, and tertiary care levels. The initiative was started with the starting of "Basic Package of Health Services" in 2005 (Alemi et al., 2023; Shoib et al., 2024) at primary care level and *National Mental Health Strategy 2019–2023* attempted to extend the services in the secondary care level (Ministry of Public Health, 2018). However, the country has been affected by a lack of adequate human resources. Currently, one psychiatrist and one psychologist are available for about half a million people as there are 129 psychiatrists and 133 psychologists in the country (Alemi et al., 2023; Shoib et al., 2024; World Health Organization, 2022). The total mental health expenditure per person is 0.3 USD, and 4.2% of the total health budget is allocated for mental health in Afghanistan (World Health Organization, 2022). Importantly, mental health services and medications are provided free of cost, and there has been a recent spike in the number of mental health workers in the country (World Health Organization, 2022). We found no supporting evidence for specialized services addressing geriatric mental health issues or specialized courses in geriatric psychiatry in Afghanistan.

2.1.4 End-of-Life Care

End-of-life care is a newer venture in Afghanistan, which is mostly related to cancer treatment. Palliative care was needed for 172,541 patients in 2015 (Krakauer et al., 2023). Being an Islamic country and due to inadequate psychosocial support, people generally seek help from Mullahs, Islamic religious persons, and spiritual healers (Abdullah et al., 2021). Hamdardi Hospice was established in 2010 as the first service center in the country.

2.1.5 Research and Gaps

According to the Mental Health Atlas (2020), only 16 articles were published on mental health in Afghanistan (World Health Organization, 2022). It indicates an extreme lack of research on mental health, and situation could be worse in case of geriatric psychiatry in the country. Local, regional, and international attention is warranted on geriatric psychiatry in Afghanistan (Lemon et al., 2023).

2.2 *Bhutan*

2.2.1 Country Profile

Bhutan is a small country in South Asia surrounded by India and China with a population of 7,70,000 (The World Bank, 2024). By the year 2020, the life expectancy in Bhutan was 72 years with a gross per capita national income of 2840 USD (WHO, 2022a). As per the WHO-Mental Health Atlas 2020, the disability-adjusted life years per 100,000 population in Bhutan is 1579.4 (WHO, 2022c). The aging population is growing in Bhutan significantly and is expected to increase further in the coming years. This will increase the healthcare needs of the geriatric population significantly in the coming days.

2.2.2 Mental Health Burden Among Older People

There is no systematic nationwide survey to estimate the burden of mental health issues in Bhutan (WHO, 2022a). As per the sources of the Ministry of Health, Royal Government of Bhutan, a total number of 36 cases of dementia were documented in Bhutan in the year 2020 (WHO, 2022a). The same source reports the number of cases of dementia in Bhutan to be 18–28 across 2016–2019 (WHO, 2022a). Due to the lack of a population-based survey in Bhutan, the exact burden of mental illnesses, age-specific burden, and illness-specific burden is not available (Gyeltshen et al., 2024; Pelzang, 2012; WHO, 2022a).

2.2.3 Available Services in Geriatric Psychiatry

In Bhutan, there are 189 community-based/non-hospital mental health outpatient facilities and 53 other outpatient facilities (mental health day care or treatment facilities) (WHO, 2022c) There is no dedicated facility for geriatric mental health care. Existing facilities provide care for all mental health-related issues. In May 2020, the Department of Medical Services, Ministry of Health, Royal Government of Bhutan designed a manual for integrated community-based screening for older adult people in Bhutan (Ministry of Health, Bhutan, 2020). Psychiatric disorders like dementia, depression, and addiction-related issues of the older adults are among the geriatric mental health conditions intended to be screened using this manual for timely intervention (Ministry of Health, Bhutan, 2020).

2.2.4 End-of-Life Care

In Bhutan, "end-of-life care" is in its infancy (Bay et al., 2019; Dorji et al., 2024; Royal Government of Bhutan, 2020). End-of-life care in Bhutan mostly deals with medical conditions and lifestyle-related disorders. There is no dedicated facility for geriatric mental health issues in Bhutan.

2.2.5 Legal and Ethical Aspects of Geriatric Psychiatry

The Royal Government of Bhutan has introduced several schemes for the social and financial protection of older adult people in Bhutan (Dorji et al., 2017).

2.2.6 Specialist Course and Training Opportunities in Geriatric Psychiatry

There is no specialist super-specialization or fellowship course in geriatric mental health in Bhutan. However, in the year 2023, to strengthen the training in geriatric psychiatry in Bhutan, a program has been initiated in the name of the "Bhutan Old Age Psychiatry Education Program 2023 webinar series" (Khesar Gyalpo University of Medical Sciences of Bhutan, 2024). This webinar series was jointly organized by Betsi Cadwaladr University Health Board, UK (BCUHB), Department of Psychiatry, Jigme Dorji Wangchuck National Referral Hospital and Khesar Gyalpo University of Medical Sciences of Bhutan (KGUMSB) (Khesar Gyalpo University of Medical Sciences of Bhutan, 2024). This program facilitated the learning in geriatric psychiatry among the participants.

2.2.7 Available Research and Gaps

As per the Mental Health Atlas 2020, there are four research articles on mental health published from Bhutan, and mental health research output constitutes approximately 7% of the total health research outputs in the country (WHO, 2022c). There is a paucity of research in geriatric psychiatry in Bhutan. As aging and old-age-related issues are emerging as a significant problem, a study was conducted in Bhutan to understand the health and social issues of the older adult population in Bhutan (Dorji et al., 2017).

2.2.8 Programs-Policies-Action Plans for Geriatric Mental Health

There is no dedicated mental health law in Bhutan; however, there is the Narcotic and Psychotropic Act, which was introduced in 2013 (WHO, 2022a). The National Health Policy in Bhutan aims to strengthen primary healthcare delivery in the country (WHO, 2022a). There are no country-specific policies or programs that exist in Bhutan exclusively meant for geriatric mental health. However, the Ministry of Health in Bhutan has initiated the Geriatric Health Support Program to emphasize on the healthcare needs of the geriatric population in the country (WHO, 2022a). The National Geriatric

Program in Bhutan provides social support to older people by facilitating shelters for the homeless older adults and those facing domestic violence (WHO, 2022a). The National Mental Health Program of Bhutan works to reduce stigma and discrimination against mental illnesses, reducing the burden of mental illnesses in the country and minimizing the treatment gap (Ministry of Health, Royal Government of Bhutan, 2020).

2.2.9 Current Challenges in Geriatric Mental Health and Ways Out

Paucity of mental health manpower and infrastructural resources is a major challenge in Bhutan (WHO, 2022a). The availability of facilities for geriatric mental healthcare in Bhutan is currently quite limited, which poses significant challenges for the aging population. Furthermore, there is a noticeable lack of comprehensive research in the field of geriatric psychiatry within the country. This gap highlights a crucial opportunity for future development and enhancement of mental health services specifically tailored for the older adults. By investing in research and expanding service offerings, Bhutan has the potential to significantly improve the mental well-being of its senior citizens.

2.3 Maldives

2.3.1 Country Profile

Maldives consists of a chain of tiny islands in the Indian Ocean with an approximate land area of 0.3 thousand square kilometers (WHO, 2006). As per the data of 2021, the total population of Maldives was 543,620 with a life expectancy of 79 years (WHO, 2022b). In Maldives, more than 5% of the total population is attributed to the older adult population (Azeez & Suzana, 2023; WHO, 2006). The economy of Maldives is largely dependent on tourism (Mohamed, 2015; Mohamed & Mansoor, 2024). The health expenditure in Maldives is about 8.04% of the GDP (WHO, 2022b). In Maldives, people believe in the concept of free-living older citizens and endorse the care of the older adults in close proximity to their family rather than in the hospital setting (Azeez & Suzana, 2023). Faith healers are one of the major stakeholders in delivery of mental healthcare in the Maldives (Mohamed & Mansoor, 2024).

2.3.2 Mental Health Burden Among Older People

A study from the Maldives reported that the majority of older people in Maldives are social, and low degree of loneliness is experienced by them; however, about 29% of the older adults experience depression (Azeez & Suzana, 2023). There is no comprehensive data to reflect the burden of mental health issues in older adult population in Maldives.

2.3.3 Available Services in Geriatric Psychiatry

The general healthcare follows a tiered referral system (Mohamed, 2015). In the first tier, the primary healthcare workers and doctors working in the community level provide the care. The second tier consists of the atoll hospitals. The third tier consists of the main tertiary referral service at the Indira Gandhi Memorial Hospital located in Male (Mohamed, 2015). No information is available regarding the mental health-related expenditures by the government (Pandey et al., 2022). No information is available regarding the government's expenses on geriatric mental health. There is a paucity of mental health resources in the country (Mohamed & Mansoor, 2024; Pandey et al., 2022). No dedicated service is available for geriatric mental health, as per the published information.

2.3.4 End-of-Life Care

The Ministry of Health, Republic of Maldives, has developed a guideline for home-based care (Jameel, 2023). This guideline documents the recommendations of home-based care for all conditions that are indicated, including those for the geriatric population and end-of-life care. Digitalization has reinforced home-based care in the Maldives by providing online healthcare support.

2.3.5 Legal and Ethical Aspects of Geriatric Psychiatry

Maldives has a mental health policy; however, there is no stand-alone policy with respect to geriatric mental health (Pandey et al., 2022). The existing mental health policy focuses on enhancing budgeting on mental health, development of leadership and enhancing coordination, quality improvement and monitoring, optimizing human resources and training, promotion of mental health and prevention of psychiatric disorders, mental health advocacy and legislation, facilitating comprehensive mental health services and treatment for drug addiction (Mohamed, 2015).

2.3.6 Specialist Course and Training Opportunities in Geriatric Psychiatry

There are no specialized courses or trainings on geriatric mental health in Maldives. The mental health professionals mostly get their training on geriatric psychiatry from abroad (mostly from Australia or the UK).

2.3.7 Available Research and Gaps

Current research in the field of geriatric psychiatry in the Maldives is limited. This shortfall in scholarly work contributes to a lack of understanding and resources available for addressing the mental health needs of the older adult population in the country. Further investigations and studies are necessary to develop effective approaches and interventions tailored to this demographic (Mohamed, 2015).

2.3.8 Programs-Policies-Action Plans for Geriatric Mental Health

Currently, the Maldives lacks a dedicated and comprehensive policy, program, or action plan specifically addressing the mental health needs of the older adult population. This absence highlights a significant gap in the healthcare framework, which is crucial for ensuring the well-being and mental health support for aging individuals in the country.

2.3.9 Current Challenges in Geriatric Mental Health and Ways Out

The mental healthcare system in the Maldives struggles with a range of substantial challenges that hinder its effectiveness. The major challenge among these is a critical shortage of skilled mental health professionals, which results in insufficient support for individuals needing care. Additionally, people find it difficult to access mental health services, particularly in remote areas, leading to a significant gap in treatment availability. The limited focus on research further compounds these issues, as there is a lack of data to inform best practices and the development of targeted interventions. Furthermore, the execution of preventive strategies remains inadequate, leaving many at risk. Finally, various administrative hurdles contribute to the inefficiency of the system, undermining efforts to provide comprehensive mental health support to the population (Mohamed & Mansoor, 2024).

There is an urgent necessity to strengthen the basic mental healthcare services available across the country, with a particular emphasis on specialized mental health programs tailored to the older adult population. This vulnerable group often faces unique challenges that require dedicated resources and attention. To effectively enhance mental healthcare for the older adults in the Maldives, it is crucial to foster collaboration between various sectors, engage in international partnerships, ensure proactive support from administrative bodies, and invest in comprehensive research initiatives. These efforts will help create a more robust framework for mental health services that meet the specific needs of the aging population.

3 Conclusions

We conducted a comprehensive literature search of geriatric psychiatry in three South Asian countries: Afghanistan, Bhutan, and the Maldives, exploring the existing literature available in English. Our findings reveal that the development of geriatric mental health services and research in these nations is currently at a rudimentary level. In particular, there appears to be a lack of specialized mental health resources existing specifically for the older adult population, which poses a significant gap in addressing their unique psychological needs. Moreover, we acknowledge that there may be important research and evidence available in local languages that we have not included in our analysis. This local literature could provide valuable insights into the cultural context of mental health among the older adults in these countries. Understanding these perspectives is crucial for developing effective interventions and policies that cater to the mental health needs of older adults in South Asia. Therefore, further exploration of indigenous sources is recommended to gain a more comprehensive understanding of the geriatric mental health landscape in these regions.

References

Abdullah, M., Niazi, N., & Pakteen, M. (2021). Palliative care: The care that is rarely practiced in health system of Afghanistan. In M. Silbermann (Ed.), *Palliative care for chronic cancer patients in the community*. Springer. https://doi.org/10.1007/978-3-030-54526-0_39

Alemi, Q., Panter-Brick, C., Oriya, S., Ahmady, M., Alimi, A. Q., Faiz, H., Hakim, N., Sami Hashemi, S. A., Manaly, M. A., Naseri, R., Parwiz, K., Sadat, S. J., Sharifi, M. Z., Shinwari, Z., Ahmadi, S. J., Amin, R., Azimi, S., Hewad, A., Musavi, Z., … Ventevogel, P. (2023). Afghan mental health and psychosocial well-being: Thematic review of four decades of research and interventions. *Bjpsych Open, 9*(4), Article e125. https://doi.org/10.1192/bjo.2023.502

Arafat, S. M. Y., & Kar, S. K. (2024). Epidemiology of psychiatric disorders and overview of access to mental health care in South Asia. In S. M. Y. Arafat, S. K. Kar, (Eds.), Access to mental health care in South Asia. Springer. https://doi.org/10.1007/978-981-99-9153-2_1

Arafat, S. M. Y., Marthoenis, M., Khan, M. M., & Rezaeian, M. (2022). Association between suicide rate and human development index, income, and the political system in 46 muslim-majority countries: An ecological study. *European Journal of Investigation in Health, Psychology and Education, 12*(7), 754–764. https://doi.org/10.3390/ejihpe12070055

Azeez, Z. A., & Suzana, M. (2023). Predictors of geriatric sociability, loneliness and depression in the maldives. *Journal of Mental Health and Aging, 7*(5), 162. https://doi.org/10.35841/aajmha-7.5.162

Bay, J., Yangden, Y., Sherpa, N. L., & Luitel, A. (2019). Palliative care: The emerging field in Bhutan. *Clinical Journal of Oncology Nursing, 23*(1), 108–111. https://doi.org/10.1188/19.CJON.108-111

Dorji, L., Jamtsho, C., Norbu, T., & Bhujel, G. D. (2017). *Understanding the situation of elderly citizens in Bhutan*. National Statistics Bureau Thimpu Bhutan. https://www.nsb.gov.bt/wp-content/uploads/dlm_uploads/2022/02/Understanding-the-situation-of-elderly-citizens-in-Bhutan.pdf

Dorji, N., Yangden, Y., Bhuti, K., Dorjey, Y., Tshering, S., Giam, C. L., & Laabar, T. D. (2024). Palliative care services in Bhutan: Current progress and future needs. *Indian Journal of Palliative Care, 0*(0), 1–7. https://doi.org/10.25259/IJPC_206_2024

ESCAP. (2024). Afghanistan. https://www.population-trends-asiapacific.org/data/AFG (Retrieved 09 December, 2024).

Gyeltshen, K., Chhetri, B., & Gyeltshen, D. (2024). Delivery of mental health services in Bhutan: Challenges and way forward. *Public Health Challenges, 3*(3), Article e211. https://doi.org/10.1002/puh2.211

Jameel, A. (2023, September 24). National guideline for home based care. Ministry of Health, Male', Republic of Maldives. https://health.gov.mv/storage/uploads/0wNNKzwA/phlhyqow.pdf

Khesar Gyalpo University of Medical Sciences of Bhutan, W. (2024). Bhutan Old Age Psychiatry Education Program 2023 | Khesar Gyalpo University of Medical Sciences of Bhutan. https://www.kgumsb.edu.bt/?p=238805, https://www.kgumsb.edu.bt/?p=238805

Krakauer, E. L., Kwete, X. J., Rassouli, M., Arreola-Ornelas, H., Ashrafizadeh, H., Bhadelia, A., Liu, Y. A., Méndez-Carniado, O., Osman, H., & Knaul, F. M. (2023). Palliative care need in the Eastern Mediterranean region and human resource requirements for effective response. *PLOS Global Public Health, 3*(11), Article e0001980. https://doi.org/10.1371/journal.pgph.0001980

Kovess Masfety, V., Sabawoon, A., & Mazzega-Grossin, A. (2018). National mental health survey and assessment of mental health services in Afghanistan. *Kabul: Conseil Santé & Governance Institute of Afghanistan.*

Lemon, C. A., Svob, C., Bonomo, Y., Dhungana, S., Supanya, S., Sittanomai, N., Diatri, H., Haider, I. I., Javed, A., Chandra, P., Herrman, H., Hoven, C. W., & Sartorius, N. (2023). Priorities for research promoting mental health in the south and east of Asia. *The Lancet Regional Health. Southeast Asia, 23*, Article 100287. https://doi.org/10.1016/j.lansea.2023.100287

Ministry of health, Bhutan. (2020). Manual for integrated community based screening for elderly people in Bhutan. Elderly Care Program Health Care & Diagnostic Division Department of Medical Services Ministry of Health. https://www.moh.gov.bt/wp-content/uploads/ict-files/2022/05/Manual-for-Integrated-Community-Based-Screening-3.pdf

Ministry of Health, Royal Government of Bhutan. (2020). National Mental Health Program | Ministry of Health. https://www.moh.gov.bt/about/who-is-who/dept-of-public-health/ncdd/national-mental-health-program/

Ministry of Public Health. (2018). National mental health strategy 2019- 2023. Minstry of Public Health. https://moph.gov.af/sites/default/files/2019-09/Mental%20Health%20Staregy%202019-2023.pdf (Retrieved on 10 December, 2024).

Mohamed, A. (2015). Resuscitating the National Mental Health Policy in the Maldives. *Australasian Psychiatry, 23*(6_suppl), 26–28. https://doi.org/10.1177/1039856215609766

Mohamed, A., & Mansoor, S. (2024). Challenges and opportunities in the mental health landscape of the Maldives. *Australasian Psychiatry*. https://doi.org/10.1177/10398562241289879

Pandey, N. M., Tripathi, R. K., Kar, S. K., Vidya, K. L., & Singh, N. (2022). Mental health promotion for elderly populations in World Health Organization South-East Asia Region: Needs and resource gaps. *World Journal of Psychiatry, 12*(1), 117–127. https://doi.org/10.5498/wjp.v12.i1.117

Pelzang, R. (2012). Mental health care in Bhutan: Policy and issues. *WHO South-East Asia Journal of Public Health, 1*(3), 339–346.

Royal Government of Bhutan. (2020). Launch of palliative care by her royal highness Ashi Kesang Wangmo Wangchuck | Ministry of Health. https://www.moh.gov.bt/launch-of-palliative-care-by-her-royal-highness-ashi-kesang-wangmo-wangchuck/

Sayed, G. D., (2011). Mental health in Afghanistan. World Bank. https://documents1.worldbank.org/curated/ar/692201467992810759/pdf/658840WP00PUBL0736B0MHinAfghanistan.pdf (Retrieved on 12 January, 2025).

Shoib, S., Hussaini, S. S., Nazari, S. K., & Saeed, F. (2024). Mental healthcare in Afghanistan. In S. M. Y. Arafat, S. K. Kar (Eds.), *Access to mental health care in South Asia*. Springer. https://doi.org/10.1007/978-981-99-9153-2_2

Trivedi, J. K., Goel, D., Kallivayalil, R. A., Isaac, M., Shrestha, D. M., & Gambheera, H. C. (2007). Regional cooperation in South Asia in the field of mental health. *World Psychiatry : Official Journal of the World Psychiatric Association (WPA), 6*(1), 57–59.

The World Bank. (2024). Bhutan. World Bank. https://www.worldbank.org/en/country/bhutan

Trani, J. F., Zhu, Y., Park, S., Khuram, D., Azami, R., Fazal, M. R., & Babulal, G. M. (2023). Multidimensional poverty is associated with dementia among adults in Afghanistan. *EClinicalMedicine, 58*, Article 101906. https://doi.org/10.1016/j.eclinm.2023.101906

WHO. (2006). WHO-AIMS report on mental health system in Maldives (pp. 1–19). WHO Regional Office for South-East Asia. https://apps.who.int/iris/bitstream/handle/10665/206158/B0768.pdf

WHO. (2022a). Addressing mental health in Bhutan. https://www.who.int/publications/i/item/9789290210153

WHO. (2022b). World health organization: Addressing mental health in Maldives (pp. 1–16). https://iris.who.int/bitstream/handle/10665/364879/9789290210191-eng.pdf

WHO. (2022c, April 15). Mental Health Atlas 2020 Country Profile: Bhutan. https://www.who.int/publications/m/item/mental-health-atlas-btn-2020-country-profile

World Health Organization. (2024). Afghanistan. https://data.who.int/countries/004 (Retrieved on 09 December, 2024).

World Health Organization. (2022). Mental Health Atlas 2020 country profile: Afghanistan. https://www.who.int/publications/m/item/mental-health-atlas-afg-2020-country-profile (Retrieved on 10 December, 2024).

Substance Use in Old Age in South Asia

Amit Singh, Shreya Shukla, and Arpit Parmar

Abstract Substance use among older adults in South Asia is a growing yet underexplored public health issue. It is posing greater challenges with the increase in the ageing population and evolving social and cultural norms. Tobacco, alcohol, areca nut, and prescription medications are among the commonly used substances. Meanwhile, illicit drug use is also reported in some regions. Contributing factors include easy accessibility to substances, chronic pain, insomnia, loneliness, and mental health issues. Cultural practices and norms regarding substances are key factors influencing their use. Limitations concerning poor awareness and help-seeking, financial adversities, frail health, and social stigma are important challenges to availing treatment and care. Inadequate research further hinders efforts to develop effective prevention and treatment strategies. Despite the major health implications of substance use and a growing need for healthcare, the facilities in South Asia often lack age-sensitive, integrated interventions to address this issue. There is a need for a comprehensive approach to managing substance use disorders in older adults, incorporating culturally adapted education, building community support systems, and providing accessible healthcare services.

Keywords Addiction · Substance-related disorders · Aged · Geriatrics · South Asia · Older adults

A. Singh
Department of Psychiatry, King George's Medical University, Lucknow, India

S. Shukla
National Drug Dependence Treatment Centre, AIIMS, New Delhi, India

A. Parmar (✉)
Department of Psychiatry, All India Institute of Medical Sciences, Bhubaneswar, India
e-mail: dr.arpitparmar@gmail.com

N. Kar et al. (eds.), *Geriatric Psychiatry in South Asia*, South Asian Perspectives in Mental Health and Psychology , https://doi.org/10.1007/978-981-96-7469-5_8

1 Introduction

South Asia is a geopolitically distinct region comprising the eight member states of India, Nepal, Pakistan, Sri Lanka, Bhutan, Bangladesh, Maldives, and Afghanistan. These nations resemble each other in terms of cultural essence and aspects related to economy and health. Around one-tenth of the world's population is 65 years or older, with the South Asian region contributing to more than 15% of this population (World Bank Group, 2024). The global share of the older adult population held by South Asia is expected to rise even further to 18.6% by 2060, emphasising the importance of health research in the geriatric population in this region (He et al., 2022).

It is seen that the population born between 1946 and 1965 had consistently high rates of substance use at all stages of life. As individuals born between this period reach old age, it will be accompanied by its own set of challenges specific to substance use in older adults with unique healthcare needs (Lin et al., 2023). It was posited at the onset of the millennia that the number of adults aged 50 years and older in need of treatment for substance use was expected to rise three-fold by 2020 in the Western population (Han et al., 2009). Similar trends are expected worldwide as the Substance Abuse and Mental Health Services Administration (SAMHSA) declares substance use in older adults an "invisible epidemic" (SAMHSA, 2020). Their presentation may be intertwined with other co-occurring neurocognitive, medical, or psychiatric comorbidities, further complicating diagnosis and intervention (Seim et al., 2020). The "older" drug-using population comprises adults anywhere between 35 and 50 years depending upon the context and geography in previous research (INCB, 2021). The United Nations defines people aged 60 years and older as older persons. Several other agencies stipulate 65 years as the cut-off minimum to be considered an older adult. However, there is no consensus definition for the "older" people who use drugs (INCB, 2021). The older adult population differs from the general population in terms of vulnerabilities, life events, physiological effects, and health consequences of drug and alcohol use (NIDA, 2020).

Substance use among the geriatric population is an overlooked entity in terms of diagnosis, research, and treatment. Although unaddressed substance use in older adults is said to have a poorer prognosis, engagement in treatment is associated with outcomes similar to or better than adult substance use (Dauber et al., 2018; Satre et al., 2004). As the physiological effects of substance use are somewhat distinct in this age group, it emphasises the need to address the issue separately. Ageism and shrinking social support are treatment barriers specific to this cohort, contributing to a substantial treatment gap (SAMHSA, 2020). This chapter aims to elucidate the predicament posed by substance use in old age in terms of epidemiology, comorbidities, diagnosis, and evidence for treatment in the South Asian population.

2 Epidemiology of Substance Use in Old Adults in South Asia

Substance use is associated with various biological, psychological, and socio-environmental factors. In many South Asian countries and their communities, socio-cultural traditions and religious sanctions play a major role in shaping substance use patterns. For instance, alcohol use is less prevalent in countries with a predominantly Muslim population (Arfken & Ahmed, 2016). Similarly, tobacco use is lower in regions predominantly inhabited by the Sikh community. Despite these variances, the use of both licit and illicit substances is prevalent among older adults.

2.1 Tobacco Use

The landscape of tobacco use in South Asia is unique since the use of smokeless tobacco forms such as *khaini, pan masala, zarda, naswar, gul, gutka/gutkha,* and other products are prominent, often predominant ways of consuming in the area. In recent years, a gradual shift in preference for smokeless tobacco over smoking has been noted, especially in India, Bangladesh, and Nepal (Suliankatchi et al., 2019). The Global Adult Tobacco Survey (GATS) reported data on adult tobacco use (including older adults) from nationally representative household surveys in Bangladesh, India, Pakistan, and Sri Lanka (Table 1). The WHO STEP surveys assess the common risk factors for non-communicable diseases (NCDs) and are another important data source regarding tobacco use in Nepal, Bhutan, and the Maldives.

In India, the second round of the GATS (GATS 2, 2016–2017) reported tobacco use prevalence of 41.4% in adults aged over 65 years. Around a fourth of all men and women in this age group consume smokeless tobacco. Meanwhile, the prevalence of smoking was only 4.4% among old women, a third of their male counterparts (TISS & MoHFW, 2018). The Longitudinal Aging Study in India (LASI) 2017–2018 reported smoking in 25.5% of men and 3.4% of women, aged 60 and above. The current use of smokeless tobacco was present in 27.5% of males and 16.2% of females (IIPS et al., 2020). In Bangladesh, GATS 2017 reported tobacco use in 63.1% of the population aged 65 and above (Bangladesh Bureau of Statistics & National Tobacco Control Cell, 2019). A similar tobacco use prevalence of 64.2% among a nationally representative sample of adults over 55 years was reported in an earlier project conducted in 2012 under the International Tobacco Control Project (ITC) Bangladesh, with smokeless tobacco use contributing a major proportion (Nargis et al., 2015). The GATS 2014 Pakistan survey reported a prevalence of 29.6% in older adults. In various provinces of Pakistan, the prevalence rates of tobacco use in old age ranged between 30.6% and 7.3% (Basit et al., 2020). In Sri Lanka, 29.6% of older adults were reported to use tobacco (NATA & DCS, 2023).

The Nepal STEPS survey 2019 found tobacco use in around 42.7% of adults between ages 55 and 69 years, with 27% currently smoking tobacco and 23% using

Table 1 Percentage of adults aged 65 and above who are current tobacco users

	Overall, tobacco use	Smoking tobacco use	Smokeless tobacco use
Bangladesh[a]	63.1	22.0	47.1
Men		38.5	33.9
Women		5.7	62.1
India[b]	41.4	15.5	29.6
Men		19.0	29.6
Women		2.0	12.8
Pakistan[c]	29.6	21.4	8.8
Men		37.3	7.9
Women		7.2	9.5
Sri Lanka[d]	26.0	6.6	20.3
Men		15.1	29.4
Women		0.0	13.2

[a]Global Adult Tobacco Survey Bangladesh 2017
[b]Global Adult Tobacco Survey 2 India 2016–2017
[c]Global Adult Tobacco Survey Pakistan 2014
[d]Global Adult Tobacco Survey Sri Lanka, 2020

smokeless tobacco. The prevalence of tobacco use in the 55–69 years age group was higher than those in the lower age groups. 80% of the geriatric population smoked tobacco cigarettes, 32% smoked *bidis*, while *hukka* use was present in 4%. When it comes to smokeless tobacco use *surti* or *khaini* use was noticed to increase with the increasing age of smokeless tobacco users. Other smokeless tobacco forms included *gutkha*, betel leaves with tobacco and snuff (Dhimal et al., 2020). The STEPS survey in Bhutan (2019), among individuals aged 55 to 69, found tobacco smoking in 3.5% and smokeless tobacco use in 17.6%. The tobacco products commonly smoked were cigarettes (65%) and bidis (51%) while the smokeless tobacco forms frequently used were chewed tobacco (83.1%) and snuff (21%) (Ministry of Health, 2020). Tobacco cultivation, manufacture, and sale were prohibited in Bhutan since 2010; however, it was legalised in 2021 (Evans-Reeves, 2023). The STEPS survey in Maldives (2020–2021) reported current tobacco use in 30.4% of adults (male, 40.3%; female, 18.2%) aged 45–69. Around 23.4% of adults were current tobacco smokers. Smoking tobacco was three times more common in males (33.9%) than in females (10.5%). The smokeless tobacco use in this age group was 9.1% (9.4% in males and 8.7% in females) (Raheem & Moosa, 2022).

Tobacco use is one of the most significant contributors to all-cause morbidity and mortality. Its continued use among the geriatric population is concerning in the face of collaborative efforts to address this issue.

2.2 Areca nut

Areca nut, also known as betel nut, is a commonly used substance with addictive properties and is classified as a Group 1 carcinogen (IARC Working Group on the Evaluation of Carcinogenic Risks to Humans, 2004). Its use is prevalent in South Asian and Western Pacific regions (Gunjal et al., 2020). It forms a key ingredient of betel quid along with betel leaves, slaked lime, and at times tobacco. Contrary to the trends reported for other substances, chewing betel quid increases significantly with age, peaking in the population over 50 years with a prevalence of 68.8% in Bangladesh (Flora et al., 2012). The Asian Betel Consortium study, however, revealed a similar trend in adults over 50 years of age among the Nepalese population and females in Sri Lanka. However, the age-specific prevalence among males in Sri Lanka declined after the age of 50 years (Lee et al., 2011). In India, areca nut usage stands at around 6.7% of the population aged 65 years and above (TISS & MoHFW, 2018). Areca nut use in any form is present in 22% of adults over 60, with "areca nut use only without tobacco" in 11.1%, "areca nut use with tobacco only" in 7.8%, and "areca nut consumption with and without tobacco, dual-use" in 3.2% (Singh et al., 2021).

Although 85% of the population presenting with oral submucosal fibrosis in dental camps in Pakistan presented with a history of areca nut and *paan* usage, no studies shed light on the issue among older adults. Little research in Afghanistan focuses on the use of areca nuts and products; the literature gap is even more glaring considering the geriatric age group. Bhutan has a high prevalence of areca nut usage, with or without tobacco. The use of betel nut peaks between the ages of 25 and 39, followed by a steady decline into old age, with 47.2% of the population above 55 years reporting its use (Tashi Penjor, 2022). Betel nut use with or without tobacco is prevalent in Maldives. Betel quid use is present in 76.6% of males and 65.8% of females aged 45–69 years and using smokeless tobacco (Raheem & Moosa, 2022).

2.3 Alcohol Use

Alcohol is one of the most commonly used substances among older adults. (Das & Sarkar, 2020; Sarkar et al., 2015). It continues to pose problems among them, even as its prevalence is observed to decrease with age (Lal & Pattanayak, 2017). In South Asia, around 9.62% of males and 0.61% of females above 65 years of age consume alcohol exceeding that of non-drinker equivalence; thus, contributing to health risks in this age group (Bryazka et al., 2022).

In India, 11.6% of the male and about 0.69% of the female population, above 65 years of age, are estimated to consume harmful amounts of alcohol (Bryazka et al., 2022). The Longitudinal Aging Study in India (LASI) 2017–2018 reported frequent non-heavy alcohol use and heavy episodic drinking in 4.9% of males aged 60 and above. Among females, frequent non-heavy alcohol use was present in 0.7% and heavy episodic drinking in 0.6% (IIPS et al., 2020). Indian studies report the prevalence of alcohol use in the population over 60 years to range anywhere from 4.1% to 42.1%, owing to diversity in the study methodology. Unsurprisingly, the alcohol use rates are higher in males over 60 compared to females, as evidenced by a 42.8% rate in a study in Indian urban slums and 30.4% in another study (Khokhar & Mehra, 2001; Pandve & Deshmukh, 2010; Srinivasan et al., 2010). Alcohol dependence is reported in 4% and 1.4% of urban and rural-dwelling older adults in India, respectively (Seby et al., 2011; Tiwari & Srivastava, 1998).

A decrease in rates of alcohol use was seen with the transition into late adulthood and old age in Nepal and around a third of the geriatric population reported alcohol consumption in the past year (Adhikari et al., 2019; Sapkota et al., 2023). Alcohol consumption in harmful amounts was reported to be 7·72% among males and 1.26% among females (Bryazka et al., 2022). Nepal STEPS survey 2019 reported the proportion of people aged 55 to 69 consuming alcohol in the past year and past month of 25% and 22%, respectively (Dhimal et al., 2020).

In Sri Lanka, alcohol use remains high in older adults, despite a decreasing trend with age. A survey conducted in 2005–2006 found alcohol use in the past 6 months in 38.2% of males and 0.7% of females in adults aged 60–69 years. In those aged 70 or older, alcohol use was present in 24.6% of males (Katulanda et al., 2014). The STEPS Survey Sri Lanka 2015 reported alcohol consumption in the past 30 days among adults aged 60–69, 17.4% (male, 33.6%; female, 1.0%) (WHO, 2015). Alcohol consumption exceeding non-drinker equivalence is estimated to be present in 14% of males and 0.48% of females (Bryazka et al., 2022).

In Bhutan STEPS survey 2019, the proportion of people aged 55–69 who consumed alcohol in the 12 months was 40.7% and in the past 30 days was 30.7% (Ministry of Health, 2020). Heavy episodic drinking was present in 53.5% of the users who consumed alcohol in the past 30 days. *Ara*, a traditional alcoholic beverage, and beer are the most commonly used forms of alcohol (Ministry of Health, 2020).

Current alcohol consumption among the older population (55–69 years) is less than 1%, according to a national survey in Bangladesh (NIPSOM & WHO, 2018). Alcohol use in the past month was present in 0.4%, while heavy episodic drinking was in only 0.2%. Similar trends in alcohol use have been reported in Pakistan and Afghanistan, which are attributable to the religious sanctions in these nations (Noormal et al., 2024). The harmful amounts of alcohol consumption among older adult men in Pakistan, Bangladesh, and Afghanistan are about 1.44%, 0.74%, and 0.05%, respectively (Bryazka et al., 2022).

Even as substance use in old age is expected to rise in the coming decades, research in the field of alcohol use in the geriatric age group is lacking both in numbers and quality. Prevalence rates have been estimated using arbitrary definitions, with only a handful of studies commenting on problematic use or alcohol dependence.

Correlates of substance use among older adults include unique life events such as the loss of a spouse, medical illnesses, and retirement from work, which make them vulnerable to alcohol use. This, coupled with possible societal acceptance of alcohol as one of the few indulgences of old age, contributes to its continued use in this age group. Both widows and recently bereaved men have been found to use alcohol and other substances more frequently compared to their married counterparts (Perkins et al., 2018). Research posits that increasing age is associated with decreasing tolerance for the effects of alcohol. The decrease in body mass and water composition also contributes to a higher blood alcohol level at comparatively lower alcohol intake. Paired with physical comorbidities, these pharmacokinetic and pharmacodynamic aspects play a crucial role in the morbidity posed by alcohol use in the geriatric population (Lal & Pattanayak, 2017).

2.4 *Prescription Drug Misuse*

Inappropriate use of prescription medications includes their use in a manner not intended by medical practitioners, which also includes use without a prescription. Although prescription drug misuse tends to decline with age, consistent with the misuse of other substances, it poses a significant challenge in the older adult population (Schepis et al., 2020). With advancing age, access to prescription medications, particularly benzodiazepines and opioids, is significantly increased due to higher rates of medical and psychiatric morbidity. This is driven by the need to self-medicate for issues of sleep disturbance, anxiety, chronic pain, and surgical procedures.

In the older age group, the use of physician sources for prescription medication is common in the absence of any prescription drug monitoring programs and unauthorised sales of these medications in certain pharmacies in South Asian member states (Schepis et al., 2020; UNODC, 2011). In the Indian population, the use of pharmaceutical opioids and sedatives in harmful patterns is present in 0.23% and 0.11%, respectively. A study conducted in an old-age home in India reported sedative use to be around 14%, with around half being self-medication (Dhikav et al., 2021). The Afghanistan National Drug Use Survey (2015) found people 60 years and older to constitute about 36% of benzodiazepine users. Benzodiazepines were suggested to be used as agents to relieve stress and pains (SGI-GLOBAL, 2015). However, its use is associated with cognitive decline, sedation, impaired coordination, and increased risk of falls (Juri et al., 2024; Liu et al., 2020). In Nepal, 33.3% of persons aged 50 and above using drugs reported lifetime use of tranquillisers (Government of Nepal, 2020). Estimates of the prevalence of harmful use of these substances are expected to be lower than in the general population; however, the morbidity associated cannot be sufficiently underscored. The lack of research on this topic in the Indian subcontinent hampers recognition and addressing of the issue.

2.5 *Use of Other Drugs*

Trends in the use of opioids have been on the rise in recent years due to the demographic ageing of the population. Around 36–16% of patients aged 60 years or older seeking treatment for substance use disorders (SUD) in India suffer from opioid use disorders (Karahda et al., 2021; Rathee et al., 2024). The South Asian subregion plays a pivotal role in the global illicit opium trade, as it includes the Golden Crescent and lies close to the Golden Triangle. Its strategic geographical position makes it vulnerable to the changing opium and stimulant landscape of the world. In contrast to the Western older adult population, natural opium products such as *afeem* and *doda* contribute a significant proportion to narcotic drug use, especially in North India (Parmar et al., 2017). In Nepal, a recent survey reported lifetime use of cannabis and opiates in 66.7% and 44.4%, respectively, of persons aged 50 and above using drugs (Government of Nepal, 2020). Also, none of them visited treatment centres in the preceding 12 months for SUD.

Cannabis has also been ratified as a narcotic and is controlled under the respective acts in all the South Asian member states. The plant, however, grows naturally in the wild across the region. Coupled with the religious acceptance of cannabis use, its exclusion from the narcotic group of substances further makes this region distinct. Across various Indian studies, the prevalence of cannabis use disorders in patients above 60 years is less than 4% in clinical populations (Grover et al., 2008; Karahda et al., 2021). Literature about the use of narcotic substances by the older adult population from other South Asian nations is scarce, while only a handful of Indian studies address the issue. At the same time, community-based research is conspicuous by its absence, posing a hindrance to our understanding of the use of cannabis in older adults.

3 Factors Influencing Substance Use in Old Age

Although it is widely recognised that substance use declines with age, recent literature highlights a concerning rise in older adults with substance use warranting further attention. Several theories have been put forth to account for the rising substance use among the geriatric population. This rise can be partly attributed to the expanding geriatric demographic, with a higher absolute number of people in this age group (Yarnell et al., 2020). At the outset of the century, it was speculated that the older adult population would surge by over 50% (World Population Prospects, 2022). The need for treatment among this cohort was also set to rise by a factor of 1.7 (Gfroerer et al., 2003). This, along with the rise in life expectancy, which is discordantly high in less developed countries, such as those in the South Asian region, contributes significantly to the burden of substance use in older adults in the region (Mangoni, 2014). Certain factors have been studied, such as the "baby-boomer" generation, which prefers personal gratification. They also have higher exposure to substance use during their younger years, contributing to a greater risk of resuming substance use in old age (Han et al., 2009). Advancements in the field of healthcare have contributed to a growing population of healthy adults, which, coupled with evolving attitudes and cultural norms surrounding substance use, shape the landscape of geriatric substance use (Yarnell et al., 2020).

Older adults have distinct life events and challenges that influence the continued use of substances in this age group (Box 1, Kuerbis, 2020). There is a shift in the long- and short-term psychological and physical needs of these individuals, only partly explained by the process of ageing. Studies have demonstrated the rise in comorbid medical conditions with age. Evidence indicates that the younger age group (under 53 years) has an average of 0.7 comorbidities, which is less than half of what is encountered by the older age group (over 74 years) (Piccirillo et al., 2008). The nature of comorbid conditions also changes from mild to moderate and severe ones, such as cancer (Piccirillo et al., 2008). Concerns about slowing down and medical comorbidities are much more common in the geriatric age group (Amarya et al., 2018). Coming to terms with the realities of ageing, cognitive challenges coupled with loss of autonomy, financial hardships, and retirement from work are common in this population (Skerrett et al., 2022). Coping with personal pain while caring for an ill significant other is a common reality among older adults. The loss of a spouse in the face of other uncertainties and poor coping further increases the risk of relapse or continuation of substance use (Yarnell et al., 2020). Engagement in religious practices is seen to help with loneliness and boredom in old age. The shift from joint and extended family setups in South Asia towards nuclear families is likely to increase this sense of loneliness and contribute to the psychological well-being of this group (Paul & Verma, 2016).

The landmark theory of maturing out of substance use, especially opioids, by Winick et al. in 1962 posits two major hypotheses. People with substance use mature out of it as a function of the length of addiction or their age (Vergés et al., 2013). Further research suggests that Winick's proposition that around two-thirds of the opioid-using population mature out after 5 years of substance use is an exaggeration. Nevertheless, the rates of 3 years of abstinence increase with the advancement of age, which may be explained by personal maturation. There are other pathways to sustained abstinence, which include adverse events and recognition of these events as a consequence of the process of drug dependence (Maddux & Desmond, 1980). Cepeda et al. (2016) proposed that with age, the stresses of a life rife with substance use take their toll, such that substance use patterns shift to more stable patterns of use supported by his support and peer networks (Cepeda et al., 2016). There is little literature about the applicability of this theory in the context of South Asia.

The South Asian region bears witness to socioeconomic and political changes in the post-colonial era, with a significant shift in culture and family structure. Most member nations have also gone through their fair share of civil unrest and internal conflicts. Coupled with rapid urbanisation, the shift from a joint family setup to a nuclear family setup is bound to impact the mental health of older adults (Paul & Verma, 2016). The Longitudinal Ageing Study in India reports that around 6% of those aged 60 years or older reside alone, and another 20% live only with their spouse (IIPS et al., 2020). Literature suggests that the older population, particularly older females, is also at risk of poverty and loss of social support (Rajwar et al., 2024). In conjunction with the general challenges of old age, these factors pose a significant mental health burden on this group, which plays a vital role in the development or continuation of substance use.

A lack of proper monitoring systems results in people including older adults overdosing or misusing pharmaceutical drugs in South Asian countries. Also, the drug regulations are only loosely implemented on the ground resulting in people without prescriptions being able to get pharmaceutical drugs (Ambekar et al., 2019).

Box 1. Risk factors associated with substance use among older adults (Kuerbis, 2020)

Demographics	
	Male gender (tobacco, cannabis, alcohol use)
	Female gender (prescription drugs)
	Poor educational status
Physical factors	
	Painful conditions
	Poor mobility
	Chronic health conditions
Psychiatric Factors	
	Cognitive impairment
	Past history of substance use
	Past history/current history of psychiatric illness
	Loneliness
	Boredom
	Poor social support
	Poor coping
Social factors	
	Bereavement
	Unexpected/forced retirement
	Social isolation
	Social network of peers
	Network of peers who use substances
	No religious affiliation
	Change in living arrangements or homelessness

4 Interplay with Comorbid Conditions

Older adults with SUD often present with comorbid psychiatric conditions, with estimates ranging anywhere from 21 to 66% globally. Depressive conditions are most often found to be comorbid with alcohol dependence, leading to greater service utilisation and an increased risk of self-harm, frequently culminating in suicide (Bartels et al., 2006). Changes in sleep architecture with age manifest as difficulties in sleep onset and maintenance (Gulia & Kumar, 2018). The prevalence of insomnia in older adults can have a detrimental effect on the quality of life for as many as a third of the Indian geriatric population (Gambhir et al., 2014). Pain conditions also form an important correlate of substance use in the older age group, leading to prescription or self-medication with opioid analgesics, which can culminate in a problem of substance use (Goyal & Mohanty, 2022).

5 Assessment of Substance Use in Older Adults

Clinical presentation of SUD might differ in the geriatric age group compared to other age groups. This population may endorse issues related to work or social interactions less frequently. On the other hand, the presence of cognitive problems may complicate the assessment using self-rated instruments that are validated for substance use evaluation. The most commonly used screening instruments in the geriatric age group include the "Cut down, Annoyed, Guilty, Eye-opener" (CAGE) questionnaire, Alcohol Use Disorder Identification Test (AUDIT), Alcohol, Smoking, and Substance Involvement Screening Test (ASSIST), and the Michigan Alcoholism Screening Test (MAST)—Geriatric version (Sarkar et al., 2021). Development and adaptation of some instruments, including CAGE, Screening Questionnaire for Detection of Alcohol Dependence, and Drug Abuse Screen Test (DAST-10) have been done in regional languages (Grover & Laxmi, 2024). However, it is important to note that no specific instruments are validated for prescription or other illicit drug use assessment in older adults. Similarly, most validated scales among adults focus on alcohol use disorders and were developed primarily for the adult population. A recent scoping review found 22 validity studies focused on the geriatric age group, but no validity studies on these scales were found in South Asian countries. Most of these studies were conducted in the USA or other Western nations (Sarkar et al., 2021).

6 Treatment Challenges

There are several challenges unique to treating SUDs in the older adult population in South Asia. These are commonly attributable to socio-cultural, economic, and healthcare system-related factors. Some of the key challenges are discussed below.

6.1 Cultural Acceptance of Substance

In some communities, certain forms of substance use are culturally normalised, particularly for older men. In some regions of India, Pakistan, and Bangladesh, hookah smoking is a popular community activity at home gatherings and celebrations. It is often linked to family traditions and observed as a symbol of brotherhood. Similarly, betel nut chewing, a practice deeply rooted in tradition, is widespread in India and Bangladesh. Additionally, opium use has traditional connotations in several parts of India and Pakistan. This cultural acceptance leads to people not recognising the substance use problem and/or delaying treatment for it.

6.2 Stigma and Misconceptions

Not only is substance use among older adults considered taboo, but seeking treatment for it is also frowned upon in many sections of society, leading to reluctance to seek help or acknowledge the problem. It may lead to even poorer help-seeking in older women (Mandal et al., 2017). Also, families may hesitate to seek treatment due to fear of societal judgment or may ignore substance use as a problem in older adult relatives. Moreover, the pessimism concerning the successful treatment of SUD, especially after prolonged use, is detrimental to treatment-seeking efforts.

6.3 Healthcare System Deficits

In South Asian countries, there is a shortage of facilities providing comprehensive treatment for SUD (Parmar et al., 2024). Moreover, there are even fewer healthcare facilities with staff trained to manage SUD treatment in older adults. In older adults, where comorbidities are common, the lack of integrated care increases the challenge. Limited mobility among older adults and the remote locations of healthcare services compound the accessibility issues. Often, they seek help from local healers and practitioners, and there is a prolonged pathway to care, increasing the burden of care. Also, the high cost of many of the evidence-based medications for SUDs alongside the financial dependence on their families limits treatment affordability.

6.4 Comorbidities and Polypharmacy

Older individuals commonly suffer from chronic diseases such as diabetes mellitus, hypertension, ischemic heart disease, and arthritis, and they are often on multiple medications. Simultaneously managing both physical illnesses and SUDs complicates the scenario. The concerns related to polypharmacy and drug interactions may place SUD management low on the priority list. Additionally, pain conditions, insomnia, and anxiety are frequent in this population, for which they take opioids, sedatives, anxiolytics, and other psychoactive medications or substances (Gambhir et al., 2014; Goyal & Mohanty, 2022). Using pharmaceutical substances without prescriptions or for prolonged periods is common. It may be difficult to establish the primary diagnosis in such patients. Furthermore, the fear of re-emergence of the illness-related primary symptoms or symptoms of substance withdrawal deters them from seeking treatment for SUD.

6.5 Inadequate Policy and Awareness

The government-supported initiatives and programs specifically aimed at addressing SUDs in older adults are lacking in many South Asian countries. Public health messaging rarely targets them or their families regarding the risks and treatments for SUDs.

7 Policies Related to the Healthcare of Older Adults

With increasing age, the treatment of SUD becomes complex due to cognitive issues, comorbidity with medical illnesses, the presence of additional psychiatric illnesses, mobility issues, and barriers to transportation. A movement to provide age-friendly care to older adults with SUD is already underway in the USA. Such age-friendly care is represented by the 5Ms of focus areas in the geriatric age group: Matters Most, Medications, Mind/Mental Health, Multi-complexity, and Mobility (Jones et al., 2023). While treating older adults with SUD, psychiatrists and addiction medicine clinicians should consider (1) Matters most: what matters most to the patient; (2) Medications: use of medications that are safe in older adults, avoid polypharmacy; (3) Mind: common comorbidities of cognitive decline and other mental illnesses; (4) Multi-complexity: the presence of other comorbid medical illnesses that may complicate treatment process; and (5) Mobility: issues with mobility, falls, etc.

In South Asia, the treatment of older adults for substance uses and related problems is usually provided along the lines of management for the adult population. There is a lack of dedicated facilities and treatment protocols in this region. A recent review on mental health promotion for the older adult population in the Southeast Asia region highlights the issues of a limited mental health budget, a severe shortage of geriatric psychiatrists, limited addiction treatment facilities, poor policy implementation, and inadequate geriatric care training (Pandey et al., 2022).

In India, there is a provision for free treatment for SUD under several state-funded schemes. Under *Ayushman Bharat Pradhan Mantri Jan Arogya Yojana* (AB

PM-JAY) launched in 2018, all senior citizens aged 70 and above, regardless of income, are provided with free health insurance coverage of up to Rs. 5 lakh per family per year (AB PM-JAY, 2024). The National Programme for Health Care of the Elderly (NPHCE) launched in 2010–11 to address various health-related problems in older adults had the provision of care through primary and secondary care service delivery through district hospitals (DH), community health centres (CHC), primary health centres (PHC), sub-centre/health and wellness centres (now known as *Ayusham Arogya Mandirs*) (DGHS & MoHFW, 2011). Also, the National Policy on Senior Citizens (2011) stressed the healthcare needs of senior citizens. It aims to provide geriatric care facilities at secondary and tertiary care levels. Though the policy does not explicitly mention substance use, it emphasises the need to increase awareness of mental health through special programs and to develop specialised geriatric care units in hospitals (Gopal et al., 2024).

Bangladesh also implemented a national policy on older persons in 2013. It emphasises the need for measures to enhance health services for older persons, training of caregivers and healthcare professionals by introducing "Geriatric Care and Medicine" as a subject in the undergraduate medicine curriculum and establishing geriatric medicine departments in various public medical colleges. However, the policy does not specifically address the mental health needs of older adults, including those related to SUD. Moreover, the policy's implementation has been largely ineffective, and public-sector geriatric care in Bangladesh continues to lag significantly behind (Dana et al., 2023).

In Pakistan, the National Policy of 1999 emphasised the need to train healthcare providers and establish a multi-tiered healthcare delivery system for older adults. Subsequent provincial policies, such as the Sindh Senior Citizens Welfare Act of 2014, mandated that geriatric medical and health services and medicines prescribed through government healthcare facilities be provided free of charge. Additionally, the Act included provisions for a 25% discount on medicines prescribed by private hospitals and clinics. Similarly, the Islamabad Capital Territory Senior Citizens Bill of 2019 proposed concessions on the purchase of medicines (SPRC, 2022). However, these initiatives tend to prioritise social protection schemes over healthcare initiatives. Furthermore, significant gaps exist in the on-ground implementation of these policies (Noreen et al., 2021; Usmani et al., 2024). As a result, a substantial disconnect persists between policy development and execution, particularly in the context of geriatric healthcare, including the management of SUD in Pakistan.

Similarly, the policies of Sri Lanka, Maldives, and Bhutan also address the mental health care needs of the population but do not explicitly mention addiction care. Countries like Nepal have a limited number of trained professionals in geriatric mental healthcare. Additionally, the population in these countries often prefers traditional healer care over conventional healthcare. Afghanistan currently lacks a formal policy related to older adults.

8 The Way Forward

In health programs, older adults with SUD should be considered a key target population. The International Narcotics Control Board (INCB) made certain key recommendations to the governments and relevant organisations regarding drug use among older adults (INCB, 2021). It includes encompassing older adult populations (65 years and above) in substance use-related epidemiological research; building and employing systems to screen for substance use/misuse, SUD and related risks and monitoring outcomes; using evidence-based strategies to prevent stigma for drug using older adults; developing effective service responses and integrated need based care policy; developing outreach services for marginalised drug using older adults; and ensuring that these services and evidence-based programmes are culturally adapted, and adhere to the principles of independence, participation, care, self-fulfilment and dignity (INCB, 2021).

Furthermore, awareness regarding SUDs and the importance of seeking help through community-based initiatives should be promoted. Families should be educated to identify signs of SUDs and support older adults in seeking care. Additionally, healthcare providers should be trained to identify and manage SUDs in older adults. To provide holistic and integrated care, age-friendly, culturally sensitive treatment programs that address physical, mental, and social health should be developed. Advocacy for policies that offer accessible, affordable, and specialised care for older adults with SUDs should be prioritised.

9 Conclusion

Substance use prevalence is reportedly lower in older adults than in the general population. However, age-related physical and psychosocial vulnerabilities make older adults particularly susceptible to substance use-related harms. Furthermore, limited treatment-seeking behaviour for SUD among older adults presents an ongoing challenge. In South Asian countries, care for SUD in older adults is either lacking or provided within broader programs and facilities targeting general geriatric health. In an initial shift from this approach, in India, geriatric mental health is being prioritised through dedicated policies, programs, and the establishment of specialised facilities for older adults. However, the large-scale implementation of healthcare initiatives addressing substance use among older adults remains elusive in India and other South Asian countries. A concerted and coordinated effort from the stakeholders is required to ensure the widespread availability of accessible, affordable, and high-quality services for SUD in the geriatric population.

References

AB PM-JAY. (2024). *Ayushman Bharat Pradhan Mantri Jan Arogya Yojana. National Portal of India*. https://www.india.gov.in/spotlight/ayushman-bharat-pradhan-mantri-jan-arogya-yojana

Adhikari, T. B., Rijal, A., Kallestrup, P., & Neupane, D. (2019). Alcohol consumption pattern in western Nepal: Findings from the COBIN baseline survey. *BMC Psychiatry, 19*(1), 283. https://doi.org/10.1186/s12888-019-2264-7

Amarya, S., Singh, K., & Sabharwal, M. (2018). Ageing process and physiological changes. In G. D'Onofrio, A. Greco, & D. Sancarlo (Eds.), *Gerontology* (Ch. 1). IntechOpen. https://doi.org/10.5772/intechopen.76249

Ambekar, A., Agrawal, A., Rao, R., Mishra, A., Khandelwal, S., & Chadda, R. (2019). *Magnitude of substance use in India*. Ministry of Social Justice and Empowerment.

Arfken, C. L., & Ahmed, S. (2016). Ten years of substance use research in Muslim populations: Where do we go from here? *Journal of Muslim Mental Health, 10*(1).

Bangladesh Bureau of Statistics and National Tobacco Control Cell. (2019). *Global Adult Tobacco Survey Bangladesh Report 2017*. Bangladesh Bureau of Statistics and National Tobacco Control Cell.

Bartels, S. J., Blow, F. C., Van Citters, A. D., & Brockmann, L. M. (2006). Dual diagnosis among older adults: Co-occurring substance abuse and psychiatric illness. *Journal of Dual Diagnosis, 2*(3), 9–30. https://doi.org/10.1300/J374v02n03_03

Basit, A., Younus, B. B., Waris, N., Fawwad, A., & Members NDSP. (2020). Prevalence of tobacco use in urban and rural areas of Pakistan; a sub-study from second National Diabetes Survey of Pakistan (NDSP) 2016—2017. *Pakistan Journal of Medical Sciences, 36*(4), 808–815. https://doi.org/10.12669/pjms.36.4.1705

Bryazka, D., Reitsma, M. B., Griswold, M. G., Abate, K. H., Abbafati, C., Abbasi-Kangevari, M., Abbasi-Kangevari, Z., Abdoli, A., Abdollahi, M., Abdullah, A. Y. M., Abhilash, E. S., Abu-Gharbieh, E., Acuna, J. M., Addolorato, G., Adebayo, O. M., Adekanmbi, V., Adhikari, K., Adhikari, S., Adnani, Q. E. S., … Gakidou, E. (2022). Population-level risks of alcohol consumption by amount, geography, age, sex, and year: A systematic analysis for the Global Burden of Disease Study 2020. *The Lancet, 400*(10347), 185–235. https://doi.org/10.1016/S0140-6736(22)00847-9

Cepeda, A., Nowotny, K. M., & Valdez, A. (2016). Trajectories of aging long-term Mexican American heroin injectors: The "maturing out" paradox. *Journal of Aging and Health, 28*(1), 19–39. https://doi.org/10.1177/0898264315585503

Dana, G. P. T., Hossain, A. H. M. K., & Hasan, S. (2023). Aging policy of Bangladesh: Issues and challenges for implementation. *Social Science Review, 40*(2), Article 2. https://doi.org/10.3329/ssr.v40i2.72207

Das, S., & Sarkar, S. (2020). Substance abuse in the elderly: A hidden behemoth. *Indian Journal of Social Psychiatry, 36*(4), 267. https://doi.org/10.4103/ijsp.ijsp_394_20

Dauber, H., Pogarell, O., Kraus, L., & Braun, B. (2018). Older adults in treatment for alcohol use disorders: Service utilisation, patient characteristics and treatment outcomes. *Substance Abuse Treatment, Prevention, and Policy, 13*(1), 40. https://doi.org/10.1186/s13011-018-0176-z

DGHS, & MoHFW. (2011). *Operational guidelines National Programme for Health Care of the Elderly (NPHCE)*. Directorate General of Health Services (DGHS) & Ministry of Health and Family Welfare (MoHFW), Government of India. https://mohfw.gov.in/sites/default/files/Operational%20Guidelines%20for%20NPHCE%202010.pdf

Dhikav, V., Chang, S., & Mor, S. (2021). Predictors of sedative–hypnotic usage among residents of old age home in northern India. *International Psychogeriatrics, 33*(12), 1333–1334. https://doi.org/10.1017/S1041610221000636

Dhimal, M., Bista, B., Bhattarai, S., Dixit, L., Hyder, M., Agrawal, N., Rani, M., & Jha, A. (2020). *Report of non communicable disease risk factors: Steps survey Nepal 2019*. Nepal Health Research Council.

Evans-Reeves, K. (2023, February 1). *Bhutan reverses sales ban on tobacco.* Blog—Tobacco Control. https://blogs.bmj.com/tc/?p=1667
Flora, M. S., Mascie-Taylor, C. G., & Rahman, M. (2012). Betel quid chewing and its risk factors in Bangladeshi adults. *WHO South-East Asia Journal of Public Health, 2*(1), 169–181.
Gambhir, I. S., Chakrabarti, S. S., Sharma, A. R., & Saran, D. P. (2014). Insomnia in the elderly—A hospital-based study from North India. *Journal of Clinical Gerontology and Geriatrics, 5*(4), 117–121.
Gfroerer, J., Penne, M., Pemberton, M., & Folsom, R. (2003). Substance abuse treatment need among older adults in 2020: The impact of the aging baby-boom cohort. *Drug and Alcohol Dependence, 69*(2), 127–135. https://doi.org/10.1016/s0376-8716(02)00307-1
Gopal, M. K., Mukherjee, R., Kumar, S., Hazra, S., Sinha, A., Joshi, D., & Sikka, H. (2024). *Senior care reforms in India final version website-compressed.pdf*. NITI Aayog Government of India. https://www.niti.gov.in/sites/default/files/2024-02/Senior%20Care%20Reforms%20in%20India%20Final%20Version%20Website-compressed.pdf
Government of Nepal. (2020). *Nepal Drug Users Survey: 2076*. Government of Nepal, Ministry of Home Affairs.
Goyal, A. K., & Mohanty, S. K. (2022). Association of pain and quality of life among middle-aged and older adults of India. *BMC Geriatrics, 22*(1), 939. https://doi.org/10.1186/s12877-022-03480-y
Grover, S., Irpati, A. S., Saluja, B. S., Basu, D., & Mattoo, S. K. (2008). Drug dependence in the geriatric age group: A clinic-based study. *International Journal of Geriatric Psychiatry, 11*, 10–15.
Grover, S., & Laxmi, R. (2024). A systematic compilation of rating scales developed, translated, and adapted in India. *Indian Journal of Psychiatry, 66*(9), 767. https://doi.org/10.4103/indianjpsychiatry.indianjpsychiatry_467_24
Gulia, K. K., & Kumar, V. M. (2018). Sleep disorders in the elderly: A growing challenge. *Psychogeriatrics: The Official Journal of the Japanese Psychogeriatric Society, 18*(3), 155–165. https://doi.org/10.1111/psyg.12319
Gunjal, S., Pateel, D. G. S., Yang, Y.-H., Doss, J. G., Bilal, S., Maling, T. H., Mehrotra, R., Cheong, S. C., & Zain, R. B. M. (2020). An overview on betel quid and areca nut practice and control in selected Asian and South East Asian countries. *Substance Use & Misuse, 55*(9), 1533–1544. https://doi.org/10.1080/10826084.2019.1657149
Han, B., Gfroerer, J. C., Colliver, J. D., & Penne, M. A. (2009). Substance use disorder among older adults in the United States in 2020. *Addiction, 104*(1), 88–96. https://doi.org/10.1111/j.1360-0443.2008.02411.x
He, W., Goodkind, D., Kowal, P., Almasarweh, I., Giang, T., Islam, M., Lee, S., Teerawichitchainan, B., & Tey, N. (2022). *Asia aging: Demographic, economic, and health transitions.* US Department of Commerce, Report, P95/22, 1.
IARC Working Group on the Evaluation of Carcinogenic Risks to Humans. (2004). Betel-quid and areca-nut chewing and some areca-nut derived nitrosamines. *IARC Monographs on the Evaluation of Carcinogenic Risks to Humans, 85*, 1.
IIPS, NPHCE, HSPH, & USC. (2020). *Longitudinal Ageing Study in India (LASI) Wave 1, 2017–18, India Report*. International Institute for Population Sciences (IIPS), National Programme for Health Care of Elderly (NPHCE), MoHFW, Harvard T. H. Chan School of Public Health (HSPH) and the University of Southern California (USC).
INCB. (2021). *Report of the International Narcotics Control Board for 2020.* United Nations: International Narcotics Control Board.
Jones, K. F., Beiting, K. J., Ari, M., Lau-Ng, R., Landi, A. J., Kelly, L., Pravodelov, V., & Han, B. H. (2023). Age-friendly care for older adults with substance use disorder. *The Lancet. Healthy Longevity, 4*(10), e531–e532. https://doi.org/10.1016/S2666-7568(23)00174-5
Juri, J., Serra, A., & Boveris, D. (2024). General considerations on psychopharmacology in older people. In N. Veronese & A. Marseglia (Eds.), *Psychogeriatrics: A clinical guide* (pp. 81–89). Springer International Publishing. https://doi.org/10.1007/978-3-031-58488-6_5

Karahda, A., Singh, P., Gupta, R., & Prasad, S. K. (2021). Pattern of substance use in the elderly: A hospital based, cross sectional study in a tertiary setting of North India. *Medical Journal of Babylon, 18*(3), 213. https://doi.org/10.4103/MJBL.MJBL_13_21

Katulanda, P., Ranasinghe, C., Rathnapala, A., Karunaratne, N., Sheriff, R., & Matthews, D. (2014). Prevalence, patterns and correlates of alcohol consumption and its' association with tobacco smoking among Sri Lankan adults: A cross-sectional study. *BMC Public Health, 14*(1), 612. https://doi.org/10.1186/1471-2458-14-612

Khokhar, A., & Mehra, M. (2001). Life style and morbidity profile of geriatric population in an urbans community of Delhi. *Indian Journal of Medical Sciences, 55*(11), 609–615.

Kuerbis, A. (2020). Substance use among older adults: An update on prevalence, etiology, assessment, and intervention. *Gerontology, 66*(3), 249–258. https://doi.org/10.1159/000504363

Lal, R., & Pattanayak, R. D. (2017). Alcohol use among the elderly: Issues and considerations. *Journal of Geriatric Mental Health, 4*(1), 4. https://doi.org/10.4103/jgmh.jgmh_34_16

Lee, C.-H., Ko, A. M.-S., Warnakulasuriya, S., Yin, B.-L., Sunarjo, null, Zain, R. B., Ibrahim, S. O., Liu, Z.-W., Li, W.-H., Zhang, S.-S., Kuntoro, null, Utomo, B., Rajapakse, P. S., Warusavithana, S. A., Razak, I. A., Abdullah, N., Shrestha, P., Kwan, A.-L., Shieh, T.-Y., … Ko, Y.-C. (2011). Intercountry prevalences and practices of betel-quid use in south, southeast and eastern Asia regions and associated oral preneoplastic disorders: An international collaborative study by Asian betel-quid consortium of south and east Asia. *International Journal of Cancer, 129*(7), 1741–1751. https://doi.org/10.1002/ijc.25809

Lin, J., Arnovitz, M., Kotbi, N., & Francois, D. (2023). Substance use disorders in the geriatric population: A review and synthesis of the literature of a growing problem in a growing population. *Current Treatment Options in Psychiatry, 1–20*,. https://doi.org/10.1007/s40501-023-00291-9

Liu, L., Jia, L., Jian, P., Zhou, Y., Zhou, J., Wu, F., & Tang, Y. (2020). The effects of benzodiazepine use and abuse on cognition in the elders: A systematic review and meta-analysis of comparative studies. *Frontiers in Psychiatry, 11*, 00755. https://doi.org/10.3389/fpsyt.2020.00755

Maddux, J. F., & Desmond, D. P. (1980). *New light on the maturing out hypothesis in opioid dependence*. UNODC—Bulletin on Narcotics—1980 Issue 1—002. www.unodc.org/unodc/en/data-and-analysis/bulletin/bulletin_1980-01-01_1_page003.html

Mandal, P., Parmar, A., Therthani, S., & Ambekar, A. (2017). Profile of elderly women seeking treatment for substance use disorders at a tertiary care treatment center. *Journal of Substance Use, 22*(3), 353–355. https://doi.org/10.1080/14659891.2016.1217092

Mangoni, A. A. (2014). Geriatric medicine in an aging society: Up for a challenge? *Frontiers in Medicine, 1*,. https://doi.org/10.3389/fmed.2014.00010

Ministry of Health. (2020). *Non-communicable disease risk factors: Bhutan STEPS Survey 2019*. Department of Public Health. https://www.who.int/publications/m/item/2019-steps-country-report-bhutan

Nargis, N., Thompson, M. E., Fong, G. T., Driezen, P., Hussain, A. K. M. G., Ruthbah, U. H., Quah, A. C. K., & Abdullah, A. S. (2015). Prevalence and patterns of tobacco use in Bangladesh from 2009 to 2012: Evidence from International Tobacco Control (ITC) Study. *PLoS ONE, 10*(11), Article e0141135. https://doi.org/10.1371/journal.pone.0141135

NATA & DCS. (2023). *Global Adult Tobacco Survey—Sri Lanka 2020 Report*. Department of Census and Statistics & National Authority on Tobacco and Alcohol. https://www.statistics.gov.lk/Resource/en/OtherCensusandSurveys/SurveyReports/GATS_Report_2020.pdf

NIDA. (2020, July 9). *Substance use in older adults drugfacts*. National Institute on Drug Abuse (NIDA). https://nida.nih.gov/publications/drugfacts/substance-use-in-older-adults-drugfacts

NIPSOM & WHO. (2018). *National STEPS Survey for Non-communicable diseases risk factors in Bangladesh 2018*. National Institute of Preventive and Social Medicine & World Health Organisation. https://cdn.who.int/media/docs/default-source/searo/bangladesh/publications/2018-national-steps-survey-for-non-communicable-diseases-risk-factors-in-bangladesh.pdf?sfvrsn=9155c4b5_3&download=true

Noormal, A. S., Winkler, V., Bhusari, S. B., Horstick, O., Louis, V. R., Deckert, A., Antia, K., Wasko, Z., Rai, P., Mocruha, A. F., & Dambach, P. (2024). Prevalence of major non-communicable diseases and their associated risk factors in Afghanistan: A systematic review and meta-analysis. *Therapeutic Advances in Chronic Disease, 15*, 20406223241229850. https://doi.org/10.1177/20406223241229850

Noreen, N., Abdullah, M., & Lalani, N. (2021). Geriatric care in Pakistan: Current realities and way forward. *Pakistan Journal of Public Health, 11*(4), Article 4. https://doi.org/10.32413/pjph.v11i4.872

Pandey, N. M., Tripathi, R. K., Kar, S. K., Vidya, K. L., & Singh, N. (2022). Mental health promotion for elderly populations in World Health Organization South-East Asia region: Needs and resource gaps. *World Journal of Psychiatry, 12*(1), 117–127. https://doi.org/10.5498/wjp.v12.i1.117

Pandve, H. T., & Deshmukh, P. (2010). Health survey among elderly population residing in an urban slum of Pune city. *Journal of the Indian Academy of Geriatrics, 6*(1), 5–8.

Parmar, A., Mohanty, D., Pal, A., & Singh, A. (2024). Substance use disorder in South Asia: Challenges and ways ahead. In S. M. Y. Arafat & S. K. Kar (Eds.), *Current perspectives on substance use disorders in South Asia: Public mental health aspects* (pp. 149–164). Springer Nature. https://doi.org/10.1007/978-981-97-6619-2_9

Parmar, A., Patil, V., & Sarkar, S. (2017). Natural opioid use in elderly in India: A case series. *Journal of Substance Use, 22*(2), 156–158. https://doi.org/10.3109/14659891.2016.1162211

Paul, A., & Verma, R. K. (2016). Does living arrangement affect work status, morbidity, and treatment seeking of the elderly population? A study of south Indian states. *SAGE Open, 6*(3), 2158244016659528. https://doi.org/10.1177/2158244016659528

Perkins, J. M., Lee, H.-Y., Lee, J.-K., Heo, J., Krishna, A., Choi, S., Nam, Y.-S., Oh, J., & Subramanian, S. V. (2018). Widowhood and alcohol, tobacco, and other drug use among older adults in India. *The Journals of Gerontology. Series B, Psychological Sciences and Social Sciences, 73*(4), 666–674. https://doi.org/10.1093/geronb/gbw134

Piccirillo, J. F., Vlahiotis, A., Barrett, L. B., Flood, K. L., Spitznagel, E. L., & Steyerberg, E. W. (2008). The changing prevalence of comorbidity across the age spectrum. *Critical Reviews in Oncology/hematology, 67*(2), 124–132. https://doi.org/10.1016/j.critrevonc.2008.01.013

Raheem, R. A., & Moosa, S. (2022). *WHO STEP survey on risk factors for noncommunicable diseases Maldives 2020–2021*. The Maldives National University, Health Protection Agency, and World Health Organization.

Rajwar, E., Pundir, P., Challa, S., Prince, A. M., Parsekar, S. S., & Vogt, T. (2024). A scoping review of income support programs offered to older adults living in South Asian countries between 2000 and 2021. *Health & Social Care in the Community, 2024*(1), 1711756. https://doi.org/10.1155/2024/1711756

Rathee, S., Joseph, J., Kumar, V., Arya, S., Taneja, K., & Gupta, R. (2024). Profile of elderly substance users-seeking treatment: A retrospective analysis from a tertiary care center in North India. *Annals of Indian Psychiatry, 8*(4), 336. https://doi.org/10.4103/aip.aip_204_23

SAMHSA. (2020). *Treating substance use disorder in older adults: Updated 2020*. Substance Abuse and Mental Health Services Administration (US). http://www.ncbi.nlm.nih.gov/books/NBK571029/

Sapkota, B. P., Baral, K. P., Rehfuess, E. A., Parhofer, K. G., & Berger, U. (2023). Effects of age on non-communicable disease risk factors among Nepalese adults. *PLoS ONE, 18*(6), Article e0281028.

Sarkar, S., Parmar, A., & Chatterjee, B. (2015). Substance use disorders in the elderly: A review. *Journal of Geriatric Mental Health, 2*(2), 74. https://doi.org/10.4103/2348-9995.174271

Sarkar, S., Sood, E., Bhad, R., & Mishra, A. (2021). Validated scales for substance use disorders in the geriatric population: A scoping review. *Journal of Geriatric Mental Health, 8*(2), 70. https://doi.org/10.4103/jgmh.jgmh_38_21

Satre, D. D., Mertens, J. R., Areán, P. A., & Weisner, C. (2004). Five-year alcohol and drug treatment outcomes of older adults versus middle-aged and younger adults in a managed care program. *Addiction, 99*(10), 1286–1297. https://doi.org/10.1111/j.1360-0443.2004.00831.x

Schepis, T. S., Klare, D. L., Ford, J. A., & McCabe, S. E. (2020). Prescription drug misuse: Taking a lifespan perspective. *Substance Abuse: Research and Treatment, 14*, 1178221820909352. https://doi.org/10.1177/1178221820909352

Seby, K., Chaudhury, S., & Chakraborty, R. (2011). Prevalence of psychiatric and physical morbidity in an urban geriatric population. *Indian Journal of Psychiatry, 53*(2), 121–127. https://doi.org/10.4103/0019-5545.82535

Seim, L., Vijapura, P., Pagali, S., & Burton, M. C. (2020). Common substance use disorders in older adults. *Hospital Practice (1995), 48*(sup1), 48–55. https://doi.org/10.1080/21548331.2020.1733287

SGI-GLOBAL. (2015). *Afghanistan National Drug Use Survey 2015*. https://colombo-plan.org/wp-content/uploads/2020/03/Afghanistan-National-Drug-Use-Survey-2015-compressed.pdf

Singh, P. K., Yadav, A., Singh, L., Mazumdar, S., Sinha, D. N., Straif, K., & Singh, S. (2021). Areca nut consumption with and without tobacco among the adult population: A nationally representative study from India. *British Medical Journal Open, 11*(6), Article e043987. https://doi.org/10.1136/bmjopen-2020-043987

Skerrett, K., Spira, M., & Chandy, J. (2022). Emerging Elderhood: Transitions from Midlife. *Clinical Social Work Journal, 50*(4), 377–386. https://doi.org/10.1007/s10615-021-00791-2

SPRC. (2022). *Legislation for older people in Pakistan*. Social Protection Resource Centre.

Srinivasan, K., Vaz, M., & Thomas, T. (2010). Prevalence of health related disability among community dwelling urban elderly from middle socioeconomic strata in Bangaluru, India. *The Indian Journal of Medical Research, 131*, 515–521.

Suliankatchi, R. A., Sinha, D. N., Rath, R., Aryal, K. K., Zaman, M. M., Gupta, P. C., Karki, K. B., & Venugopal, D. (2019). Smokeless Tobacco use is "replacing" the smoking epidemic in the South-East Asia region. *Nicotine & Tobacco Research: Official Journal of the Society for Research on Nicotine and Tobacco, 21*(1), 95–100. https://doi.org/10.1093/ntr/ntx272

Tashi Penjor. (2022). *Prevalence of betel or areca nut (AN) use and its associated factors among Bhutanese population aged 15–69 years old: An analysis of national health data of non-communicable disease (NCD) survey in 2019*. Chulalongkorn University.

TISS, & MoHFW. (2018). *Global Adult Tobacco Survey GATS 2 India 2016–17*. Tata Institute of Social Sciences (TISS) & Ministry of Health and Family Welfare (MoHFW), Government of India. https://ntcp.mohfw.gov.in/assets/document/surveys-reports-publications/Global-Adult-Tobacco-Survey-Second-Round-India-2016-2017.pdf

Tiwari, S. C., & Srivastava, S. (1998). Geropsychiatric morbidity in rural Uttar Pradesh. *Indian Journal of Psychiatry, 40*(3), 266–273.

UNODC. (2011). *Misuse of prescription drugs: A South Asia perspective*. United Nations Office on Drugs and Crime (UNODC) Regional Office for South Asia.

Usmani, B. A., Lakhdir, M. P. A., Sameen, S., Batool, S., Odland, M. L., Goodman-Palmer, D., Agyapong-Badu, S., Hirschhorn, L. R., Greig, C., & Davies, J. (2024). Exploring the priorities of ageing populations in Pakistan, comparing views of older people in Karachi City and Thatta. *PLoS ONE, 19*(7), Article e0304474. https://doi.org/10.1371/journal.pone.0304474

Vergés, A., Haeny, A. M., Jackson, K. M., Bucholz, K. K., Grant, J. D., Trull, T. J., Wood, P. K., & Sher, K. J. (2013). Refining the notion of maturing out: Results from the National Epidemiologic Survey on alcohol and related conditions. *American Journal of Public Health, 103*(12), e67–e73. https://doi.org/10.2105/AJPH.2013.301358

WHO. (2015). *Sri Lanka—Steps 2014*. World Health Organization. https://extranet.who.int/ncdsmicrodata/index.php/catalog/614/related-materials

World Bank Group. (2024). *World Development Indicators*. DataBank. https://data.worldbank.org/indicator/SP.POP.65UP.TO.ZS

World Population Prospects. (2022). *World population prospects—Population division—United Nations*. https://population.un.org/wpp/

Yarnell, S., Li, L., MacGrory, B., Trevisan, L., & Kirwin, P. (2020). Substance use disorders in later life: A review and synthesis of the literature of an emerging public health concern. *The American Journal of Geriatric Psychiatry: Official Journal of the American Association for Geriatric Psychiatry, 28*(2), 226–236. https://doi.org/10.1016/j.jagp.2019.06.005

Social Determinants and Cultural Aspects of Geriatric Mental Health in South Asia

Hitesh Khurana and Sujata Sethi

Abstract South Asia is a region marked by significant geographic and cultural diversity. With around 7% of the world's land area, South Asia is home to about 25% of the global population. Political conflicts, poor education levels, poverty, and economic disparities are some of the cultural peculiarities of South Asian countries. The number of older adults in the region has risen, currently totaling around 126 million. South Asian families traditionally respect older adults, involve them in decision making and consider their welfare as the primary family responsibility. But the migration of younger generations due to inadequate employment opportunities in hometowns has weakened family ties, leaving older adults more vulnerable. Along with this loneliness, abuse is another important mental health issue that the older adults are facing in the region. This puts pressure on governments to develop stronger health and social policies for older adults' welfare. There is paucity of data on mental health of older people from South Asia, except India. The chapter reviews existing literature to shed light on cultural issues impacting on the mental health of older people in the region.

Keywords Cognitive decline · Common mental disorders · Culture · Dementia · Depression · Elder · Loneliness · Mental health · Older adults · South Asia

1 Introduction

As defined by the World Bank, Bangladesh, Bhutan, India, the Maldives, Nepal, Pakistan, and Sri Lanka constitute South Asia (World Bank Group, 2023). This region has some cultural commonalities. These countries were the colonies of one or the other European countries, gaining freedom in the later half of the twentieth century. The World Bank considers these all as developing countries with Maldives as a low-income country and the rest as low-middle-income countries. However, there is a feeling that some of these countries, especially India, are the emerging economic

H. Khurana · S. Sethi (✉)
Department of Psychiatry, Pandit. B.D. Sharma Post Graduate Institute of Medical Sciences, Rohtak, India
e-mail: reachsujatasethi@gmail.com

N. Kar et al. (eds.), *Geriatric Psychiatry in South Asia*, South Asian Perspectives in Mental Health and Psychology , https://doi.org/10.1007/978-981-96-7469-5_9

superpower. Internal political and communal conflicts mark some countries, e.g. Afghanistan, Bangladesh, India, and Sri Lanka. Agriculture and tourism are the main sources of livelihood in these countries. The younger population is often looking for high-paid public and skilled jobs leading to their migration to metropolitan cities and other countries, leaving behind the older adults in the native home. Joint families are still more prevalent as compared to Western countries. In South Asia, primary health care facilities are still the backbone of health care delivery. Besides the Western system of medicine, Ayurveda, Unani and Siddha systems are also quite popular in this region (Kafczyk & Hämel, 2023). However, when it comes to mental health, the resources are too meager making it quite difficult for the older adults to access these in these countries. With planned reduction in fertility rates, South Asian countries are likely to have a large population of older adults that may choke the resources and existing social and health care facilities (Ashraf et al., 2013).

2 South Asia: Region of Poor Development and Socio-Cultural Diversities

South Asia has about 7% of the total land area of the globe with 25% of the world population. About 95% of the population of South Asia is living in three countries namely, Bangladesh, India, and Pakistan. Population growth is quite variable within South Asia, with 0.4% growth for Sri Lanka to 3.5% for Afghanistan within 5 years (Véron et al., 2008). Sri Lanka, India, Bangladesh, and Pakistan rank among the top 50 nations with a high proportion of population aged 65 years and above. As per UN criteria Sri Lanka with 7.8% older adults in its population is already an aging country (Population Reference Bureau, 2020).

There are marked geographical variations and natural disasters like cyclones, droughts, floods are quite common. Economic growth is slow in this part of the world and not providing an adequate number of jobs (*South Asia,* 2024). Examining the most relevant indices for a country's development namely, literacy, GDP, and urbanization, reveals sharp contrasts between these countries. Literacy rates for women were much lower (around 60%) in 2011 for India and 50% for Pakistan. After sub-Saharan Africa, South Asia is the second least developed region of the world with a human development index of 0.6 against the world average of 0.74. South Asian countries are generally considered low- and middle-income countries (Véron et al., 2008). Emigration to European and American countries for employment is quite common in these countries.

The South Asian region finds its place among the countries with fast-growing populations with a fertility rate of 3.2 children per woman against the world average of 2.7. The average life expectancy at birth is 3.6 years below the world average. The health indices of South Asian countries rank among the lowest in the world. Infant mortality was 11‰ in Sri Lanka in the early 2000s and even higher, i.e. 16% in Afghanistan, and the fertility rate ranges from 2–7% (Véron et al., 2008).

In South Asia, the increasing population of older adults is a health management problem just because of its huge absolute number. The current projections suggest that adults aged 60 years and over will constitute over 13% of the population in India by 2031. But going by the absolute number, India already has more older adults than any of the aged countries like Japan. The communicable diseases, and infant and maternal mortality are common health challenges for South Asian countries and these countries are dealing with these issues with some success. However, the older adults population poses unique health problems due to degenerative disorders and other non-communicable diseases and these countries do not have effective working models or policies to address these problems.

3 Epidemiology of Mental Disorders in South Asia

Though South Asia is home to about one-third of older people of the world. Yet, there is inadequate focus on mental health issues. In this chapter, we present the review of some studies selected for this chapter. Compared to India, data from the rest of South Asia is much less. Hence, to focus better on these regions, Indian research is dealt with separately. After India, we could find epidemiological studies primarily from Sri Lanka, followed by Nepal. No research originating from Maldives could be located.

A survey of Tables 1 and 2 reflects prevalence of dementia ranging between lowest 1.93% (Banerjee et al., 2017) to highest 14.5% among older people in the community in India (Nagoor et al., 2018). Prevalence in other countries also varies from 3.98% in Sri Lanka (Silva et al., 2003) to 8.9% in Nepal (Aich et al., 2017). These prevalence figures are very close to 7% reported in the Longitudinal Ageing Study in India (Lee et al., 2023). Most of the studies available are cross-sectional, and some are even retrospective chart reviews (Aich et al., 2017). Except for a few studies (Naheed et al., 2023; Silva et al., 2003) most of the studies have small samples. Mini Mental State Examination (MMSE) is most commonly used for detecting dementia. This tool is best used for the screening purpose and indicates the vulnerability to dementia in association with other risk factors such as age >90 years (Naheed et al., 2023), female gender (Lee et al., 2023; Naheed et al., 2023), lesser education (Philip & Johns, 2024), cognitive decline (Acharya et al. 2023), and depressive symptoms (Thapa et al., 2014). Most of the research has been on identifying depressive illnesses. After dementia, depressive illnesses are most associated with disability during late age (Bamonti et al., 2024). A large number of studies are reported from India, Nepal, and Sri Lanka. The prevalence of depressive symptoms in South Asia varied from 15.4% (Thapa et al., 2020) to as high as 53.1% (Manandhar et al., 2019). The prevalence seems to be higher in institutionalized settings at 76% (Abeysekera & De Zoysa, 2021; Ramesh et al., 2023) to 89%, as well as in the community setting (60%) (Thapa et al., 2018). Higher age (Farooq et al., 2019; Ogbo et al., 2018) and female gender (Sabzwari et al., 2019) increase the odds of getting depressive symptoms. Most of the community based studies are carried out in a large representative sample (Farooq et al., 2019; Sabzwari et al., 2019; Senarath et al., 2014; Thapa et al., 2018), but have used different tools leading to varying rates. Common mental disorders (CMD) also showed wide variations in prevalence ranging from 7% (Nagoor et al., 2018), 18% (Patel et al., 2024; Thapa et al., 2020) in Nepal and India, respectively, to 44% in Bhutan (Sithey et al., 2018). Higher prevalence was seen among the hospital attendees and those with comorbidities (Grover et al., 2021). Symptoms of stress (Thapa et al., 2020) and Post-Traumatic Stress Disorder (PTSD) were also commonly observed among the older persons especially those who were displaced due to migration and conflict (Frounfelker et al., 2023; Thapa et al., 2003).

Sexual disorders (Rao et al., 2015) and sleep disorders (Abeysekera & De Zoysa, 2021) among the older adults are less emphasized upon in the South Asian research. It is worth noting that most of the studies used the screening questionnaires to detect the prevalence of common mental disorders as well as severe illness such as dementia and depression. For the purpose of diagnosis, these tools may not be very suitable. And also, as pointed out by Fotheringham et al. (2022), without cultural validation these tools may not be suitable for use in the South Asian community.

4 Socio-cultural Determinants of Geriatric Mental Health

The health status of any country depends not just on the availability of health infrastructure and manpower but also other socioeconomic conditions such as literacy, income, sex ratio, income and social protection, unemployment and job security, working life conditions, food insecurity, housing, basic amenities, and the environment, social inclusion, and non-discrimination, determine the service utilization and outcome of health-related conditions. There is little information available on the socio-cultural issues of the older adults in South Asia countries.

South Asia has a good adult literacy rate of about 74.19%, ranging between 97.86% for Maldives to 71.15% for Nepal and improving with time (*South Asia Literacy Rate 1975–2024*, 2024). However, these rates do not reflect the lower literacy among older adults, ranging from 29.5% for females and 59.47% for males as projected by the world bank for year 2019 (Trading Economics, 2024). Literacy among older adults reported from studies from Nepal varies between 23–32%. In Bhutan and India too, the majority of the older adults have low education and have low income mostly through state welfare policies, and a small proportion earns through participation in manual jobs (Dorji et al., 2017; Moneer et al., 2012). Pakistan and Afghanistan have even lower literacy rates (13–37%) (Hussain et al., 2020). India fares slightly better with literacy rates of 45.38% for those aged 65 years or more. Of all the south Asian countries, Maldives can boast of high literacy rates among those aged 65+ (91.7% as in 2014) (National Bureau of Statistics, 2014).

Economically, the older adults are generally grouped among the poorer strata of any nation. In South Asia (LMIC countries), 40% older adults categorized as the poorest. Nearly 20% older adults have no income at all (Andrea Wojnar, 2023). As people enter late adulthood, they lose physical strength. There are no policies for

Table 1 Epidemiological studies of prevalence of mental disorders among older adults in South Asia (other than India)

Country	Author	Study type	Sample	Tools used	Results
Bangladesh	Naheed et al. (2023)	Cross-sectional	2795 individuals aged > 60	MMSE	Dementia prevalence = 8.0% Odds of dementia was two times higher in females than males and nine times higher in people aged ≥ 90 years than people aged 60–69. Poor education was a significant risk factor for dementia
Bhutan	Sithey et al. (2018)	Cross-sectional	$N = 7041$ (612 subjects aged 65 + years)	GHQ-12	Common mental disorders Among 65 + 44.3% Among younger = 26.9–34.4%
Nepal	Khattri et al. (2020)	Cross-sectional	$N = 392$ older adults in outpatient clinic	ICD-10 based clinical interview	Neurotic disorders = 37.0% Mood disorders = 28.3% 66–75 years age group was most affected
Nepal	Thapa et al. (2020)	Cross-sectional	$N = 794$ older adults living in community	DASS-21	Depression = 15.4% Anxiety = 18.1% Stress = 12.1% Risk factors identified were female gender, working in agriculture, lower household wealth, perceived poor health, smoking, chronic conditions, migration of adult children, and exposure to adverse life events
Nepal	Devkota et al. (2019)	Cross-Sectional	$N = 124$ Age > 60 years	UCLALS GDS-15	Depression = 49.2% Moderate to severe Loneliness was reported by about 45% subjects
Nepal	Manandhar et al. (2019)	Cross-sectional	$N = 439$ older adults	GDS-15	Depression = 53.1%
Nepal	Thapa et al. (2018)	Systematic Review	26 studies on the prevalence of depression among older adults	–	Depression: Prevalence Community = 25.5%–60.6% Aged-care facilities 17.3%–89.1% Hospital settings:53.2%–57.1%, Anxiety symptom:21.7%–32.3%

(continued)

Table 1 (continued)

Country	Author	Study type	Sample	Tools used	Results
Nepal	Aich et al. (2017)	Retrospective	$N = 257$ Age > 60 years	Chart review	Psychosis = 27.6% Depression = 15.2% Alcohol dependence = 10.5% Anxiety = 9.7% Dementia = 8.9% Mania = 4.3%
Nepal	Lam et al. (2017)	Cross-sectional	$N = 1{,}073$ adults Number of older adults not mentioned	CES	21.3% had CES-D score 16 or greater. Age over 60 and lack of formal education were associated with increased risk of depressive symptoms
Nepal	Thapa et al. (2014)	Retrospective	$N = 120$ subjects Age > 65 years	Chart review	Depressive disorder = 26.7% Risk for dementia higher in those aged 75 years and above
Nepal	Shakya (2012)	Cross-sectional	$N = 100$ Age > 55 years	Open clinical interview	mood disorder = 46% anxiety disorders = 22%, substance use disorders = 19% Organic disorders = 12% Somatoform disorders = 10%
Nepal	Thapa et al. (2003)	Cross-sectional	$N = 418$ (92 were aged 55–85) Bhutanese refugee in Nepal	Specific modules of CIDI (GAD, PTSD, Somatoform Pain Disorders, Depression)	28.3% of those aged 55 years and above reported disability
Nepal	Koirala et al. (2000)	Retrospective	$N = 75$ Psychiatric Out Patients, Age range = 60–88 years	Chart Review	Mood disorder = 30.7% Organic brain disorder = 28%
Pakistan	Farooq et al. (2019)	Cross-sectional	2867 older adults	AKUADS	27.4% reported having anxiety and depressive symptoms Odds ratio for anxiety and depressive symptoms among older adults was 1.02(60–69 years) to 1.26(70 years and above)

(continued)

Table 1 (continued)

Country	Author	Study type	Sample	Tools used	Results
Pakistan	Sabzwari et al. (2019)	Cross-sectional with multi-stage cluster sampling	$N = 1200$ urban older adults	PHQ-2, 6-CIT, IADL, ADL	55.3% participants were female 51.8% were screened positive for depression 63.1% had cognitive impairment
Sri Lanka	Alwis et al. (2024)	Meta-Analysis	52,778 subjects from 33 studies		Depressive disorders Pooled prevalence = 19.4% young persons = 39% Adults = 8.7% Older persons = 18.4%
Sri Lanka	Abeysekera and De Zoysa (2021)	Cross-sectional	$N = 310$ Age = 60–103 years	GDS, PCS, PSQI	Depression = 76.5% Sleep Disorders = 55.5% Catastrophizing Pain = 29%
Sri Lanka	Gamage et al. (2019)	Cross-Sectional	$N = 421$ subjects living in old age home age: 71.9 ± 6.7 years with 65.8% females	MMSE	Being educated, married, and coming to old age facility on own will were protective against cognitive decline
Sri Lanka	Senarath et al. (2014)	Cross-sectional	$N = 1{,}2841$	PHQ-9 with 10 as cut off score	Major depression = 4.5% Mild depression = 13.3% Prevalence in older adults = 11.6%
Sri Lanka	Malhotra et al. (2010)	Cross-Sectional	$N = 1{,}181$ Age > 65 years	GDS	Overall depression = 27.8% Women = 30.8% Men = 24.0%
Sri Lanka	Rodrigo et al. (2010)	Cross-Sectional	$N = 100$ Age > 55 years Out door attendees	GDS, MMSE	Very likely depressed = 31% MMSE < 23 With less than secondary education = 24/42 (57.1%) Secondary and higher level of education = 32/58 (55.2%)
Sri Lanka	Silva et al. (2003)	Cross-sectional Two stage sampling	$N = 703$ Age > = 65 years	SMMSE	Screened positive for dementia = 42(5.97%) Diagnosed dementia = 28(3.98%)
Sri Lanka	Wijeratne et al. (2010)	Cross-sectional	$N = 100$ Inmates of Old Age Homes Age = > 60 years	GDS	Depressive symptoms = 56%(of which 23.2% had severe depression). Female sex, chronic diseases, family conflicts, and lack of psychological support were significantly associated with depression

(continued)

Table 1 (continued)

Country	Author	Study type	Sample	Tools used	Results
Srilanka	Rajapakshe et al. (2019)	Cross-sectional	$N = 1283$ Age $= 60–74$ years	GDS	prevalence of depression = 13.9% (mild depression: 11.2%; moderate to severe depression: 2.7%)
South Asia region	Ogbo et al. (2018)	Cross-sectional	Population 18 years and above	GBD 2016 data DSM-IV and ICD-10 diagnoses	Burden of depressive disorders was highest among older age groups (75–79 years) in all countries India had largest DALY due to depressive disorders followed by Bangladesh and Pakistan

Abbreviations AKUADS: Aga Khan University Anxiety Depression Scale; ADL: Katz Index of Activities of daily living; CES-D: Center for Epidemiologic Studies Depression Scale; CIDI: Composite International Diagnostic Interview; CIT: Cognitive Impairment test; DALY: Disability-Adjusted Life Years; DASS-21: Depression Anxiety and Stress Scale-21; GAD: Genralised Anxiety Disorder: GBD: Global Burden of Disease; GDS: Geriatric Depression Scale, GDS-15: Geriatric Depression Scale-15; GHQ-12: General Health Questionnaire-12; IADL: Lawton's Instrumental Activities of Daily Life; MMSE: Mini Mental State Examination; PCS: Pain Catastrophizing Scale; PHQ-9: Patient Health Questionnare-9; PSQI: Pittsburgh Sleep Quality Index; PTSD: Post-Traumatic Stress Disorder; SMMSE: Sinhalese Mini Mental State Examination UCLALS: University of California Los Angles Loneliness Scale; YLD: Years Lived with Disability

older adults in most of the countries for their re-employment. Most of the older adults in South Asian countries live on their pension or the financial assistance from the government schemes. Particularly for the South Asian older adults, where their population is growing with a higher rate than the rest of the world, they might face poverty, neglect and other hardship due to no or little income and growing inflation. In Nepal, the older persons live either on old age allowance (94%) or depend upon farming. The majority of the older adults have some disability but their access to the health care system is poor and many times because of lack of any source of income (Gupta et al., 2016; Paudel, 2022). In Afghanistan, the older adults have to face hardships to get their pension and other dues from government agencies. There is a possibility that pensions, which is the only source of income for many older adults, may be cut down by 90% during the current regime (Ehsan, 2023). Inflation, difficulties with the pension system, and financial assistance were rated as serious difficulties toward health attainment in Pakistan (Usmani et al., 2024). Poor awareness (29%) and inadequate pension amount, corruption, and non-poor getting the benefit are commonly reported difficulties by the Indian senior citizens (Kulkarni et al., 2011).

Work status wise as noted in the Building Knowledge base on Population Ageing in India (BKPAI) survey (Moneer et al., 2012), work participation was low among the older adults with 39% for men and 11% for women. Most of them (71%) felt pressured

Table 2 Epidemiological studies of prevalence of mental disorders among older adults in India (2014–2024)

Place (Indian state)	Author	Study Design	Sample	Tools	Results
Kerala	Pranav et al. (2024)	Cross-Sectional	$N = 320$ post retiree Mean age 69.5 years	WEMWBS and WHO QoL BREF	Higher QoL and well-being was seen among those retiring from public sector and living in rural areas
Kerala	Philip and Johns (2024)	Cross-Sectional	$N = 535$ inmates of Old Age Homes	MMSE, PMIS	17–31% older adults had cognitive impairment. Lesser education and increasing age were significantly associated with cognitive decline
Rajasthan	Patel et al. (2024)	Systematic review with Meta-Analysis	23 studies	MeSH word Seach on Scopus and PubMed of Indian studies with older adults sample	Anxiety = 18.7% High hetergeniety in the included studies
Uttar Pradesh	Pandit et al. (2024)	Cross-sectional Multistage Cluster Sampling	$N = 350$ Age 70.66 ± 9.53 years, Rural	HMSE	24.9% of subjects were screened positive for cognitive decline
Various states of India	Basu et al. (2024)	Cross-sectional data from wave 1 from Longitudinal Ageing Study of India	$N = 28{,}150$ women Age = 50+ years	CIDI-SF, ADL, IADL	21.76% women aged 50+ reported depression compared to 17.60% among those aged below 50
Tamil Nadu	Devaraj et al. (2024)	Cross-Sectional	$N = 114$ Age = 60+ years	ADL, DSSI, MMSE	self-neglect was reported by 21.1% Medical help was refused by 47.38% Low literacy, low SES and situational impairments were significantly associated

(continued)

Table 2 (continued)

Place (Indian state)	Author	Study Design	Sample	Tools	Results
Tamil Nadu	Ramesh et al. (2023)	Cross-Sectional	$N = 311$ Old age home inmates	DASS-21	Depression = 84.2%, Anxiety = 49.2%, Stress = 55.9%
New Delhi	Acharya et al. (2023)	Cross-Sectional	$N = 365$ Age = 60+	BADL, MoCA-B	Subjects with dementia were screened out using MMSE Overall MCI = 9.3% Among males = 13.3% Among females = 6.5%
Various states of India	Muhammad (2023)	Secondary analysis of Longitudinal Ageing Study in India	$N = 28{,}027$ Age = 60+ years	multivariable logistic and linear regression models	Odds ratio suggested that rural background was associated with depressive symptoms in women and cognitive symptoms among men
Various states of India	Lee et al. (2023)	Secondary analysis of Longitudinal Ageing Study in India	$N = 28{,}949$ Age = 60+	Logistic modeling and imputation	Dementia = 7.4% Dementia is more prevalent among females and in rural areas
Various states of India	Sharma and Pradhan (2023)	Longitudinal Ageing Study in India (2017–18)	$N = 31{,}646$	Analysis of Health, Economic, & Social determinants of dimensions of aging	Cognitive Impairment = 16% Old age, females, less educated, economically weak were more at risk of developing dementia

(continued)

Table 2 (continued)

Place (Indian state)	Author	Study Design	Sample	Tools	Results
	Muhammad et al. (2021)	Longitudinal Ageing Study in India wave 1 (2017–2018)	$N = 31{,}464$	Analysis of Health, Economic, & Social determinants of dimensions of aging	Unsafe neighbourhood = 14.3% Violent crimes = 1.3% Depression = 8.6% Elder abuse = 5.2%
Maharashtra	Goswami and Deshmukh (2021)	Cross-sectional	$N = 290$ Rural Age 60+ years	GDS	Depression = 41.7%
Punjab	Grover et al. (2021)	Cross-sectional	$N = 311$ Age = 60+ years Secondary data analysis Subjects were attending Non-communicable disease clinic in the hospital	VASS, PHQ-9, GAD-7, UCLAS	Abuse = 24% Anxiety (39%), Depression (54%), Loneliness (38.6%)
Jammu	Kumari et al. (2021)	Cross-sectional	$N = 425$ Age = 67.47 ± 6.43 years Rural	MMSE GDS-15	Cognitive impairment = 36% Depression = 29.1%
Various states of India	Sinha et al. (2021)	National Mental Health Survey of India Multi stage cluster sampling	$N = 34{,}802$ older adults = 6.6–12.8% in various states of India	MINI	Older adults had a higher lifetime (6.93%) and current (3.53%) than younger population Specific phobia (1.72%) was most common anxiety disorder. All CMD were more common among females
Karnataka	Khanna and Metgud (2020)	Cross-sectional	$N = 770$ Age = 60+ Urban	MMSE, ZCBS	Cognitive impairment = 8.4%

(continued)

Table 2 (continued)

Place (Indian state)	Author	Study Design	Sample	Tools	Results
NewDelhi	Sudan et al. (2020)	Cross-Sectional	$N = 300$ Age = 65+ years	EASI, AAT	Abuse among psychiatric patients = 21.3% Among physical illness = 4%
Rajasthan	Patel et al. (2020)	Cross-sectional	$N = 331$ Age = 67.9 ± 7.8	GAD,GDS, MMSE	severe depression = 17% severe anxiety = 10.3%, Cognitive impairment = 51.2% Prevalence more in rural areas and females
Tamil Nadu	Ramalingam et al. (2019)	Cross-sectional	$N = 243$ M:F::1:1.63	HSEABST	Elder abuse = 50.3%
Karnataka	Akila et al. (2019)	Cross-sectional House to house survey in rural and urban areas	$N = 510$	GDS, BADL, IADL, HMSE	A higher proportion of older adults in rural areas (32.6%) are at risk of depression than in urban (30.4%)
Odisha	Ashe and Routray (2019)	Cross-sectional Simple random sampling	$N = 354$ Urban Slum Dwellers	GDS, IADL, KIDL	Severe depression = 44.9% Mild depression = 36.2%
Punjab	Mehra et al. (2019)	Cross-sectional	$N = 125$ Age = 55+ years	VASS	58.4% had psychiatric morbidity. Depression was most common disorder. 41.6% complained of abuse
Andhra Pradesh	Nagoor et al. (2018)	Cross-sectional Community based	$N = 416$ Age = 60+	MMSE, GDS, BADL	Cognitive impairment = 47.7% Depression = 27.7% Dementia = 14.9% Anxiety = 7.2%
Maharashtra	Rathod et al. (2019)	Cross-sectional Probability proportionate Sampling House to house Survey	$N = 400$ Age = 60+ years	MDIS	Depression = 16.5% Lack of adequate sleep and leisure time, staying alone and illiteracy were significant predictors of depression

(continued)

Table 2 (continued)

Place (Indian state)	Author	Study Design	Sample	Tools	Results
Pudduchery	Ramalingam et al. (2018)	Cross-sectional	$N = 243$ Age 60+ years Rural	GHQ-12	Almost 50% of older adults suffered from common mental disorders. CMD were more prevalent among lesser educated, having lesser income and widowed
Gujarat	Patel and Singh (2018)	Cross-sectional Community based	$N = 560$ Age = 50+ years Rural & Urban	MMSE	Cognitive Impairment = 25% Age 60 years of above, not living with spouse or children, lesser education were significantly associated with cognitive impairment
Maharashtra	Goswami et al. (2017)	Cross-Sectional Community based Convenient Sampling	$N = 290$ Rural	GDS-15	Depression = 41.7% Female sex, living without spouse, abuse, not having right to make decisions were the risk factors
Karnataka	Bharath et al. (2017)	Cross-sectional Hospital Based	$N = 7469$ Age = 60+ years	Petersen Criteria for MCI	MCI = 0.007% Primary males were affected
West Bengal	Banerjee et al. (2017)	Cross-sectional Community based Random sampling 2007–08	$N = 100{,}802$ (males = 53,209)	YLL, YLD, DALY	Dementia = 1.53% among those aged 65 + years Men had higher mortality adjusted for diagnosis of dementia

(continued)

Table 2 (continued)

Place (Indian state)	Author	Study Design	Sample	Tools	Results
Kerala	Nakulan et al. (2015)	Cross-sectional Community based	$N = 220$ Age = 60+ years	MADRS, ICD-10-based SCL	ICD-10 Depressive episode = 36.1% Female gender and life events in the previous year were significant risk factors
Karnataka	Rao et al. (2015)	Cross-sectional Community based	$N = 259$ Age = 60+ years	ASES, IIEF, PEDT, HSDD, FSFQ	Sexually active –27.4% Among males: Erectile Dysfunction = 43.5% Premature ejaculation = 10.9% Hypoactive Sexual Desire = 0.77% Anorgasmia = 0.38% Among females: Arousal Dyspareunia = 8% Anorgasmia = 20% disorder = 28%, HSSD = 16%

Abbreviations: AAT: Actual Abuse Tool; ADL: Katz Index of Activities of daily living; ASES: Arizona Sexual Experience Scale; BADL: Barthel's Index of Activities of Daily Living; CIDI-SF: Composite International Diagnostic Interview-Short Form; CMD: Common Mental Disorder; DASS-21: Depression Anxiety and Stress Scale-21; DSSI: Duke Social Support Index; EASI: Elder Abuse Suspicion Index; FSFQ: Female Sexual Function Questionnaire; GAD-7: Generalized Anxiety Disorder-7 Scale; GDS: Geriatric Depression Scale; HMSE: Hindi Mental State Examination; HSEABST: Hwalek-Sengstock Elder Abuse Screening Test; HSSD: Hypoactive sexual desire disorder; IIEF: International Index of Erectile Function; KIDL: Katz Index of daily living; LADL: Lawton's Instrumental Activities of Daily Life; MCI: Mild Cognitive Impairment; MDIS: Major Depression Inventory Scale; MINI: Mini International Neuro-Psychiatric Interview; MADRS: Montgomery Asberg Depression Rating Scale; MoCA-B: Montreal Cognitive Assessment-Basic; PEDT: Premature ejaculation diagnostic tool; PHQ-9: Patient Health Questionnaire; PMIS: Picture Memory Impairment Screen; UCLA: University of California, Los Angeles Loneliness Scale; SCL: Symptom Checklist; VASS: Vulnerability to Abuse Screening Scale; WEMWBS: Warwick-Edinburgh Mental Well-being Scale; WHO QoL BREF: World Health Organizations Quality of Life Scale-Brief Version; YLD: Years lived with Disability; YLL: Years of life lost from mortality; ZCBS: Zarit Caregiver Burden Scale to work to fulfill their financial needs. They were primarily engaged in manual or unskilled low wages work. Even among the oldest older adults (80 years and above) work participation was high (males = 13% females = 3%). In the neighboring countries, Nepal (Gupta et al., 2016) and Bhutan (Dorji et al., 2017) also older people were involved in manual work in the farms. In Bhutan older persons preferred to work voluntarily at religious places (Dorji et al., 2017).

Building a Knowledge Base on Population Ageing in India (BKPAI) survey (Moneer et al., 2012) and HelpAge India survey 2024 revealed a dismal condition of the older adults in India. Sixty to sixty-six percent of the older adults in these surveys were financially insufficient. The living conditions of older adults in the BKPAI survey were below satisfactory. Twenty-five percent lived in mud-thatched (*kachcha*) houses. Wood was the most common household fuel. Water and sanitation conditions were inadequate. About one-third of the older adults had monthly expenditure of less than 1000 rupees (22 USD). Only 16% received financial support from their children, relatives, or family members (Moneer et al., 2012).

The older adults in South Asia living in a family have better life despite financial constraints. They are often involved in decision making, taking care of the toddlers in joint families. As per religious traditions, particularly Hinduism and Islam, the eldest son in the family is expected to perform the holy duty of caring for parents. South Asia still has predominantly patrilineal families, with the senior most male being the nominal head in the family. In the absence of a male, widowed mothers or/grandmothers play the same role. It is seen that with a female as head, whether by choice or mostly unwillingly (Habib, 2020; Thampi & Mathew, 2024; Watt et al., 2014), children achieve better educational milestones (Chudgar, 2011). Most of the older adults prefer to engage in voluntary work such as serving at religious places or get taken care of by the family. In the SA countries, taking care of the older adults is considered a family responsibility but not many older adults find a healthy environment in the families (Gulzar et al., 2008; Gupta et al., 2016; Paudel, 2022; Usmani et al., 2024). Poor socioeconomic status is the prime determinant of the poor quality of life among older adults (Ghosh & Dinda, 2020; Santhalingam et al., 2022).

In spite of good social values and the attitude of family toward older people, the intergenerational relationships are slowly eroding away and more and more reports about elder abuse are pouring in recently. Migration, kinship disputes, abuse by the children for property inheritance are also common in these countries (Skirbekk & James, 2014; Thomas, 2023). Children of many older adults do not live with them (Dorji et al., 2017). Even in the Maldives, a country with a small population and high literacy, the intergenerational gap is high. The older people find it difficult to communicate with the younger generation due to technical illiteracy, linguistic gap, and antisocial or abusive behavior of younger ones. The children in Maldives leave their sick older parents totally to the state to care (Aminath, 2023), unlike India where maintenance of parents and senior citizen acts are in force. High proportion of older adults (55%), particularly the oldest of the older adults, poor, illiterate, and widows reported poor physical and mental health. Acute as well as chronic morbidities were reported by about 13% older adults' women and 9% older adult men (Moneer et al., 2012).

In the South Asian countries, people have a poor understanding of the symptoms of mental illness and the need for treatment. A mental health survey carried out in India highlighted that there was a long latency between the onset of disorder and the patient being brought to the care facility; this being 2.5 months and one year for epilepsy and depressive episode, respectively. The treatment gap for various disorders ranged from 70 to 90%. The treatment gap was larger in the rural areas.There were wide variations in reporting symptoms from the culturally similar regions. Overall, the survey suggested poor mental health awareness among people (Murthy, 2017). Under such circumstances, extending mental health care to older adults is even more challenging. Multiple reasons are likely for such latency. Most of the time, especially at the first instance of mental illness, the symptoms are normalized and attributed to one or the other social or physical cause. It is not uncommon to see that the patients in South Asia receive their first consultation from a 'wise man' of the family or locality. Following that, they visit multiple doctors (Murthy, 2017). To the best of our efforts, no study for other South Asian countries regarding mental health literacy was retrieved. This area remains highly under-researched.

5 Loneliness Among Older Adults

Loneliness is a *perceived social isolation* and discontent with the *quality* of their relationships rather than the *quantity* of relationships they have (Shah, 2021). Living alone or feeling alone both arouse sympathetic activity and act as stressors. Thus, loneliness is a risk factor for many chronic diseases, including such as heart disease, depression, anxiety, and cognitive decline (Mushtaq et al., 2014). Older adults in South Asia are particularly vulnerable to loneliness. Younger generations migrating to other places within or out of the country is not a new phenomenon. In recent years, migration has become a problem for the older people due to the inversion of the population pyramid with more older adults than children. Till a few decades ago, primarily the males (or sons) were migrating, with whom the older people preferred to stay for cultural and religious reasons. Now, young females also prefer to migrate for better education and employment (Migration and Migrants: Regional Dimensions and Developments, 2021; UNICEF, 2022), giving the older persons a Hobson's choice to live alone. Youth also migrate to neighboring countries due to political conflicts. Youth emigrating for refuge, death of family members in the conflicts also give rise to loneliness and consequent depressive and anxiety symptoms (Dost et al., 2024). These data suggest a strong causal connection of social isolation leading to loneliness among the South Asian older adults. With disabilities and physical weakness due to ageing, loneliness puts them in double jeopardy (Rajan, 2023). The feminization of the older population can be considered as the third dimension of jeopardy. If senior citizens at all choose to migrate, they get acculturation difficulties and often feel lonely after migration (Ali et al., 2021). With all these etiological factors, physical loneliness or isolation is emerging as an epidemic. Nearly 13% older adults report being lonely (Srivastava & Srivastava, 2023). In the

10/66 Dementia Research Group on adults aged over 65 years from one rural and one urban location in India ($n = 1001$ at baseline), it was found that 18.3% of participants reported feeling lonely (Gao et al., 2021). Perceived loneliness in South Asia is associated with female gender, being widowed, lower income and education (Grenade & Boldy, 2008; Srivastava & Srivastava, 2023). Unfamiliarity with technology, not able to make effective use of mobile phone (Aminath, 2023; Grey et al., 2024; Petersen et al., 2016), lack of social networks, deaths, lack of friends, increasing nuclear families, generation gap, lack of children or migrating to other cities or countries especially from rural areas for various reasons (Berg-Weger & Morley, 2020) and children engaged with electronic gadgets (MacDonald & Schermer, 2021) also add to the loneliness among older adults. Health problems such as poor functional status, cognitive impairment, urinary incontinence, illness, depression increase loneliness among older adults (Singh & Misra, 2009). Stigma of mental illness may also lead to feelings of isolation and loneliness (Grover et al., 2019). Loneliness is a health hazard and the person suffering from it may be prone to various infections, heart disease, anxiety and depression, dementia, and even suicide (Hussain et al., 2023; Knight, 2022). The problem is rampant in South Asia, however, the focus of research on loneliness and its determinants is primarily being reported from the US and European countries (Ali et al., 2021; B. Hussain et al., 2023). Loneliness complicates the outcome of any other concomitant disease. Some researchers have equated loneliness itself to disease (Tiwari, 2013; WHO, 2022). Loneliness exposes older adults to committing crimes and also makes them vulnerable to criminal activities (Hindustan Times, 2019; Srivastava & Srivastava, 2022). Being employed is inversely associated with loneliness. Thus, being in employment offers two-fold advantages for older adults (Shankar & Kidd, 2022). But it is a matter of debate and choice if one should seek employment or be looked after at the senescence of life.

During the UN decade of older adults (2021–2030), the WHO also has made loneliness among older adults as its health priority and focused on developing guidelines so as to improve international collaboration to prevent loneliness by making it a political priority, too (Knight, 2022; Mohan, 2021). Local governments are encouraged to create old age-friendly communities, transportation, use of digital devices, and appropriate information technology to reduce loneliness among older adults (WHO, 2022).

6 Substance Use Disorders among Geriatric Populations

The South Asian sub-region, also colloquially known as the Golden Crescent (Pakistan, Iran, & Afghanistan) and Golden Triangle (Thailand, Myanmar, & Laos), is the world's most prolific area of opiate production. Traditionally, there has been significant cannabis and opium use within the sub-region used for social, religious, and medicinal purposes (Aroonsrimorakot et al., 2020).

Not much of recent data about the health risk behaviors is available among older adults from South Asian countries. Data from the study on Adult Health and Global

Ageing (SAGE) wave-I revealed about 1/3rd of the older adults indulged in smoking tobacco and being physically less active (Oduro et al., 2023). Bhutan banned the sale and use of any form of tobacco in 2005, even then as per a survey, 20.5% of older adults between age 55–69 years were smokers (Gurung et al., 2016). Prevalence of smoking among 55–69-year-old showed a declining trend from 70% in 2007 to 42% in 2019 in Nepal (Ghimire et al., 2019; Mandal, 2022). Nearly 18% of the adults attending outdoor services of a hospital had a positive history of smoking. Low literacy, male gender, being unemployed, living alone were strong determinants of smoking. Opium use was common among those who were chronic smokers (Hamrah et al., 2019). Subgroup analysis of Longitudinal Ageing Study in India data revealed smoking increasing the odds for non-communicable diseases such as hypertension, heart disease, and cancer among older adults (Boro & Saikia, 2024). A mental health survey carried out in India highlights high prevalence of mental disorders among the older adults. Substance use disorders were the most prevalent in the age group 50–59 years. Tobacco use was prevalent in 5–40% of the participants (Gururaj et al., 2016).

Research from India has looked at the epidemiology of substance use, mostly alcohol use and related disorders in older adults (Nadkarni et al., 2013). Also, these studies have used different definitions for substance use and abuse disorders, have heterogeneous populations, and samples from different settings. According to the National Mental Health Survey 2015–2016 (Gururaj et al., 2016) prevalence of alcohol and nicotine use disorders in the older adults (above 60 years of age) was 4.07% and 26.3%, respectively. The prevalence of any substance use disorder was 27.8% compared to 22.4% in all populations. The prevalence of alcohol use in the older population was around 4.5% in a community sample (Alam & Karan, 2011). In another nationwide survey, older adults aged 65+ years, 41.4% were found to be current tobacco users (Tata Institute of Social Sciences (TISS), 2017). Most older adults with substance abuse are likely to be those with onset of substance abuse at a younger age. Mental health issues such as depression, anxiety, or psychosocial problems (loneliness, stress, role/identity loss), can contribute to late-onset substance abuse (Emiliussen et al., 2017).

Older people have more physical comorbidities such as chronic pain, diabetes, hypertension, along with psychiatric comorbidities like anxiety, depression, or sleep difficulties. Many of these patients may get prescriptions of psychotropic agents such as benzodiazepines from general practitioners and may develop dependence for prescription drugs (Franchi et al., 2019). Various factors associated with excessive use of prescription drugs include female gender, social isolation, and comorbid psychiatric illness (Sarkar et al., 2015).

Older adults with substance abuse had an increased risk for neglect. Many older adults live alone or with their spouses. The older adults with substance abuse have an increased risk of being violent and physically aggressive toward the spouse and other family members. About 4.4% of victims and 26.9% of perpetrators of elder abuse had been using one or another psychoactive substance (Conrad et al., 2019).

To cope with loneliness and on the other hand, post-retirement over-involvement in social life, bereavement, and availability of pension money may put this group at risk for substance abuse (Kuerbis et al., 2014).

7 Older Adults and Suicide

The geriatric population has unique issues such as physical illness, retirement, loss of job, dependency on others for daily needs, loss of spouse/close friends and loneliness, making them vulnerable for high levels of distress (De Leo, 2022).

About 10% of world's suicides take place in India, Pakistan, and Sri Lanka (Khan, 2002). Jordan et al. cited in their scoping review that the suicide rates in South Asia can be compared to the global average and males committing suicide outnumber females. The suicide rate among the South Asian population ranges between 0.43/100,000 (general population) to 331.0/100,000 (suicides of older adults in India) of the population and the rate varies between countries, and is mainly linked to the development levels of the country. Suicidal deaths are underreported from the South Asia. The actual rates are likely to be much higher than reported in the studies. Data on suicide behavior by the older persons is very limited (Jordans et al., 2014).

The rate of suicide in the older adults is much higher than the adult population and the incidence of suicide across the various regions of South Asia (Vijayakumar et al., 2020). Hanging is found to be the common mode of suicide in older adults (Crestani et al., 2019).

National mental health survey data from India and reported that India accounts for 26.6% of global suicide deaths, and that the prevalence was higher among those over 60 years of age (Amudhan et al., 2020). However, Philip et al. (2022) found that there is a slight modest increase in the suicidal rates among people 60 years and above, and the rates were higher among older adult women compared to older adult men in India (Philip et al., 2023). In India, most suicides are reported to be due to personal or social reasons, followed by health and other reasons (Dandona et al., 2016). Chandrasekaran (2008) investigated the predictors of repeated suicide attempts of 348 samples from India and found that repeat suicide attempts are associated with depression, hopelessness, and suicidal intent, and that the presence of major depressive disorder and social dissidence are predictive factors for repeat attempts (Chandrasekaran, 2008).

A scoping review by Arafat et al. (2022) concluded that the prevalence of depression seems to be lower in South Asian countries as compared to other regions of the world among fatal (37.3%) and nonfatal suicidal attempts (32.7%). Presence of preexisting psychiatric morbidities and stressful life events are the most common risk factors for suicide in older adults in South Asian countries (Arafat et al. 2022).

Not much work has been done in Bangladesh regarding the suicidal behavior among older adult population. One review assessed depression and suicidal thoughts among 625 rural older adults of Bangladesh (Greig & Kabir, 2022) and reported that 23% of participants had suicidal thoughts. The frequency of suicidal thoughts was significantly higher among illiterate persons, women, and those living without partners. Living with family members and having a good contact with them were identified as protective factors in Bangladesh (Wahlin et al., 2015). Shoib et al. (2021) identified depression along with hopelessness as the key contributing factors of suicidal behaviors among the geriatric population in Kashmir, India. In Sri Lanka, about 23.6% of all deaths among the older adults were reported to be suicides (Seneviratne et al., 2022).

A recent review concluded that lack of social integration or interaction along with some psychiatric disorders leads to suicidal ideation and completed suicide in the older adults in these countries. South Asia has unique characteristics in several aspects like religious and cultural diversity, poverty, unemployment, demographic structure of the region, migration, natural disasters and calamities, political environment, poor policy implementation, and easy access to suicide means (e.g. pesticides) that may contribute to high suicide rates in older adults of South Asian region (Kar et al., 2022).

8 Old Age Women's Mental Health in South Asia

Numerous studies from South Asian countries unanimously agree to the fact that except substance use disorders other psychiatric disorders like common mental disorders, depression, and cognitive disorders are more prevalent among older women as compared to their men counterparts. This can be due to two reasons. Firstly, women outlive men as the result of that there are more older females than males living in the world. There are certain biological changes such as musculoskeletal weakness, hearing and visual disabilities which act as stressors evoking anxiety, depression, and cognitive difficulties as the age advances. And secondly, there are certain social and cultural factors prevalent in South Asia that make older women more vulnerable to these disorders.

Culturally and religiously women hold a prestigious position in the society. Particularly in Hinduism there is a big number of women deities, and no religious ceremony is considered complete without participation of wife. Woman's role traditionally becomes more and more powerful as she becomes older (Regmi, 1982). However, women's condition is today's South Asian countries is quite different.

Women in South Asia are lesser educated than men, particularly in India, Pakistan, Nepal, and Afghanistan (Sheikh & Loney, 2018). Only 29% of women aged 65 years and above are educated as compared to 59% literacy among older males in South Asia (Trading Economics, 2024).

As long as fathers or the older men are the heads of the family, the women are generally engaged in household chores, rearing grandchildren with little role in decision making. This lack of autonomy is independent of educational status (Acharya et al., 2010). Economic insecurity, dependency, lack of assets are some remarkable characteristics of older women. Living alone is almost a norm for them and about 20% of them start living alone for the first time due to the death of their spouse and children migrating away for jobs. The cultural values, especially in India and Nepal favor parents to stay with sons and not with the daughters, which also promotes the trend of older women living alone (Acharya et al., 2023). Those living with children frequently report abuse. Many of the older adult ladies find spirituality as a way of networking with others.

Widowhood increases their economic insecurity and dependency as in many cultures particularly Pakistan, women at the time of marriage are asked to transfer their share of ancestral property by swearing Holy Quran (Niaz & Hassan, 2006) and as per sharia law an Afghani widow would inherit only one-eighth to one-fourth of her husband's wealth on his death and the rest would be divided among the relatives. Her remarriage is also possible with her brother-in-law, who would always treat her as a brother's wife despite marrying her. She and her daughters (not son) will not be financially supported by him if he is facing financial constraints. Many times, the widows in Afghanistan are shifted to a geographically and culturally secluded area where *the wakil* (male head of that area) drives them into prostitution (Carter, 2015).

The primary concerns of the older adult women, as evident from the epidemiological studies, are common mental disorders, depression, and cognitive decline and these are rarely addressed. Even after migrating from South Asia, older women continue to face health-related challenges (Bailey et al., 2018).

9 Elder Abuse in South Asia

In addition to the other social and mental health problems, older adults are often susceptible to abuse. Abuse is said to occur when there is any kind of harm that occurs in a relationship based on trust. It was first reported as 'granny battering' in 1975 from UK (Paranitheran & Edirisinghe, 2009). The International Network for the Prevention of Elder Abuse (World Health Organization, 2002) has adopted the definition of elder abuse as "a single or repeated act, or lack of appropriate action that causes harm or distress to an older person, occurring within any relationship where there is an expectation of trust." Neglect in various forms such as ignoring the person's need to socialize, nutritional needs, avoiding health care, etc. is also very common forms of mistreatment against older persons.

It is widely prevalent around the world, both over and under-reported. Again, it seems quite likely that the elder abuse or mistreatment is most likely to occur in South Asia in comparison to the rest of the world simply due to the massive population of older adults in this region. One among 6 older adults report having suffered abuse of neglect. The prevalence of different kinds of abuse varies from 0.9% (sexual abuse) to 11.6% for psychological abuse (World Health Organization, 2024). However, the literature on this aspect is quite limited from the South Asian countries. Most of the work is reported from India and some from Nepal, Sri Lanka, and Bangladesh. We could not access any data from Afghanistan. Maldives reported 39 cases (59% males) of elder abuse between January to April 2020 (PSM News, 2020). Abusive behaviors against older people are common from family members, especially sons and daughters-in-law, who are culturally expected to look after their parents (Chandanshive et al., 2022), relatives, as well as the community (Shankardass, 2013). The prevalence rates vary from country to country and within the countries. Within Nepal, in a study of 353 subjects aged 60 and more, 54.4% reported one or the other kind of abuse (S. R. Acharya et al., 2021). A survey of abuse reports published in newspapers of Nepal reported that physical abuse and neglect were quite common, and resultant death was reported in about 49% of cases (Dhakal & Yashohangmarai, 2011). Out of 109 old age home inmates in Nepal, 11% of were forced to leave home by their family members, and about 60% reported one or the other kind of neglect or abuse by the caregivers before they shifted their location (Adhikari Baral et al., 2021). A Longitudinal Ageing Study in India also reported 52.8% of older adults reporting abuse a few times, and 14.4–32.8% reported frequent to occasional abuse (Sathya et al., 2022). In the other studies from India, rates of elderly abuse varied widely between 5.2% (Chandanshive et al., 2022; Pengpid & Peltzer, 2021) to 50.2% in the rural areas (Ramalingam et al., 2019). Even in the hospital outdoor and indoor settings, 9.8% older adults reported disrespect and abuse by the staff (Krishnamoorthy et al., 2023). In the Nepalese study, neglect (23.1%) and physical abuse (20.6%) were the most common kinds of abuse. Sri Lankan data suggest prevalence of abuse of older persons between 5.6% (physical abuse) to 45% (neglect) (Edirisinghe et al., 2014). Still higher figures of physical abuse (41%) and social neglect (68%) are reported from some areas of Pakistan (Mushtaq & Ali, 2020). These prevalence rates are much higher than the global prevalence figures making it a reason to worry and take action for the South Asian countries. The factors contributing to abusive patterns of behaviors across different studies from South Asia are quite similar. Lower caste, tobacco use, lesser education, being retired, poor financial status, female gender, particularly widowed and having a chronic disease were common victim related factors associated with abuse (Acharya et al., 2021; Krishnamoorthy et al., 2023; Masih et al., 2024; Ramalingam et al., 2019; Tareque et al., 2015). An Indian review (Bambawale, 1997) highlighted the pervasive nature of abuse including legal transactions and helplessness of the older adults in abusive relationships. A need for legal literacy as well as social and public health reforms (Shankardass, 2013) were suggested to prevent elder abuse.

While staying in abusive relations the older people experience lower life satisfaction, depression, poor physical health, poor health care utilization (Pengpid & Peltzer, 2021), and increased mortality risk (Dong et al., 2011).

The United Nations Principle 17 and the International Plan of Action on Ageing states that "Older persons should be able to live in dignity and security and be free of exploitation and physical or mental abuse" acknowledged elder abuse as a serious obstacle to the fulfillment of healthy living by the older adults and recommended all countries to have a policy to prevent it (Paranitheran & Edirisinghe, 2009).

Many South Asian Countries formulated or revised their policy for the care of older adults and prevention of their abuse. Sri Lanka passed the Protection of the Rights of Elders Act, No. 9 of 2000 and created the National Council for Elders for their welfare. This act made the offspring legally responsible for the care of their old parents (Paranitheran & Edirisinghe, 2009). This act has provisions to check violence and abuse against older adults. But there are problems in its implementation due to inadequate knowledge about it among the citizens (Maduwage, 2020).

The Senior Citizens Act (2063) of Nepal has provisions for social security and protection from abuse and human rights (Senior Citizens Act (2063), 2006). India also passed an act for the protection of senior citizens from abuse (The Maintenance and Welfare of Parents and Senior Citizens Act, 2007). This act makes it illegal for the sons, sons-in-law, daughters, and daughters-in-law to neglect or abuse their parents and other older adults living with or away from them. Bangladesh also formulated and implemented the Maintenance of Parents Act in 2013 based on the preaching of Holy Quran and holds sons and daughters responsible for the care of their parents even when they are living away (Yasmin, 2019). Pakistan also approved its Islamabad Capital Territory Senior Citizens Act 2019 to ensure dignity and care of its older citizens. The Parental Protection Ordinance 2021 instructs the children to protect their parents. Legally there have been significant efforts to prevent elder abuse in the South Asian countries. However, there is little impact of these legislations because of poor enforcement and awareness (Karim, 2021; Mandal, 2011).

10 Welfare Policies for Older Adults in South Asia

Keeping in view that the health problems of the older adults are emerging as public health problems for the concerned nation, all countries in South Asia have formulated their policies.

Article 53 of the Afghanistan constitution is committed to the welfare of older adults. If an older person has only one son, then he is exempted from essential military services. Any criminal aged above 65 is given non-detention punishment only instead of imprisonment in Afghanistan. However, the country's policy is yet lacking in its social security benefits to the older adults. Health services in Afghanistan are largely run by the private sector, therefore not easily accessible to most of the older adults (Langari, 2011).

In Bangladesh, the National Health Policy (2008) and the National Policy on Older Persons and Maintenance of Parents Act (2013) make the State and adult children responsible for providing food, financial, and social security to the older adults. The welfare of older foundation rules 2018 act was made to develop old friendly communities and surroundings (Social Protection Resource Centre, n.d.).

Bhutan's national health policy is based on the principle of gross national happiness (GNH). The GNH policy works to ensure dignity of Bhutanese older persons by working toward ensuring psychological well-being, health, education, time use, cultural diversity and resilience, good governance, community vitality, ecological diversity and resilience, and living standards (McClaflin, 2017).

The Article 9 of the constitution of Bhutan directs the government to secure protection of extended family systems that ensures safety of older people. The country's National Pension and Provident Fund Plan provides financial support to the retired old age person. Those retiring from private companies are looked after by the Royal Insurance Corporation of Bhutan Limited (RICBL) (Dorji et al., 2017). To ensure good mental health to older persons Bhutan has also launched Bhutan Old Age Psychiatry Education Program in 2023 (*Bhutan Old Age Psychiatry Education Program 2023*, 2024). In the year 2020, Bhutan prioritized mental health of the older adults by including screening of dementia and depression in its community health program guidelines for the health care workers visiting homes, residence health care facilities for the older adults (Elderly Care Program, 2020).

The National Policy for Older Persons in India (1999) and the National Policy for senior citizens (2011) direct the state governments to ensure dignity and well-being of older persons by providing them financial security, health care, shelter, and protection against abuse. In an analysis of the policies and legislation for the older people through the primary health care system of the country, it was felt that the policies are aimed to support the families in a family-led approach through integrating community health workers. Besides that, the policies also empower the community in integrating traditional Ayurveda, Yoga and Naturopathy, Unani, Siddha, and Homeopathy (AYUSH) services into Primary Mental Healthcare (PMHC) (Kafczyk & Hämel, 2023).

Keeping in view of growing issues related to older adults, Maldives launched its health policy for older people in 2017 (Ministry of Gender Family & Social Services, 2017). The policy focuses on four key areas, namely, Care and protection, Independence and participation, Health and well-being, and Preparation for old age. There are provisions for pension and universal health insurance under this policy, and various bills and acts are drafted to ensure dignified care and protection of the rights of older people. A 3-module certificate course is also launched under this policy (Maldives, 2022).

Nepal's senior citizen policy advocates care for all senior citizens with dignity. It identifies the 'helpless' and 'incapable' senior citizens to prioritize its health and social welfare schemes for the older adults. The policy definition of family members includes son/daughter-in-law also. It makes it mandatory for the family members to provide food, shelter, and financial support to the older adults. The policy prohibits the community from forcing older people to live away from the families. This policy also has provision for care centers (similar to old age homes) and day care centers, as well as senior citizen clubs to ensure the care and welfare of its senior citizens (Acharya et al., 2023).

Pakistan has well-documented policies on the welfare of senior citizens (Social Protection Resource Centre, n.d.). The National Policy for older adults' health 1999 aims to provide training and awareness to the primary doctors in gerontology and multi-tiered health care delivery system for older people. Relief package for older people (2004) provides awareness among the young students regarding the respect and care for elder citizens in the society. The Senior Citizen Bill 2007 ensures concessional traveling, feasibility of pension and legal services and separate counters and free entry of senior citizens at public places. Punjab Senior Citizens Welfare and Rehabilitation Bill 2013 proposes to provide health care facilities, social security, and support in case of any emergency and disability is the province of Punjab.

Health policy for older adults in Sri Lanka reflects its commitment to provide comprehensive and dignified health care services to its older adults. It aims to minimize disease and disability at old age by encouraging participation of all health care providers including non-governmental organizations and private sector in providing preventing, promotive, and curative, palliative and rehabilitative services in an equitable manner. The policy advocates providing health care to the older adults by the well-trained man power (National Elderly Health Policy Sri Lanka, 2017). With enactment of Protection of the Rights of Elders Act in 2000, the government established a National Council for Elders to develop and implement programs to protect and promote the rights of elders (Samaraweera & Maduwage, 2016).

Despite having policies for older persons in all South East countries, there are gaps in the policy recommendation and implementation. There is a huge resource limitation in these countries. In Afghanistan, services to older adults are almost non-existent. No geriatric training facilities exist in Afghanistan, Bangladesh, Nepal, Pakistan, Maldives, and Sri Lanka. In Bangladesh, there are two indoor units for geriatric patients and few non-governmental organizations providing care to geriatric patients. Only India and Sri Lanka have geriatric training facilities. India has national geriatric centers (8 out of 20 are functional) and training facilities in geriatric mental health too but the number of trained people is too small to look after a huge geriatric population. Data available from Bangladesh, India, Pakistan, and Sri Lanka suggest less than 10 geriatricians in each of these countries (Matthews et al., 2023).

Further, social security to older persons is also limited. The monthly benefit given to the older person in Bangladesh, India, Pakistan, and Sri Lanka is meager and keeps the older person below poverty line only as per the World Bank standards. Pension benefits reach only 2.5% of the target population. Out-of-pocket health expenditure among older persons in these countries is very high (Matthews et al., 2023).

11 Way Forward

With more of population greying and inevitable social changes happening in South Asia, it is time to stop considering older adults as an extension of adult population. This population is different psychologically, socially, and biologically and their needs are different. This realization brings us to face the fact that robust research in the field of mental health needs of the older adults is must to obtain accurate information and design programs that fit the needs of this special population. Focused epidemiological studies for older adults can help not only to assess the existing gap between geriatric mental health service needs and available services but also help the governments to formulate effective national policies for the older adults. The future needs for this sector require a focus on developing infrastructure and resources as per need analysis, integration of geriatric mental health in National Mental Health Policy and traditional health delivery systems, creating appropriate training opportunities in geriatric mental health including training of paramedical personnel and setting up specialized psychogeriatric services. It is prudent to develop culturally appropriate measures and services with a special focus on strengthening family and community support systems.

Despite having national policies for older adults in place, most of the South Asian countries face a major challenge in its implementation in a true sense. Till the benefits of these schemes reach beneficiaries, services for older adults will remain a dream.

12 Conclusions

This chapter is an attempt to analyze the epidemiology of various mental health issues of older adults in South Asian countries. With fast-growing population of older adults, mental health services in this region pose an extra challenge to the already strained health care system. In addition to diverse cultural norms and prevailing poverty, the changing family and social structure is adding a new dimension. Not only the greying population is on the increase but also the older adults are being left alone by the younger family members who are migrating to bigger cities or other countries for better job and living opportunities. Lack of research into the needs of older adults, low literacy rate, poor mental health literacy, and lack of services increase the mental health gap. Factors like loneliness, substance abuse, and elder abuse further complicate the mental health issues. No wonder the suicide rate among older adults in South Asia is much higher than the adult population. Older women in South Asia face even bigger issues because of the gender bias in social position and power.

National health policies for the older adults in South Asian countries underscore the family-based support, training community health workers, and integration with traditional medicine. However, the effective implementation is far from reality because of different local and social reasons.

References

Abeysekera, N. W. B. Y., & De Zoysa, E. (2021). Higher prevalence of geriatric depression, catastrophizing pain and sleep disorders in institutionalized elders: A cross-sectional study in Galle District, Sri Lanka. *BMC Geriatrics, 21*(1), 685. https://doi.org/10.1186/s12877-021-02536-9

Acharya, D. R., Bell, J. S., Simkhada, P., Van Teijlingen, E. R., & Regmi, P. R. (2010). Women's autonomy in household decision-making: A demographic study in Nepal. *Reproductive Health, 7*(1), 1–12. https://doi.org/10.1186/1742-4755-7-15

Acharya, S. R., Suman, B. K., Pahari, S., Shin, Y. C., & Moon, D. H. (2021). Prevalence of abuse among the elderly population of Syangja, Nepal. *BMC Public Health, 21*(1), 1348. https://doi.org/10.1186/s12889-021-11417-0

Acharya, T., Dhungana, G. K., Traille, K., & Dhakal, H. (2023). Senior citizens in Nepal: Policy gaps and recommendations. *Gerontology & Geriatric Medicine, 9*, 23337214231179904. https://doi.org/10.1177/23337214231179902

Adhikari Baral, M., Khatri Chhetri, B., & Bhandari, P. (2021). Abuse of older adults before moving to old age homes in Pokhara Lekhnath Metropolitan City, Nepal: A cross-sectional study. *PLoS ONE, 16*(5), Article e0250639. https://doi.org/10.1371/journal.pone.0250639

Aich, T. K., Shah, S., & Subedi, S. (2017). Pattern of neuropsychiatric illnesses in geriatric population: An outpatient study report. *Journal of Psychiatrists' Association of Nepal, 4*(1), 12–19. https://doi.org/10.3126/jpan.v4i1.16737

Akila, G., Arvind, B., & Isaac, A. (2019). Comparative assessment of psychosocial status of elderly in urban and rural areas, Karnataka, India. *Journal of Family Medicine and Primary Care, 8*(9), 2870. https://doi.org/10.4103/jfmpc.jfmpc_536_19

Alam, M., & Karan, A. (2011). *Elderly health in India: Dimension, differentials and determinants BKPAI Working Paper No. 3.* https://www.isec.ac.in/wpcontent/uploads/2024/02/BKPAI%20Working%20paper%203.pdf

Ali, S. H., Islam, T., Pillai, S., Kalasapudi, L., Mammen, S., Inala, S., Kalasapudi, V., Islam, N. S., & Gunness, H. (2021). Loneliness and mental health outcomes among South Asian older adult immigrants in the United States: A cross-sectional study. *International Journal of Geriatric Psychiatry, 36*(9), 1423–1435. https://doi.org/10.1002/gps.5549

Alwis, I., Baminiwatta, A., & Chandradasa, M. (2024). Prevalence and associated factors of depression in Sri Lanka: A systematic review and meta-analysis. *Social Psychiatry and Psychiatric Epidemiology, 59*(2), 353–373. https://doi.org/10.1007/s00127-023-02495-z

Aminath, J. (2023). *Aged care and intergenerational solidarity in Small Island Developing States (SIDS): A case of the Maldives.* https://social.desa.un.org/sites/default/files/inline-files/Aminath%20Jameel_Aged%20care%20and%20inergenerational%20solidarity%20im%20SIDS%20A%20case%20of%20the%20Maldives.pdf

Amudhan, S., Gururaj, G., Varghese, M., Benegal, V., Rao, G. N., Sheehan, D. V., Kokane, A. M., Chavan, B. S., Dalal, P. K., Ram, D., Pathak, K., Lenin Singh, R. K., Singh, L. K., Sharma, P., Saha, P. K., Ramasubramanian, C., Mehta, R. Y., & Shibukumar, T. M. (2020). A population-based analysis of suicidality and its correlates: Findings from the National Mental Health Survey of India, 2015–16. *The Lancet Psychiatry, 7*(1), 41–51. https://doi.org/10.1016/S2215-0366(19)30404-3

Arafat, S. M. Y., Menon, V., Varadharajan, N., & Kar, S. K. (2022). Psychological autopsy studies of suicide in South East Asia. *Indian Journal of Psychological Medicine, 44*(1), 4–9. https://doi.org/10.1177/02537176211033643

Arafat, S. M. Y., Saleem, T., Menon, V., Ali, S.A.-Z., Baminiwatta, A., Kar, S. K., Akter, H., & Singh, R. (2022). Depression and suicidal behavior in South Asia: A systematic review and meta-analysis. *Global Mental Health, 9*, 181–192. https://doi.org/10.1017/gmh.2022.20

Aroonsrimorakot, S., Laiphrakpam, M., & Metadilogkul, O. (2020). Social, religious, recreational and medicinal usage of cannabis in India and Thailand. *Interdisciplinary Research Review, 14*, 43–50. https://doi.org/10.14456/jtir.2019.37

Ashe, S., & Routray, D. (2019). Prevalence, associated risk factors of depression and mental health needs among geriatric population of an urban slum, Cuttack, Odisha. *International Journal of Geriatric Psychiatry, 34*(12), 1799–1807. https://doi.org/10.1002/gps.5195

Ashraf, Q. H., Weil, D. N., & Wilde, J. (2013). The effect of fertility reduction on economic growth. *Population and Development Review, 39*(1), 97–130. https://doi.org/10.1111/j.1728-4457.2013.00575.x. PMID: 25525283; PMCID: PMC4267474.

Bailey, C., Sattar, Z., & Akhtar, P. (2018). Older south Asian women sharing their perceptions of health and social care services and support: A participatory inquiry. *Health Science Reports, 1*(8). https://doi.org/10.1002/hsr2.55

Bambawale, U. (1997). The abused elderly. *The Indian Journal of Medical Research, 106*, 389–395. http://www.ncbi.nlm.nih.gov/pubmed/9361473

Bamonti, P. M., Kennedy, M. A., Ward, R. E., Travison, T. G., & Bean, J. F. (2024). Association between depression symptoms and disability outcomes in older adults at risk of mobility decline. *Archives of Rehabilitation Research and Clinical Translation, 6*(2). Article 100342. https://doi.org/10.1016/j.arrct.2024.100342

Banerjee, T. K., Dutta, S., Das, S., Ghosal, M., Ray, B. K., Biswas, A., Hazra, A., Chaudhuri, A., Paul, N., & Das, S. K. (2017). Epidemiology of dementia and its burden in the city of Kolkata,

India. *International Journal of Geriatric Psychiatry, 32*(6), 605–614. https://doi.org/10.1002/gps.4499
Basu, S., Maheshwari, V., Sodhi, B., Mannan, P., & Kukreti, P. (2024). The prevalence of depression, determinants, and linkage with functional disability amongst postmenopausal women in India: Evidence from the longitudinal ageing study in India. *Asian Journal of Psychiatry, 96*. Article 104030. https://doi.org/10.1016/j.ajp.2024.104030
Berg-Weger, M., & Morley, J. E. (2020). Loneliness in old age: An unaddressed health problem. *Journal of Nutrition, Health and Aging, 24*(3), 243–245. https://doi.org/10.1007/s12603-020-1323-6
Bharath, S., Sadanand, S., Kumar, K. J., Balachandar, R., Joshi, H., & Varghese, M. (2017). Clinical and neuropsychological profile of persons with mild cognitive impairment, a hospital based study from a lower and middle income country. *Asian Journal of Psychiatry, 30*, 185–189. https://doi.org/10.1016/j.ajp.2017.10.007
Bhutan Old Age Psychiatry Education Program 2023. (2024). https://www.kgumsb.edu.bt/?p=238805
Boro, S., & Saikia, N. (2024). The effects of substance use on non-communicable diseases among older adults aged 60 and above in the North-eastern States of India. *PLoS ONE, 19*(9), Article e0307603. https://doi.org/10.1371/journal.pone.0307603
Carter, W. (2015). *Widowhood in Afghanistan—Lacuna Magazine*. https://lacuna.org.uk/equality/widowhood-in-afghanistan/
Chandanshive, P., Subba, S. H., Parida, S. P., & Mishra, S. (2022). Prevalence patterns and associated factors of elder abuse in an urban slum of eastern India. *BMC Geriatrics, 22*(1), 317. https://doi.org/10.1186/s12877-022-02986-9
Chandrasekaran, R. (2008). Predictors of repeat suicidal attempts after first-ever attempt: A two-year follow-up study. *Hong Kong Journal of Psychiatry, 4*, 18–21.
Chudgar, A. (2011). Female headship and schooling outcomes in rural India. *World Development, 39*(4), 550–560. https://doi.org/10.1016/j.worlddev.2010.08.021
Conrad, K. J., Liu, P.-J., & Iris, M. (2019). Examining the role of substance abuse in elder mistreatment: Results from mistreatment investigations. *Journal of Interpersonal Violence, 34*(2), 366–391. https://doi.org/10.1177/0886260516640782
Crestani, C., Masotti, V., Corradi, N., Schirripa, M. L., & Cecchi, R. (2019). Suicide in the elderly: A 37-years retrospective study. *Acta Bio-Medica: Atenei Parmensis, 90*(1), 68–76. https://doi.org/10.23750/abm.v90i1.6312
Dandona, R., Bertozzi-Villa, A., Kumar, G. A., & Dandona, L. (2016). Lessons from a decade of suicide surveillance in India: Who, why and how? *International Journal of Epidemiology*, https://doi.org/10.1093/ije/dyw113
De Leo, D. (2022). Late-life suicide in an aging world. *Nature Aging, 2*(1), 7–12. https://doi.org/10.1038/s43587-021-00160-1
Devaraj, V., Rose, A., & Abraham, V. J. (2024). Nature, prevalence, and risk factors for self-neglect among older people: A pilot study from Vellore, South India. *BMC Public Health, 24*(1), 948. https://doi.org/10.1186/s12889-024-18029-4
Devkota, R., Mishra, K., & Shrestha, S. (2019). Loneliness and depression among older people living in a community of Nepal. *Journal of Nepal Health Research Council, 17*(2), 185–192. https://doi.org/10.33314/jnhrc.v0i0.1561
Dhakal, D., & Yashohangmarai. (2011). *A baseline study on reported cases of elder abuse in Nepali Press*. https://un.info.np/Net/NeoDocs/View/History/Default.aspx?RefId=3388&fbclid=IwAR326VbYtNwghK9x-O0XiRzUc4ZxsUhnBwiCqNfVahq4otHxC4yogYe-_9U
Dong, X. Q., Simon, M. A., Beck, T. T., Farran, C., McCann, J. J., Mendes de Leon, C. F., Laumann, E., & Evans, D. A. (2011). Elder abuse and mortality: The role of psychological and social wellbeing. *Gerontology, 57*(6), 549–558. https://doi.org/10.1159/000321881
Dorji, L., Jamtsho, C., Norbu, T., & Dhoj Bhujel, G. (2017). *Understanding the situation of elderly citizens in Bhutan* (Issue 10). www.nsb.gov.bt.

Dost, N. A., Stanikzai, M. H., & Jafari, M. (2024). Depression and anxiety symptoms among Afghan war widows and their associated factors: A cross-sectional analytical study. *Indian Journal of Psychiatry, 66*(12), 1145–1149. https://doi.org/10.4103/indianjpsychiatry.indianjpsychiatry_339_24

Edirisinghe, P., Paranitharn, P., Perera, W., & Willams, S. (2014). Elder abuse among outpatient department attendees in a tertiary care hospital in Sri Lanka. *Ceylon Medical Journal, 59*(3), 84. https://doi.org/10.4038/cmj.v59i3.6527

Ehsan, K. (2023). *Poverty and old age: The struggle of Afghanistan's senior citizens.* Kabul Now. https://kabulnow.com/2023/03/poverty-and-old-age-the-struggle-of-afghanistans-senior-citizens/

Elderly Care Program. (2020). *Manual for integrated community based screening for elderly people in Bhutan.* https://www.moh.gov.bt/wp-content/uploads/ict-files/2022/05/Manual-for-Integrated-Community-Based-Screening-3.pdf

Emiliussen, J., Nielsen, A. S., & Andersen, K. (2017). Identifying risk factors for late-onset (50+) alcohol use disorder and heavy drinking: A systematic review. *Substance Use & Misuse, 52*(12), 1575–1588. https://doi.org/10.1080/10826084.2017.1293102

Farooq, S., Khan, T., Zaheer, S., & Shafique, K. (2019). Prevalence of anxiety and depressive symptoms and their association with multimorbidity and demographic factors: A community-based, cross-sectional survey in Karachi, Pakistan. *BMJ Open, 9*(11). https://doi.org/10.1136/bmjopen-2019-029315

Fotheringham, L., Paddick, S.-M., Barron Millar, E., Norman, C., Lukose, A., Walker, R., & Varghese, M. (2022). Screening tools for common mental disorders in older adults in South Asia: A systematic scoping review. *International Psychogeriatrics, 34*(5), 427–438. https://doi.org/10.1017/S1041610220003804

Franchi, C., Rossio, R., Ardoino, I., Mannucci, P. M., & Nobili, A. (2019). Inappropriate prescription of benzodiazepines in acutely hospitalized older patients. *European Neuropsychopharmacology, 29*(7), 871–879. https://doi.org/10.1016/j.euroneuro.2019.05.004

Frounfelker, R. L., Mishra, T., Holmes, K. B., Gautam, B., & Betancourt, T. S. (2023). Mental health among older Bhutanese with a refugee life experience: A mixed-methods latent class analysis study. *American Journal of Orthopsychiatry, 93*(4), 304–315. https://doi.org/10.1037/ort0000684

Gamage, M. W. K., Hewage, C., & Pathirana, K. D. (2019). Associated factors for cognition of physically independent elderly people living in residential care facilities for the aged in Sri Lanka. *BMC Psychiatry, 19*(1), 10. https://doi.org/10.1186/s12888-018-2003-5

Gao, Q., Prina, A. M., Prince, M., Acosta, D., Luisa Sosa, A., Guerra, M., Huang, Y., Jimenez-Velazquez, I. Z., Llibre Rodriguez, J. J., Salas, A., Williams, J. D., Liu, Z., Acosta Castillo, I., & Mayston, R. (2021). Loneliness among older adults in Latin America, China, and India: Prevalence, correlates and association with mortality. *International Journal of Public Health, 66*, Article 604449. https://doi.org/10.3389/ijph.2021.604449

Ghimire, S., Mishra, S. R., Baral, B. K., Dhimal, M., Callahan, K. E., Bista, B., & Aryal, K. K. (2019). Noncommunicable disease risk factors among older adults aged 60–69 years in Nepal: Findings from the STEPS survey 2013. *Journal of Human Hypertension, 33*(8), 602–612. https://doi.org/10.1038/s41371-019-0161-7

Ghosh, D., & Dinda, S. (2020). Determinants of the quality of life among elderly: Comparison between China and India. *The International Journal of Community and Social Development, 2*(1), 71–98. https://doi.org/10.1177/2516602620911835

Goswami, S., & Deshmukh, P. R. (2021). The prevalence of depression among the elderly people living in rural Wardha. *Industrial Psychiatry Journal, 30*(1), 90–95. https://doi.org/10.4103/ipj.ipj_43_17

Goswami, S., Deshmukh, P., Pawar, R., Raut, A., Bhagat, M., & Mehendale, A. (2017). Magnitude of depression and its correlates among elderly population in a rural area of Maharashtra: A cross-sectional study. *Journal of Family Medicine and Primary Care, 6*(4), 803. https://doi.org/10.4103/jfmpc.jfmpc_97_17

Greig, A., & Kabir, R. (2022). Assessing the risk factors for suicide and appropriate intervention as a prevention method among older adults. *Interações: Sociedade e as Novas Modernidades, 42*, 70–89. https://doi.org/10.31211/interacoes.n42.2022.a4

Grenade, L., & Boldy, D. (2008). Social isolation and loneliness among older people: Issues and future challenges in community and residential settings. *Australian Health Review, 32*(3), 468. https://doi.org/10.1071/AH080468

Grey, E., Baber, F., Corbett, E., Ellis, D., Gillison, F., & Barnett, J. (2024). The use of technology to address loneliness and social isolation among older adults: The role of social care providers. *BMC Public Health, 24*(1), 108. https://doi.org/10.1186/s12889-023-17386

Grover, S., Verma, M., Singh, T., Dahiya, N., & Nehra, R. (2019). Loneliness and its correlates amongst elderly attending non-communicable disease rural clinic attached to a tertiary care centre of North India. *Asian Journal of Psychiatry, 43*(March), 189–196. https://doi.org/10.1016/j.ajp.2019.06.001

Grover, S., Verma, M., Singh, T., Dahiya, N., & Nehra, R. (2021). Screening for abuse of older adults: A study done at primary health care level in Punjab, India. *Indian Journal of Psychological Medicine, 43*(4), 312–318. https://doi.org/10.1177/0253717620928782

Gulzar, F., Zafar, M. I., Ahmad, A., & Ali, T. (2008). *Socio-economic problems of senior citizens and their adjustment in Punjab, Pakistan.* https://api.semanticscholar.org/CorpusID:154475261

Gupta, A. A., Lall, A. K., Das, A., Saurav, A., Nandan, A., Shah, D., Agrahari, A., & Yadav, D. K. (2016). Health and socioeconomic status of the elderly people living in hilly areas of Pakhribas, Kosi Zone, Nepal. *Indian Journal of Community Medicine: Official Publication of Indian Association of Preventive & Social Medicine, 41*(4), 273–279. https://doi.org/10.4103/0970-0218.193333

Gurung, M. S., Pelzom, D., Dorji, T., Drukpa, W., Wangdi, C., Chinnakali, P., & Goel, S. (2016). Current tobacco use and its associated factors among adults in a country with comprehensive ban on tobacco: Findings from the nationally representative STEPS survey, Bhutan, 2014. *Population Health Metrics, 14*, 28. https://doi.org/10.1186/s12963-016-0098-9

Gururaj, G., Varghese, M., Benegal, V., Rao, G., Pathak, K., Singh, L., Mehta, R., Ram, D., Shibukumar, T., Kokane, A., Lenin Singh, R., Rhavan, B., Sharma, P., Ramasubramanian, C., Dalal, P., Saha, P., Deuri, S., Giri, A., Kavishvar, A., … NMHS Collaborators Group. (2016). *National Mental Health Survey of India, 2015–2016—Mental Health Systems*, 130.

Habib, T. Z. (2020). Becoming female head of a household: By force or by choice? *Oalib, 07*(10), 1–12. https://doi.org/10.4236/oalib.1106825

Hamrah, M. S., Hamrah, M. H., Hamrah, M. H., Hamrah, A. E., Dahi, T., Pahlavanzade, B., Charkazi, A., & Hamrah, M. H. (2019). The prevalence and associated factors of cigarette smoking and its association with opium use among outpatients in Afghanistan: A cross-sectional study in Andkhoy city. *Avicenna Journal of Medicine, 9*(4), 129–133. https://doi.org/10.4103/ajm.AJM_40_19

Hindustan Times. (2019, January 28). Delhi elderly couple death: Under police watch, yet lonely, vulnerable. *Hindustan Times.* https://www.hindustantimes.com/delhi-news/delhi-elderly-couple-death-under-police-watch-yet-lonely-vulnerable/story-a5HA86gZShU5RwX4v0MMLJ.html

Hussain, B., Mirza, M., Baines, R., Burns, L., Stevens, S., Asthana, S., & Chatterjee, A. (2023). Loneliness and social networks of older adults in rural communities: A narrative synthesis systematic review. *Frontiers in Public Health, 11*,. https://doi.org/10.3389/fpubh.2023.1113864

Hussain, N., Said, A. S. A., & Khan, Z. (2020). Influence of health literacy on medication adherence among elderly females with Type 2 diabetes in Pakistan. *International Quarterly of Community Health Education, 41*(1), 35–44. https://doi.org/10.1177/0272684X19896724

Jordans, M. J., Kaufman, A., Brenman, N. F., Adhikari, R. P., Luitel, N. P., Tol, W. A., & Komproe, I. (2014). Suicide in South Asia: A scoping review. *BMC Psychiatry, 14*(1), 358. https://doi.org/10.1186/s12888-014-0358-9

Kafczyk, T., & Hämel, K. (2023). Primary mental healthcare for older people in India: Between stigmatization and community orientation. *Discover Mental Health, 3*(1), 14. https://doi.org/10.1007/s44192-023-00040-7

Kar, S. K., Arafat, S. M. Y., Pandey, N. M., Kabir, R., & Singh, S. (2022). Suicide in the geriatric population of South East Asia—Contexts and attributes. *F1000Research, 11*, 1223. https://doi.org/10.12688/f1000research.126744.1

Karim, M. R. (2021). Protection of elderly parents in Bangladesh. *International Islamic University of Malaysia Law Journal, 29*, 221–248. https://journals.iium.edu.my/iiumlj/index.php/iiumlj/article/download/592/319/2476

Khan, M. M. (2002). Suicide on the Indian subcontinent. *Crisis, 23*(3), 104–107. https://doi.org/10.1027//0227-5910.23.3.104

Khanna, A., & Metgud, C. (2020). Prevalence of cognitive impairment in elderly population residing in an urban area of Belagavi. *Journal of Family Medicine and Primary Care, 9*(6), 2699. https://doi.org/10.4103/jfmpc.jfmpc_240_20

Khattri, J. B., Godar, S. T., Subedi, A., & Tirkey, S. (2020). Psychiatric morbidities of elderly out-patients attending various outreach clinics in gandaki province of Nepal: A descriptive cross-sectional study. *Journal of Nepal Medical Association, 58*(225). https://doi.org/10.31729/jnma.4996

Knight, B. E. N. (2022). Loneliness: Unpacking the silent epidemic damaging our health. *UNSW Newsroom*, 1–5. https://www.unsw.edu.au/news/2022/11/loneliness--unpacking-the-silent-epidemic-damaging-our-health

Koirala, N. R., Mahat, P., Nepal, M. K., Ojha, S. P., Sinha, U. K., Pokhrel, A., & Sharma, V. D. (2000). Geriatric psychiatry: Socio-demographic characteristics and diagnostic profile among senior citizens attending the psychiatric outpatient department of a tertiary health care facility in Nepal. *Journal of Institute of Medicine Nepal, 22*(3, 4). https://doi.org/10.59779/jiomnepal.133

Krishnamoorthy, Y., Elangovan, V., Krishnan, M., Sinha, I., Samuel, G., & Kanth, K. (2023). Institutional disrespect and abuse during health-care utilization in public health facilities of Tamil Nadu: A facility-based cross-sectional survey. *Indian Journal of Public Health, 67*(1), 47–53. https://doi.org/10.4103/ijph.ijph_888_22

Kuerbis, A., Sacco, P., Blazer, D. G., & Moore, A. A. (2014). Substance abuse among older adults. *Clinics in Geriatric Medicine, 30*(3), 629–654. https://doi.org/10.1016/j.cger.2014.04.008

Kulkarni, S., Raju, S., & Bammidi, S. (2011). *Social security for the elderly in India. Thematic Paper*, 1–56.

Kumari, R., Langer, B., Gupta, R. K., Bahl, R., Akhtar, N., & Nazir, H. (2021). Prevalence and determinants of cognitive impairment and depression among the elderly population in a rural area of North India. *Indian Journal of Community Medicine: Official Publication of Indian Association of Preventive & Social Medicine, 46*(2), 236–240. https://doi.org/10.4103/ijcm.IJCM_475_20

Lam, M. S., Fitzpatrick, A. L., Shrestha, A., Karmacharya, B. M., Koju, R., & Rao, D. (2017). Determining the prevalence of and risk factors for depressive symptoms among adults in Nepal. *International Journal of Noncommunicable Diseases, 2*(1), 18–26. https://doi.org/10.4103/jncd.jncd_34_16

Langari, A. Z. (2011). Older persons and multiple discrimination. *Welcome to United Nations.* https://social.un.org/ageing-working-group/documents/Olderperson%20(Afghanistan).pdf

Lee, J., Meijer, E., Langa, K. M., Ganguli, M., Varghese, M., Banerjee, J., ... & Dey, A. B. (2023). Prevalence of dementia in India: National and state estimates from a nationwide study. *Alzheimer's & Dementia, 19*(7), 2898–2912. https://doi.org/10.1002/alz.12928

MacDonald, K. B., & Schermer, J. A. (2021). Loneliness unlocked: Associations with smartphone use and personality. *Acta Psychologica, 221*, Article 103454. https://doi.org/10.1016/j.actpsy.2021.103454

Maduwage, S. (2020). Situational overview of elder abuse in Sri Lanka. In *International handbook of elder abuse and mistreatment* (pp. 427–437). Springer Singapore. https://doi.org/10.1007/978-981-13-8610-7_24

Maldives. (2022). http://www.searo.who.int/maldives/mediacentre/ental-health-policy-2015-2025.pdf

Malhotra, R., Chan, A., & Østbye, T. (2010). Prevalence and correlates of clinically significant depressive symptoms among elderly people in Sri Lanka: Findings from a national survey. *International Psychogeriatrics, 22*(2), 227–236. https://doi.org/10.1017/S1041610209990871

Manandhar, K., Risal, A., Shrestha, O., Manandhar, N., Kunwar, D., Koju, R., & Holen, A. (2019). Prevalence of geriatric depression in the Kavre district, Nepal: Findings from a cross sectional community survey. *BMC Psychiatry, 19*(1), 271. https://doi.org/10.1186/s12888-019-2258-5

Mandal, A. K. (2022). Trend of tobacco use: Reviewing the STEPS surveys conducted in Nepal. *Journal of Health Promotion, 10*(1), 89–100. https://doi.org/10.3126/jhp.v10i1.50990

Mandal, S. N. (2011). Protection of rights of oldage person in India: A challenging facet of human rights. *SSRN Electronic Journal*. https://doi.org/10.2139/ssrn.1880956

Masih, M., Wagstaff, C., & Kaur-Aujla, H. (2024). The global psychological and physical effects of domestic abuse and violence on South Asian women: A qualitative systematic review. *Frontiers in Global Women's Health, 5*, 1365883. https://doi.org/10.3389/fgwh.2024.1365883

Matthews, N. R., Porter, G. J., Varghese, M., Sapkota, N., Khan, M. M., Lukose, A., Paddick, S.-M., Dissanayake, M., Khan, N. Z., & Walker, R. (2023). Health and socioeconomic resource provision for older people in South Asian countries: Bangladesh, India, Nepal, Pakistan and Sri Lanka evidence from NEESAMA. *Global Health Action, 16*(1). https://doi.org/10.1080/16549716.2022.2110198

McClaflin, C. (2017). *Dignity rights, aging, & the law in modern day Bhutan.*

Migration and Migrants: Regional Dimensions and Developments. (2021). In *World Migration Report*. https://worldmigrationreport.iom.int/what-we-do/world-migration-report-2024-chapter-3/asia

Mehra, A., Grover, S., Agarwal, A., Bashar, M., & Avasthi, A. (2019). Prevalence of elder abuse and its association with psychiatric morbidity in a rural setting. *Journal of Neurosciences in Rural Practice, 10*(02), 218–224. https://doi.org/10.4103/jnrp.jnrp_338_18

Ministry of Gender Family and Social Services. (2017). *Maldives inaugurates first-ever National Elderly Policy*. https://gender.gov.mv/en/?p=1748

Mohan, R. (2021, March 14). Japan's Ministry of Loneliness, UAE's Ministry of Happiness: A look at some offbeat govt posts. *The Economic Times.*

Moneer, A., James, K. S., Giridhar, G., Sathyanarayana, K. M., Kumar, S., Raju, S. S., Syamala, T. S., Subaiya, L., & Bansod, D. W. (2012). *Report on the status of elderly in Select States of India, 2011*. https://india.unfpa.org/sites/default/files/pub-pdf/AgeingReport_2012_F.pdf

Muhammad, T. (2023). Life course rural/urban place of residence, depressive symptoms and cognitive impairment among older adults: Findings from the longitudinal aging study in India. *BMC Psychiatry, 23*(1), 391. https://doi.org/10.1186/s12888-023-04911-9

Muhammad, T., Meher, T., & Sekher, T. V. (2021). Association of elder abuse, crime victimhood and perceived neighbourhood safety with major depression among older adults in India: A cross-sectional study using data from the LASI baseline survey (2017–2018). *BMJ Open, 11*(12):e055625. https://bmjopen.bmj.com/lookup/doi/10.1136/bmjopen-2021-055625

Murthy, R. S. (2017). National Mental Health Survey of India 2015–2016. *Indian Journal of Psychiatry, 59*(1), 21–26. https://doi.org/10.4103/psychiatry.IndianJPsychiatry_102_17

Mushtaq, N., & Ali, R. (2020). Challenges to elderly people in Quetta City (Balochistan) Pakistan. *Elderly Health Journal, 6*(2), 91–97. https://doi.org/10.18502/EHJ.V6I2.5015

Mushtaq, R., Shoib, S., Shah, T., & Mushtaq, S. (2014). Relationship between loneliness, Psychiatric disorders and physical health? A review on the psychological aspects of loneliness. *Journal of Clinical and Diagnostic Research, 8*(9), WE01–WE04. https://doi.org/10.7860/JCDR/2014/10077.4828

Nadkarni, A., Murthy, P., Crome, I. B., & Rao, R. (2013). Alcohol use and alcohol-use disorders among older adults in India: A literature review. *Aging & Mental Health, 17*(8), 979–991. https://doi.org/10.1080/13607863.2013.793653

Nagoor, K., Darivemula, S. B., Reddy, N. B., Patan, S. K., Deepthi, C. S., & Chittooru, C. S. (2018). Prevalence of mental illness and their association with sociodemographic factors in the rural geriatric population in Chittoor, Andhra Pradesh, India: A community-based study. *Journal of Education and Health Promotion, 7*, 165. https://doi.org/10.4103/jehp.jehp_193_18

Naheed, A., Hakim, M., Islam, M. S., Islam, M. B., Tang, E. Y. H., Prodhan, A. A., Amin, M. R., Stephan, B. C. M., & Mohammad, Q. D. (2023). Prevalence of dementia among older age people and variation across different sociodemographic characteristics: A cross-sectional study in Bangladesh. *The Lancet Regional Health - Southeast Asia, 17*. Article 100257. https://doi.org/10.1016/j.lansea.2023.100257

Nakulan, A., Sumesh, T. P., Kumar, S., Rejani, P. P., & Shaji, K. S. (2015). Prevalence and risk factors for depression among community resident older people in Kerala. *Indian Journal of Psychiatry, 57*(3), 262–266. https://doi.org/10.4103/0019-5545.166640

National Bureau of Statistics. (2014). *Maldives population and housing census statistical release III: Education*. https://statisticsmaldives.gov.mv/nbs/wp-content/uploads/2016/02/StatisticalReleaseII-Education.pdf

National Elderly Health Policy Sri Lanka. (2017). https://extranet.who.int/countryplanningcycles/sites/default/files/planning_cycle_repository/sri_lanka/srl_natioanl_elderly_health_policy.pdf

Niaz, U., & Hassan, S. (2006). Culture and mental health of women in South-East Asia. *World Psychiatry, 5*(2), 118. https://pmc.ncbi.nlm.nih.gov/articles/PMC1525125/

Oduro, J. K., Okyere, J., & Nyador, J. K. M. T. (2023). Risky health behaviours and chronic conditions among aged persons: Analysis of SAGE selected countries. *BMC Geriatrics, 23*(1), 145. https://doi.org/10.1186/s12877-023-03836-y

Ogbo, F. A., Mathsyaraja, S., Koti, R. K., Perz, J., & Page, A. (2018). The burden of depressive disorders in South Asia, 1990–2016: Findings from the global burden of disease study. *BMC Psychiatry, 18*(1), 333. https://doi.org/10.1186/s12888-018-1918-1

Pandit, P., Kumari, R., Tripathi, A., & Mishra, P. (2024). Cognitive functioning among community-dwelling older adults in rural population of lucknow and Its association with comorbidities. *Indian Journal of Psychological Medicine, 46*(4), 338–343. https://doi.org/10.1177/02537176231225838

Paranitheran, P., & Edirisinghe, P. (2009). Elder abuse—A wake up call. *Ceylon Medical Journal, 54*(1), 1. https://doi.org/10.4038/cmj.v54i1.463

Patel, R., & Singh, U. (2018). Prevalence study of cognitive impairment and its associated sociodemographic variables using mini-mental status examination among elderly population residing in field practice areas of a medical college. *Indian Journal of Community Medicine, 43*(2), 113. https://doi.org/10.4103/ijcm.IJCM_102_17

Patel, M., Bhardwaj, P., Nebhinani, N., Goel, A. D., & Patel, K. (2020). Prevalence of psychiatric disorders among older adults in Jodhpur and stakeholders perspective on responsive health system. *Journal of Family Medicine and Primary Care, 9*(2), 714–720. https://doi.org/10.4103/jfmpc.jfmpc_1016_19

Patel, M., Mantri, N., Joshi, N., Jain, Y., Goel, A. D., Gupta, M., ... & Bhardwaj, P. (2024). Is anxiety a public health problem among older adults in India: Results from a systematic review and meta-analysis. *Journal of Family Medicine and Primary Care, 13*(7), 2545–2554. https://doi.org/10.4103/jfmpc.jfmpc_1664_23

Paudel, B. B. (2022). Socio-economic and health status of elderly people in Nepal. *Journal of Development and Social Engineering, 4–8*, 1–8.

Pengpid, S., & Peltzer, K. (2021). Elder abuse and health outcomes among community-dwelling older adults in India: Results of a national survey in 2017–2018. *Journal of Elder Abuse & Neglect, 33*(4), 327–341. https://doi.org/10.1080/08946566.2021.1970683

Petersen, J., Thielke, S., Austin, D., & Kaye, J. (2016). Phone behaviour and its relationship to loneliness in older adults. *Aging & Mental Health, 20*(10), 1084–1091. https://doi.org/10.1080/13607863.2015.1060947

Philip, A. J., & Johns, F. (2024). Prevalence of cognitive defects among senior inmates of old-age homes in a district of South Kerala. *Cureus*. https://doi.org/10.7759/cureus.65082

Philip, S., Mukherjee, N., & Shekhar, A. (2023). Rise in suicide related deaths in minors during the pandemic in a LAMI country. *International Journal of Social Psychiatry, 69*(4), 1057–1058. https://doi.org/10.1177/00207640221117019

Population Reference Bureau. (2020). *Countries with the oldest populations in the World.*

Pranav, M. K., Francis, P. T., Olickal, J. J., Rose, B. M., Sarma, P. S., & Thankappan, K. R. (2024). Mental well-being and the quality of life among retired public and private sector employees: A comparative study from Kerala, India. *Cureus.* https://doi.org/10.7759/cureus.71663

PSM News. (2020, June 15). Gender minister calls for nation-wide efforts to build a safer society for the elderly. *Public Service Media.* https://psmnews.mv/en/69964

Rajan, S. I. (2023). Migration in South Asia: Old and new mobilities. In S. I. Rajan (Ed.), *Migration in South Asia. IMISCOE Research Series* (pp. 3–15). Springer Nature Singapore. https://doi.org/10.1007/978-3-031-34194-6_1

Rajapakshe, O. B. W., Sivayogan, S., & Kulatunga, P. M. (2019). Prevalence and correlates of depression among older urban community-dwelling adults in Sri Lanka. *Psychogeriatrics, 19*(3), 202–211. https://doi.org/10.1111/psyg.12389

Ramalingam, A., Sarkar, S., Premarajan, K., Rajkumar, R., & Subrahmanyam, D. (2018). Prevalence and correlates of common mental disorders among the rural elderly in Puducherry, South India: A cross-sectional community-based study. *International Journal of Preventive Medicine, 9*(1), 65. https://doi.org/10.4103/ijpvm.IJPVM_386_15

Ramalingam, A., Sarkar, S., Premarajan, K., Rajkumar, R., & Subrahmanyam, D. (2019). Prevalence and correlates of elder abuse: A cross-sectional, community-based study from rural Puducherry. *The National Medical Journal of India, 32*(2), 72. https://doi.org/10.4103/0970-258X.275344

Ramesh, S., Kosalram, K., & Srinivas, V. (2023). Non-communicable diseases and their impact on depression, anxiety, and stress among the geriatric population residing in old age homes in Chennai, Tamil Nadu. *Journal of Family Medicine and Primary Care, 12*(9), 1931–1937. https://doi.org/10.4103/jfmpc.jfmpc_801_23

Rao, T. S., Ismail, S., Darshan, M. S., & Tandon, A. (2015). Sexual disorders among elderly: An epidemiological study in south Indian rural population. *Indian Journal of Psychiatry, 57*(3), 236–241. https://doi.org/10.4103/0019-5545.166618

Rathod, M. S., Dixit, J. V., Goel, A. D., & Yadav, V. (2019). Prevalence of depression in an urban geriatric population in marathwada region of Western India. *Indian Journal of Psychological Medicine, 41*(1), 32–37. https://doi.org/10.4103/IJPSYM.IJPSYM_234_18

Regmi, R. K. R. (1982). Socio-economic and cultural aspects of ageing in Nepal. *Digital Himalaya.* https://himalaya.socanth.cam.ac.uk/collections/journals/opsa/pdf/OPSA_03_03.pdf

Rodrigo, C., Perera, S., Adhikari, M., Rajapakse, A., & Rajapakse, S. (2010). Cognitive impairment and symptoms of depression among geriatric patients in a tertiary care unit in Sri Lanka. *Indian Journal of Psychiatry, 52*(3), 279–280. https://doi.org/10.4103/0019-5545.71000

Sabzwari, S. R., Iqbal, R., Fatmi, Z., & Azam, I. (2019). Factors associated with geriatric morbidity and impairment in a megacity of Pakistan. *PloS One, 14*(6). Article e0218872. https://doi.org/10.1371/journal.pone.0218872

Samaraweera, D., & Maduwage, S. (2016). Meeting the current and future health-care needs of Sri Lanka's ageing population. *WHO South-East Asia Journal of Public Health, 5*(2), 96. https://doi.org/10.4103/2224-3151.206259

Santhalingam, S., Sivagurunathan, S., Prathapan, S., Kanagasabai, S., & Kamalarupan, L. (2022). The effect of socioeconomic factors on quality of life of elderly in Jaffna district of Sri Lanka. *PLOS Global Public Health, 2*(8), Article e0000916. https://doi.org/10.1371/journal.pgph.0000916

Sarkar, S., Parmar, A., & Chatterjee, B. (2015). Substance use disorders in the elderly: A review. *Journal of Geriatric Mental Health, 2*(2), 74. https://doi.org/10.4103/2348-9995.174271

Sathya, T., Selvamani, Y., & Nagarajan, R. (2022). Elder abuse/mistreatment and associated covariates in India: Results from the Longitudinal Aging Study in India wave 1, 2017–2018. *Epidemiology and Health, 44*, Article e2022017. https://doi.org/10.4178/EPIH.E2022017

Senarath, U., Wickramage, K., & Peiris, S. L. (2014). Prevalence of depression and its associated factors among patients attending primary care settings in the post-conflict Northern Province in Sri Lanka: a cross-sectional study. *BMC Psychiatry, 14*, 85. https://doi.org/10.1186/1471-244X-14-85

Seneviratne, V. L., Ranaweera, S., & Atkins, M. (2022). Elder suicides: A reminder from the forgotten generation. *Asian Journal of Psychiatry, 71*, Article 103028. https://doi.org/10.1016/j.ajp.2022.103028

Senior Citizens Act (2063). (2006). https://nepal.unfpa.org/sites/default/files/pub-pdf/senior_citizens_act.pdf

Shah, S. (2021). Loneliness as a risk factor for chronic disease. In *A prescription for healthy living* (pp. 111–120). Elsevier. https://doi.org/10.1016/B978-0-12-821573-9.00009-6

Shakya, D. (2012). Psychiatric morbidities of elderly psychiatry out-patients in a tertiary-care hospital. *Journal of College of Medical Sciences-Nepal, 7*(4), 1–8. https://doi.org/10.3126/jcmsn.v7i4.6735

Shankar, A., & Kidd, T. (2022). Loneliness in older Indian dyads. *International Journal of Environmental Research and Public Health, 19*(9). https://doi.org/10.3390/ijerph19095302

Shankardass, M. K. (2013). Addressing elder abuse: Review of societal responses in India and selected Asian countries. *International Psychogeriatrics, 25*(8), 1229–1234. https://doi.org/10.1017/S104161021300063X

Sharma, M., & Pradhan, M. R. (2023). Socioeconomic inequality in cognitive impairment among India's older adults and its determinants: A decomposition analysis. *BMC Geriatrics, 23*(1), 7. https://doi.org/10.1186/s12877-022-03604-4

Sheikh, S. M., & Loney, T. (2018). Is educating girls the best investment for South Asia? Association between female education and fertility choices in South Asia: A systematic review of the literature. *Frontiers in Public Health, 6*, 172. https://doi.org/10.3389/fpubh.2018.00172

Shoib, S., Islam, S. M. S., Arafat, S. Y., & Hakak, S. A. (2021). Depression and suicidal ideation among the geriatric population of Kashmir, India. *International Journal of Social Psychiatry, 67*(6), 651–655. https://doi.org/10.1177/0020764020968592

Silva, H. A. de, Gunatilake, S. B., & Smith, A. D. (2003). Prevalence of dementia in a semi-urban population in Sri Lanka: Report from a regional survey. *International Journal of Geriatric Psychiatry, 18*(8), 711–715. https://doi.org/10.1002/gps.909

Singh, A., & Misra, N. (2009). Loneliness, depression and sociability in old age. *Industrial Psychiatry Journal, 18*(1), 51. https://doi.org/10.4103/0972-6748.57861

Sinha, P., Hussain, T., Boora, N. K., Rao, G. N., Varghese, M., Gururaj, G., Benegal, V., & NMHS India Collaborators Group. (2021). Prevalence of common mental disorders in older adults: Results from the national mental health survey of India. *Asian Journal of Psychiatry, 55*. https://doi.org/10.1016/j.ajp.2020.102463

Sithey, G., Li, M., Wen, L. M., Kelly, P. J., & Clarke, K. (2018). Socioeconomic, religious, spiritual and health factors associated with symptoms of common mental disorders: A cross-sectional secondary analysis of data from Bhutan's gross national happiness study, 2015. *BMJ Open, 8*(2). Article e018202. https://doi.org/10.1136/bmjopen-2017-018202

Skirbekk, V., & James, K. S. (2014). Abuse against elderly in India—The role of education. *BMC Public Health, 14*, 336. https://doi.org/10.1186/1471-2458-14-336

Social Protection Resource Centre. (n.d.). *Legislation for older people in Pakistan.* Retrieved January 3, 2025, from https://www.sprc.org.pk/wp-content/uploads/2022/03/SPRC-POLICY-BRIEF-updated.pdf

South Asia Literacy Rate 1975–2024. (2024). https://www.macrotrends.net/global-metrics/countries/SAS/south-asia/literacy-rate

South Asia. (2024). https://www.worldbank.org/en/region/sar/overview#2

Srivastava, M., & Srivastava, P. (2022). "Loneliness scares": Crime against elderly. In *Handbook of aging, health and public policy* (pp. 1–11). Springer Nature Singapore. https://doi.org/10.1007/978-981-16-1914-4_174-1

Srivastava, P., & Srivastava, M. (2023). Prevalence and correlates of loneliness in the later life—Insights from Longitudinal Ageing Study in India (LASI) Wave-1. *Indian Journal of Psychiatry, 65*(9), 914–921. https://doi.org/10.4103/indianjpsychiatry.indianjpsychiatry_594_22

Sudan, A., Shahi, P., & Julka, D. (2020). Prevalence of abuse in elders with psychiatric morbidity and its sociodemographic association. *Cureus*. https://doi.org/10.7759/cureus.7906

Tareque, M. I., Islam, T. M., Koshio, A., & Kawahara, K. (2015). Economic well-being and elder abuse in Rajshahi district of Bangladesh. *Research on Aging, 37*(2), 200–224. https://doi.org/10.1177/0164027514527833

Tata Institute of Social Sciences (TISS). (2017). *Global Adult Tobacco Survey GATS 2 India 2016–17*. https://ntcp.mohfw.gov.in/assets/document/surveys-reports-publications/Global-Adult-Tobacco-Survey-Second-Round-India-2016-2017.pdf

Thampi, K., & Mathew, L. M. (2024). Aging in place for community-dwelling older adults in India: A qualitative exploration of prospects and challenges. *Gerontology & Geriatric Medicine, 10*, 23337214231223636. https://doi.org/10.1177/23337214231223636

Thapa, D. K., Visentin, D., Kornhaber, R., & Cleary, M. (2018). Prevalence of mental disorders among older people in Nepal: A systematic review. *Kathmandu University Medical Journal (KUMJ), 16*(62), 181–190. http://www.ncbi.nlm.nih.gov/pubmed/30636762

Thapa, D. K., Visentin, D. C., Kornhaber, R., & Cleary, M. (2020). Prevalence and factors associated with depression, anxiety, and stress symptoms among older adults: A cross-sectional population-based study. *Nursing & Health Sciences, 22*(4), 1139–1152. https://doi.org/10.1111/nhs.12783

Thapa, P., Chakraborty, P., Khattri, J., Ramesh, K., & Sharma, B. (2014). Psychiatric morbidity in elderly patients attending OPD of tertiary care centre in western region of Nepal. *Industrial Psychiatry Journal, 23*(2), 101. https://doi.org/10.4103/0972-6748.151673

Thapa, S. B., Van Ommeren, M., Sharma, B., de Jong, J. T. V. M., & Hauff, E. (2003). Psychiatric disability among tortured Bhutanese refugees in Nepal. *American Journal of Psychiatry, 160*(11), 2032–2037. https://doi.org/10.1176/appi.ajp.160.11.2032

The Maintenace and Welfare of Parents And Senior Citizens Act. (2007). https://www.indiacode.nic.in/bitstream/123456789/6831/1/maintenance_and_welfare_of_parents_and_senior_citizens_act.pdf

Thomas, S. E. (2023). Law and its discontents: Ageing and family law in India. *Journal of Social and Economic Development, 1–16*,. https://doi.org/10.1007/s40847-022-00211-2

Tiwari, S. C. (2013). Loneliness: A disease? *Indian Journal of Psychiatry, 55*(4), 320–322. https://doi.org/10.4103/0019-5545.120536

Trading Economics. (2024). *South Asia—Elderly literacy rate, Population 65+ years, female*. Trading Economics. https://tradingeconomics.com/south-asia/elderly-literacy-rate-population-65-years-female-percent-wb-data.html

UNICEF. (2022). Children on the move in South Asia regional brief. In *Children on the move in Africa*. https://www.unicef.org/rosa/media/17711/file/Children%20on%20the%20Move%20in%20South%20Asia:%20Regional%20Brief.pdf

United Nations Population Fund. (2016). *Caring for our elders: Early responses-india ageing*.

Usmani, B. A., Lakhdir, M. P. A., Sameen, S., Batool, S., Odland, M. L., Goodman-Palmer, D., Agyapong-Badu, S., Hirschhorn, L. R., Greig, C., & Davies, J. (2024). Exploring the priorities of ageing populations in Pakistan, comparing views of older people in Karachi City and Thatta. *PLoS ONE, 19*(7), Article e0304474. https://doi.org/10.1371/journal.pone.0304474

Véron, J., le groupe CSF, Kneipp, R., & Rogers, G. (2008). The demography of South Asia from the 1950s to the 2000s. A summary of changes and a statistical assessment. *Population, 63*(1), 9–89. https://shs.cairn.info/journal-population-2008-1-page-9?lang=en

Vijayakumar, L., Daly, C., Arafat, Y., & Arensman, E. (2020). Suicide prevention in the Southeast Asia region. *Crisis, 41*(Supplement 1), S21–S29. https://doi.org/10.1027/0227-5910/a000666

Wahlin, Å., Palmer, K., Sternäng, O., Hamadani, J. D., & Kabir, Z. N. (2015). Prevalence of depressive symptoms and suicidal thoughts among elderly persons in rural Bangladesh. *International Psychogeriatrics, 27*(12), 1999–2008. https://doi.org/10.1017/S104161021500109X

Watt, M. H., Perara, B., Osbyte, T., Ranabahu, S., Rajapakse, H., & Maselko, J. (2014). Care-giving expectations and challenges among elders and their adult children in Southern Sri Lanka. *Ageing and Society, 34*(5), 838–858. https://doi.org/10.1017/S0144686X12001365

WHO. (2022). *Reducing social isolation and loneliness among older people.* https://www.who.int/activities/reducing-social-isolation-and-loneliness-among-older-people

Wijeratne, M. D. M., Wijerathne, S. A., Wijesekara, S. G., & Wijesingha, I. (2010). Prevalence of depression among institutionalized elders in the Colombo district. *Students Medical Journal Faculty of Medicine Colombo*, 27–31. https://www.med.cmb.ac.lk/SMJ/VOLUME-1-DOWNLOADS/Page-27-31-Research-papers-Prevalence-of-depression-among-institutionalized-elders-in-the-Colombo-district.pdf

World Bank Group. (2023). *Population ages 65 and above, total—South Asia.* https://data.worldbank.org/indicator/SP.POP.65UP.TO?locations=8S&name_desc=false

World Health Organization. (2002). Missing voices. Views of older persons on elder abuse. *Revista Espanola de Geriatria y Gerontologia, 37*(6), 319–331. https://doi.org/10.1016/s0211-139x(02)74838-5

World Health Organization. (2024). *Abuse of older people.* Factsheet. https://www.who.int/news-room/fact-sheets/detail/abuse-of-older-people

Wojnar, A. (2023). India's ageing population: Why it matters more than ever. *Hindustan Times.*

Yasmin, S. (2019). The rights of parents to maintenance in Bangladesh: An overview of the Parents Maintenance Act, 2013. *Scholars International Journal of Law, Crime and Justice*, *2*(10), 309–313. https://doi.org/10.36348/SIJLCJ.2019.v02i10.003

Public Mental Health Aspects of Geriatric Psychiatry in South Asia

Abhinav Tewari, Aditya Agrawal, and Anuranjan Vishwakarma

Abstract South Asia comprises eight countries that share significant socio-cultural and economic backgrounds. The countries in this region: India, Pakistan, Bangladesh, Afghanistan, Sri Lanka, Nepal, Maldives, and Bhutan, account for nearly a quarter of the world's total population. There is a considerable treatment gap for mental health services, which is further exacerbated among the older adults (aged over 60 years). The lack of awareness, stigma, limited mental healthcare infrastructure, and the presence of medical conditions in old age, combined with rapidly changing demographics and societal conditions in the region, render the older adults highly vulnerable to the ill effects of untreated mental illnesses. A collaborative effort, including policy changes and shifts in attitude, is necessary to mitigate this risk. This chapter seeks to explore the existing public health aspects of psychiatric illness.

Keywords South Asia · Public mental health · Old age psychiatry · Policy · Psychiatric services

1 Introduction

Public mental health refers to the application of principles of public health to mental health issues with the aim of enhancing psychological well-being across communities rather than at the individual level (Cadeddu et al., 2015). The key principles applied are those related to the prevention of mental health problems, promotion of psychological well-being, access to care, equity to prevent disparity in mental health outcomes, and policy-related aspects.

The world is experiencing a substantial demographic shift, and South Asia is no exception. The region's ageing population is growing rapidly, with the proportion of older adults (aged 60 and above) expected to increase from 143 million in 2015 to nearly 488 million by 2050 (Bloom & Luca, 2016). The number and percentage

A. Tewari (✉) · A. Agrawal · A. Vishwakarma
Department of Psychiatry, Ram Manohar Lohia Institute of Medical Sciences (RMLIMS), Lucknow, India
e-mail: abhinav.aiims08@gmail.com

N. Kar et al. (eds.), *Geriatric Psychiatry in South Asia*, South Asian Perspectives in Mental Health and Psychology , https://doi.org/10.1007/978-981-96-7469-5_10

of older individuals in developing countries have surged significantly within just one generation, contrasting sharply with developed nations. Data indicates that the growth of the older population in developing East and Southeast Asia is occurring at a faster rate compared to other Western nations (Cheng & Heller, 2009). This notable rise underscores the urgent need for comprehensive public mental health services for the ageing population among developing countries in the South Asia region.

Despite the increasing prevalence of mental health conditions such as depression, dementia, and anxiety among older adults, mental healthcare in the region remains insufficient. Factors including social stigma, inadequate healthcare infrastructure, and economic constraints contribute to this gap (Kohli et al., 2020). India constitutes a significant portion of South Asia's population. According to recent demographic data, the older adult population (aged over 60 years) comprises approximately 10% of the nation's population. By 2026, the older adult population (over 60 years) is expected to make up 14% of the total population, and by 2050, it will comprise 19% (Srivastava, 2021). The second-largest country, Pakistan, is also predicted to have 15.1% of its population as older adults by 2050 (Murad & Siraj, 2024).

2 Need for Public Mental Health Services for Older Adults in the South Asia

The region's population is ageing due to several factors, the most prominent being increasing life expectancy and declining fertility rates. All countries face significant challenges in ensuring that their social and health systems are prepared to accommodate this substantial shift. Approximately 1 in 6 people over the age of 60 worldwide reported experiencing a mental health condition (WHO, 2023).

There is limited data on this aspect from developing countries, including South Asia, due to stigma, limited resources, challenges in accessing healthcare, and a lack of high-quality health reporting systems. It is also notable that most studies involving the older adult age group focus either on depression or anxiety. Other disorders, such as schizophrenia and substance use disorders, are often under-researched or go undiagnosed, raising concerns that the currently available information on older adults' mental health issues represents only the tip of the iceberg (Kabir et al., 2024).

In a study of self-reported depression among South Asian countries involving over 7,000 individuals aged 50 and above, the prevalence across various nations ranged from 11.4% to 47.7% (Bishwajit et al., 2017). In India, the National Mental Health Survey (NMHS) reported a prevalence of depressive disorders of up to 7% among older adults, which is higher compared to younger adults (5%). Data from the Longitudinal Ageing Study in India (LASI), which comprises over 30,000 older adults aged 60 and above, found the prevalence of major depression to be 8.5% (7.4% in men, 9.5% among women) (Paul et al., 2023). Regional surveys within India have yielded similar results. A study from north India of over 3000 older adult participants estimated the prevalence of depression to be 8.9% (Sengupta & Benjamin, 2015). A systematic review of 23 studies involving over 24,000 participants revealed that the prevalence of anxiety among older adults in India is 18.7% (Patel et al., 2024).

Concerning Bangladesh, a search for literature focusing on geriatric mental health yielded limited results. A nationwide survey found that the prevalence of mental health disorders among individuals aged 60 and above is 28.1% (Arafat & Mazumder, 2025). A study of over 1000 respondents from both urban and rural settings in Bangladesh indicated a high prevalence of depression, with over half of the respondents experiencing mild to severe depression (Hossain et al., 2024).

In Sri Lanka, findings from a national survey among older adults reported that almost 1/3rd of this population had depressive symptoms (Malhotra et al., 2010). Individual studies from various areas have reported rising rates of mental health conditions such as dementia and substance use. Data from the nationwide prevalence of common mental health disorders and suicidality in Nepal indicated the lifetime prevalence of any mental disorder in the age group of 60 to 69 years to be 11.5% (Dhimal et al., 2022). The prevalence of geriatric depression in a cross-sectional survey of 460 older adult participants in Nepal was 53.1% (Manandhar et al., 2019).

No studies focusing on geriatric mental health from Afghanistan could be found. This may be attributed to the long-term political and societal turmoil in the region. Bhutan has many studies related to mental health among various age groups, but none have focused on public mental health aspects of old age mental healthcare.

No nationally representative study on old age mental health problems was available from Pakistan. The prevalence of depression in the older adults has been reported to be as high as 40%. Various studies focusing on the prevalence of mental health disorders locally among older adults are available, but the lack of comparability makes it difficult to get a holistic view (Bhamani et al., 2013; Mubeen et al., 2012).

3 Current State of Public Mental Health Services for Older Adults

The public health approach to mental healthcare involves two main themes: mental health promotion and the prevention of mental illness. Promotion implies creating conditions at the individual, community, social, and environmental levels that foster optimal psychological development. Prevention concerns itself with aspects of mental disorders in terms of reducing incidence, prevalence, and risk factors, thereby decreasing the impact of illness on families and societies (Rangarajan et al., 2021).

The South Asia region's population is ageing, and life expectancy is rising. The significant mental health morbidity among older adults leads to an increased demand for mental healthcare services, resulting in a corresponding rise in mental healthcare needs. All countries face substantial challenges to ensure that their social and health systems are prepared to accommodate this considerable shift (Chomik & Piggott, 2015).

In many areas of healthcare, models or solutions developed in Western countries are applied to specific populations to address pressing issues. While Western nations have already experienced a demographic shift towards an ageing population and have implemented public health policies to tackle mental health challenges among older adults, these approaches are not directly applicable in the context of South Asian countries. These nations face unique challenges, necessitating the development of affordable, acceptable, and suitable solutions for this culturally distinct environment population.

As recommended by the WHO, the mental health budget should constitute 5% to 15% of the country's total healthcare expenditures. Unfortunately, the actual spending on healthcare and that dedicated to mental healthcare represents a minuscule portion of the region's healthcare budget. The range of healthcare spending in these countries in 2021 ranged from 0.4 to 2.2% of GDP, except for the Maldives, which spent 7.2% of its GDP on healthcare. The WHO recommendation suggests a pyramid model for mental health delivery that prioritises care which is accessible, effective, comprehensive, coordinated, continuous, and respectful of human rights (Funk & Pathare, 2003). Emphasis is placed on personal care and community-based informal services. The integration of mental healthcare with physical health is encouraged from the primary healthcare level. Continuity of care is maintained by providing further specialised services for individuals with severe mental health issues.

Recent trends indicate that policymakers have recognised the urgent need for mental health programmes, as reflected in policies and legislation related to mental healthcare. India led the way by initiating its mental health plan (MHP) in 2014, followed by other countries in the region. Upon closer inspection, most of these policies contain limited provisions specifically aimed at addressing the mental health issues faced by older adults. In fact, many mental health programmes tend to address these concerns within the broader context of the adult population (Matthews et al., 2023). The downside of this approach is that it neglects to consider the specific factors affecting the older age group, which differ from those of the general adult population, influencing both the risk of mental health problems and the course of illness, thus necessitating tailored measures to address them.

3.1 Afghanistan

Afghanistan has limited mental health facilities. The availability of psychiatrists is 0.34 per 100,000 population, and there are barely 100 psychologists in the whole country (Shoib et al., 2024). The country's mental health policy was enacted in 1987 but did not see implementation due to long-standing political and economic turmoil (Afghanistan, 2024; Shoib et al., 2024). The current mental healthcare is provided mainly via WHO initiatives and by the NGOs operating in the region. The country has a long way to go in terms of manpower training and mental health policies before old age public mental health aspects can receive adequate attention.

3.2 *Bangladesh*

In Bangladesh, as in many South Asian member states, mental health issues among the older adults are often underdiagnosed and receive insufficient treatment. This situation stems from several factors, including a lack of awareness, stigma, and the threats of neglect, discrimination, and mistreatment faced by the senior population. As a developing nation, there is a prevalent shortage of appropriate geriatric mental health services due to limited focus on this issue, inadequate planning, and financial constraints (Arafat et al., 2024).

Mental healthcare for older adults involve various healthcare professionals skilled in both allopathic and alternative treatment methods. The lack of an established geriatric psychiatry curriculum for specialised training underscores the urgent need for qualified practitioners. The Department of Geriatric and Organic Psychiatry at the National Institute of Mental Health (NIMH) in Dhaka offers tertiary-level mental health services (Karim et al., 2024). While other tertiary medical institutions can address psychiatric conditions across all age groups, they lack dedicated facilities specifically for older adults' mental health concerns. In addition, there are limited or non-existent mental health services for the older adult at both primary and district levels. Recently, physicians and nurses trained in mental health issues under the WHO's mhGAP initiative have been providing mental healthcare to a broader area and across all age groups, including older adults.

Private medical practitioners, NGOs, and informal caregivers significantly contribute to managing mental health concerns among the older adult population in the country. Psychiatrists and psychologists working privately provide outpatient services, while various NGOs, such as the Subatra Trust and the Sir William Beveridge Foundation, deliver extensive care and rehabilitation for seniors. However, these organisations often struggle with a shortage of specialised mental health professionals due to an insufficient number of trained geriatric psychiatrists (Arafat et al., 2024). Families who can afford it often hire informal caregivers to look after their older adults relatives.

3.3 *Bhutan*

There is a huge unmet need of psychiatry services in general in the nation. Lack of manpower, trained clinicians, very short training period of health workers are among the major lacunas. In Bhutan, the PHC doctors, nursing staff, and workers are trained to diagnose and deliver care for mental health problems such as anxiety, depression, alcohol, and drug use. The country is late to introduce psychiatry in its postgraduate education programme with the first batch of psychiatry residents passing out in 2022 only (Gyeltshen et al., 2024).

Of these the only particular training on geriatric mental health has started in the last 5 years. This includes an older adults care programme and a manual for integrated community-based screening published in 2020. This manual is for screening and care of older adults by healthcare workers in Bhutan at home, residence, community setting, or hospitals. Among mental health problems, it covers the important topics of Depression and Dementia. National Mental Health Program was implemented in 1997, and it aims to incorporate mental healthcare at the primary level (Masaki & Tshering, 2021).

3.4 India

India has multiple policies and legislations to promote care and protect the rights of the older adults population (Philip et al., 2021). The National Policy for Older Persons was established in 1999. Its aim is to encourage individuals to make provisions for their old age, to ensure they are fully independent and capable. Additionally, it promotes the role of the family in caring for older adult members, which may be supported by assistance from NGOs. This has been since followed up by multiple frameworks such as Maintenance and Welfare of Parents and Senior citizens Act (2007), National Programme for Health Care of the Elderly (2010), National Health policy (2017), and Mental Health Care Act (2017).

The Integrated Programme for Older Persons (IPSrC) provides financial aid to NGOs to set up and run old age homes, daycare centres, and mobile medical units, ensuring essential services like food, shelter, and medical care for older adults. The Central Government Health Scheme allows pensioners from Central government offices to obtain medications for chronic conditions for periods of up to three months. Seniors can choose from health insurance options like the Varistha Mediclaim Policy from National Insurance and Navprabhat through Life Insurance Corporation. These plans cover hospitalisation, domiciliary expenses, and, if chosen, critical illnesses, providing affordable risk coverage and support for disabilities caused by accidents or illnesses (Chakrapani & Bharat, 2023). Critical illnesses include coronary artery surgery, cancer, renal failure, stroke, multiple sclerosis, and organ transplants; however, paralysis and blindness necessitate an additional premium. Notably, these policies exclude mental illness from the covered conditions. Very few insurance plans extend coverage for mental health issues, and those that do often come with a higher premium. Regrettably, as reported by the media and suggested by anecdotal evidence, many claims related to mental health are often denied due to policy language and technicalities.

Mental healthcare for older adults is greatly inadequate, with conditions like dementia often unrecognised. The matter of geriatric mental healthcare is often addressed peripherally, lacking the necessary mechanisms for enforcement or integration with the current health infrastructure (Kaur et al., 2023). Key barriers include a lack of awareness about dementia and depression as medical issues and a critically short workforce to treat mental disorders. This scarcity affects all mental health throughout life and has been highlighted in a recent Lancet series on Global

Mental Health. We lack the necessary economic and human resources for comprehensive specialist service coverage. Specialist services, focused on medical treatments, might have limited roles in long-term care for older adults, especially those with dementia (WHO, 2017). Developing services should prioritise home-based care, addressing the diverse medical and psychosocial needs of individuals and caregivers, and enhancing community acceptance of mental healthcare. Sustainable services must align with community aspirations, ensuring culturally relevant and affordable interventions provided by public and low-cost entities. It's important to acknowledge that mental illness among the older adults often co-occurs with other health issues like vision and hearing impairments, hypertension, diabetes, arthritis, and cardiovascular diseases. Thus, an ideal care model must consider both mental and physical health needs (Mirza & Singh, 2019). Raising awareness about late-life mental disorders for both the community and health professionals is urgent, including improving access to healthcare for older adults with mental illness. Health education should train workers and the community to recognise signs of mental disorders, reinforcing that depression and dementia are legitimate conditions, not merely effects of ageing.

3.5 *Maldives*

The Maldives faces a unique challenge due to its diverse island geography, along with economic and political instability, as well as the threat posed by rising sea levels. The mental health infrastructure consists of only one outpatient facility, one day care facility, and one community hospital, but there is no specialised mental hospital (WHO & Ministry of Health, Male, 2006). Maldives has implemented the National Mental Health Policy 2015–2025, which highlights a need for focus on healthy ageing and the well-being of older adults but the primary focus remains on pension scheme and financial assistance only.

3.6 *Nepal*

Nepal has a single health policy that includes mental health in one of its sections. There is no separate mental health policy. In 2018, the Epidemiology and Disease Control Division (EDCD) of the Department of Health Services (DHS) was designated as the focal unit to oversee mental health in Nepal (Rai et al., 2021). Recently, the government has introduced a National Mental Health Strategic and Action Plan (2020), which includes provisions for free primary mental health services nationwide and advocates for the integration of mental health within existing infrastructure. However, there is limited access to psychosocial services outside a few tertiary hospitals, and it fails to address mental health issues in the older adults.

Faith healing and traditional healing systems are deeply rooted in Nepal's cultural identity, often creating a framework around which individuals' understanding of psychological factors is based. This is particularly important to note when formulating a geriatric mental healthcare plan, as traditional and faith-based healers are often the first point of contact for this population (WHO, 2022).

The government has initiated community-based programmes, but mental healthcare is not yet fully integrated into primary care. NGOs play a significant role in delivering mental health services to the community. As part of WHO's Special Initiative for Mental Health in 2021, Nepal was selected to participate in the transformation and scaling up of its mental health services (WHO, 2021). In terms of geriatric mental healthcare, it mentions establishing a dementia care plan, but no specific strategies are outlined for other geriatric mental health issues (Shoib et al., 2024).

3.7 *Pakistan*

The political and economic instability in Pakistan since independence has led to significant neglect of public healthcare services, resulting in 90% out-of-pocket expenditure among the population (Noreen et al., 2022). Pakistan has 1000 government hospitals and about 300 private hospitals. The overall status of mental healthcare services in the public sector is not adequate, and the private sector offers expensive care. Pakistan lacks specialists in Geriatric Mental Health, and as a result, mental illness in older adults is often treated by psychiatrists, neurologists, or physicians. The goal of the 1999 national policy was to train healthcare practitioners for older adults; however, this has not been implemented. Only a few geriatricians and clinicians trained in Geriatric Psychiatry are available, and almost none of the nurses have received training in Geriatric Mental Health (Khan et al., 2018). The nation lacks specific programmes or policies addressing older adults with mental health issues, and the general mental health policy does not explicitly discuss the mental well-being of older adults (Murad & Siraj, 2024).

At a regional level, there is a provision for the establishment of one old facility in every district of Sindh province, yet its implementation remains lacking. Conversely, Islamic laws and councils have deemed such welfare homes to be contrary to religious obligations. This creates a conflict among the Pakistani population, thereby hindering the development and acceptance of geriatric mental healthcare in the country (Dayani et al., 2024).

3.8 *Sri Lanka*

Sri Lanka was one of the first countries to recognise the impact of mental illness and actively endeavoured to implement its Mental Health Policy in 2005. It progressed towards a community model of mental health service delivery, which involved the training of medical officers, psychiatric nurses, and psychologists. Consequently, the number of medical officers and paramedical staff trained and engaged in psychiatric care delivery has increased rapidly over the past decade. Community clinics, residential facilities, and an emergency helpline are being operated by the government in the country (Rajasuriya et al., 2021). In addition, to compensate for the shortage of human resources, non-medical personnel known as Community Support Officers are also trained to offer mental health services and coordinate with medical staff. Despite the progress made, the country falls behind in having an updated mental health law, as the current mental health policy was only valid until 2015.

In the older adult population, Sri Lanka faces challenges such as male suicide among older adults and abuse, alongside issues like dementia and depression. A psychogeriatric postgraduate curriculum has also commenced in the past few years (Kathriarachchi et al., 2019). The National Institute of Mental Health also has a psychogeriatric unit that specifically addresses the issues faced by this age group. The Sri Lankan Association of Geriatric Medicine publishes care pathways to assess, diagnose, and treat medical and psychiatric problems in older adults for both specialists and non-specialists. Sri Lanka has been proactive in implementing mental health policies, but there is still much more to address regarding geriatric mental healthcare as the country confronts an advancing ageing problem (Rajapakshe et al., 2019).

4 Challenges in Geriatric Public Mental Health in South Asia

The South Asia region faces many challenges in the promotion of mental health across all age groups. These include various social, cultural, and economic barriers that are common among different countries in the region (Rajkumar, 2024). There exists a substantial "unmet need" for mental healthcare, characterised by a widespread lack of understanding that psychological distress requires medical attention. Moreover, there is low acceptance of contemporary medical approaches to mental disorders among the public, along with significant limitations in the availability of mental health services within public health frameworks. Affected individuals and their families often underutilise these services, and there are considerable challenges in facilitating recovery and reintegration for those with mental health issues (Murthy, 2015). Additionally, numerous countries lack sufficient institutional frameworks—such as supportive policy, legislation, and funding—to effectively organise mental healthcare. Table 1 summarises the existing literature on the challenges confronted by mental health services that diminish the effectiveness of public mental health measures for all age groups, including older adults.

Furthermore, older adults face unique challenges in obtaining mental healthcare, adversely affecting their quality of life and reducing the effectiveness of public mental health initiatives (Mazumder et al., 2023). One of the unique challenges arises from the social construct of "ageism" (Gilleard, 2023). There is a misplaced belief that older individuals are not capable of contributing to society or their families and are

Table 1 Challenges of public mental health in South Asia

Challenge	Implication on public mental health
Lack of mental health policy	Lack of long-term vision to improve mental health
Lack of mental health legislation	No enforceability of directives aimed at improving mental health
Integration of mental health into disability-related legislation	Insufficient budget allocation to mental health, compared to physical disabilities
Low health budget	Mental health gets a minuscule part of the already insufficient health budget
Institution-based services	Lack of community care and poor long-term prognosis
Available treatment is limited to psychotropic medications	Lack of holistic treatment involving psychosocial interventions
Lack of trained psychiatric team approach	Understaffed health facilities can only provide limited care
Lack of health monitoring systems	The effectiveness and acceptability of existing interventions are not reviewed

Source Carbonell et al. (2020), Semrau et al. (2016) and Votruba et al. (2018)

often seen as a burden. This can lead to a variety of problems that infringe upon their rights and liberties, making treatment even more challenging.

The shift from joint families to nuclear families in South Asia, where extended families were once more common, has affected older adults. The traditional family structure is evolving alongside globalisation and economic changes. Historically, older adults have been revered and respected in this part of the world, with the corresponding concept of "filial piety" demanding respect and a duty of care towards the older adults (Prince et al., 2007). With the change in family structure due to the migration of children away from their parents, there is a shortage of caregivers and family members to support the geriatric population in their struggles with ageing and mental health issues.

Elder mistreatment (EM), previously an uncommon issue among South Asian communities, is on the rise as well (Talpur et al., 2018). The pilot study of the Longitudinal Ageing Study in India (LASI) found that around 26 per cent of older adults had experienced some form of violence (Berkman et al., 2012). When families and caregivers view older adults as a burden, it may cause stress and resentment, potentially leading to violence and neglect against them. Older adults are often dependent on family or children for daily expenses, including treatment-related costs. This limits their participation in decision-making regarding their health (Giebel et al., 2022).

Violence heightens the risk of declines in psychological and physical health among older adults. The negative associations between violence and both physical and mental health are well-documented in various studies (Berkman et al., 2012; Dahal et al., 2021; Edirisinghe et al., 2014). It can leave mistreated older adults stripped of their fundamental meaning in life (Chokkanathan et al., 2014). Evidence also suggests that violence is linked to distress and increased mortality among older individuals (Kosberg et al., 2003).

Studies have indicated gender differences in the prevalence of mental illness among older adults in South Asia. Women generally remain at home and encounter fewer opportunities for socialisation, employment, and independent functioning. This predisposes them to isolation and depression; when combined with their longer lifespan, early spousal deaths, financial insecurities, and children moving away from home, it creates a high-risk environment for mental health issues (Bohra et al., 2015; Srivastava & Muhammad, 2020).

South Asia is also particularly susceptible to chronic illnesses such as diabetes, hypertension, coronary artery disease, stroke, and cancer (Afshar et al., 2015). Physical illnesses like osteoarthritis can significantly affect mental health and overall well-being by limiting mobility and hindering an individual's independence in daily activities. These illnesses not only increase the physical health burden but also predispose individuals to other mental health problems, leading to a predicted rise in mental illness rates among the older adults if basic physical health needs are not addressed (Arokiasamy et al., 2015).

Isolation is a prevalent issue that exacerbates mental health problems among older adults. It can stem from a variety of factors. Many individuals report a loss of social contact with their peers and a diminished sense of purpose following retirement from the workforce (Bulut, 2022). A change of location or city can also have similar effects, as individuals become estranged from their familiar surroundings. The death of a spouse can profoundly impact the survivor psychologically, leading to negative mental health outcomes (Srivastava, 2021).

5 Suggested Measures and Future Directions

5.1 Integration of Mental Health into Primary Care

The World Health Organization (WHO) advocates for integrating mental health into primary healthcare. Incorporating mental healthcare into primary healthcare services is a powerful strategy for enhancing community mental health. This approach is particularly beneficial for older individuals who frequently seek treatment for chronic conditions like diabetes and hypertension in primary care settings. In India, the collaborative care model has demonstrated success in providing mental health services within primary health centres. The MANAS trial, which means "promoting mental health," compared collaborative stepped care with enhanced usual care in a cluster-randomised study. The stepped care involved initial recognition of mental health issues and resolution by advice and education delivered via a health counsellor. The provisions provided a step up in the level of care for those with complex needs via pharmacological treatment by a primary care physician and supervision and referral intake by a mental health specialist. The MANAS trial in India demonstrated that lay health counsellors trained in mental health interventions improved depression outcomes (Chatterjee et al., 2008). "Ayushman Bharat" is a vital nationwide initiative aimed at improving primary healthcare at sub-health centres and primary health centres. These facilities are evolving into "health and wellness centres," which offer health promotion and chronic condition prevention services, including mental health support. The initiative also provides health insurance for economically disadvantaged populations, including the older adults (Mahapatra & Seshadri, 2024).

5.2 Use of Technology in Geriatric Mental Health

Health technologies make use of personal technologies such as smartphones to work around factors hindering access to care (Torous et al., 2021). This is particularly beneficial in areas where levels of mobile device ownership and internet usage are sufficient but access to or utilisation of in-person services is minimal. WHO's online "Step-by-Step" initiative is a recent illustration of employing DHTs in resource-constrained environments. It provides psychoeducation and training in stress management techniques through an internet-enabled device. A recent trial found that the programme was associated with significant reductions in depression, anxiety, post-traumatic stress, and personal problems among at-risk populations (Cuijpers et al., 2022).

A significant portion of South Asia has gained access to mobile technology over the past decade. Research on health technologies for mental health has been limited for the population in the South Asian region. However, India has launched telepsychiatry guidelines and established tele-mental health centres of excellence. As technology evolves and internet access increases, mental health services for the older adults can reach those who are unable to access care physically. Global research has shown that AI-based chatbots represent a promising avenue to supplement the mental health needs of older adults (Chou et al., 2023). Similar research and advancements are necessary in this region to address the mental health treatment gap, particularly among older adults who can access these from the comfort of their homes.

5.3 Social Engagement Activities

Global evidence indicates the positive impacts of activities like intergenerational programmes (Aekwarangkoon & Noonil, 2020), visits by local volunteers, group activities, and community-based daycare (Jacob et al., 2007).

Evidence indicates that integrating these activities with other interventions, including exercise, peer counselling, dietary counselling, and psychoeducation, may yield additional beneficial effects (Rana et al., 2009). Comprehensive studies from other Asian regions have demonstrated the positive effects of social interaction through laughter therapy in alleviating depressive symptoms and enhancing the quality of life among older adults (Ko & Youn, 2011). India has many laughter clubs in urban areas, which can be linked with primary care psychiatry services for early recognition of cases and prompt intervention.

Religious beliefs and activities form a core part of daily life in the South Asia region (Coelho-Júnior et al., 2022). They also serve as a significant source of social engagement for older adults and shape many behavioural and mental health-related beliefs. Consequently, religious organisations and faith healers are often the first point of contact, and their role in connecting patients with community psychiatry must not be overlooked (Saha et al., 2021). The Dava-Dua project in Gujarat, India, exemplifies a synthesis of "magical-religious ailments" and "modern psychiatric interventions" in the treatment of mental illness. This initiative provides psychiatric care to individuals visiting the Mira Datar Dargah in search of a cure, thereby enhancing accessibility to psychiatric services while promoting the equitable treatment of patients through the sensitisation and training of faith healers (Pandya et al., 2020).

5.4 Expanding Geriatric Mental Health Workforce

Governments should invest in training programmes for geriatric psychiatrists and psychologists. Many nations lack training in age-related disorders. Basic needs and ailments of the older adults should come into the undergraduate curriculum, and specialised knowledge and application should be provided with postgraduate psychiatry and geriatric medicine programmes.

Super-specialisation in geriatric mental health in India can also be envisaged in other nations. Specialist clinicians, equipped with a comprehensive understanding of the mental health needs of older adults, can ensure high-quality care. These clinicians can contribute to the research aspects in the domain of older adults' mental health, which is currently scarce (Matthews et al., 2023). Furthermore, the presence of experts in the field will ensure that existing policies can be modified and any new policies can be designed with consideration for the specific mental health needs of older adults. This approach will allow for greater efficiency and improved resource allocation to enhance public health outcomes for older adults.

Beyond the regular courses, short-term mental health training for primary care doctors and community health workers currently serving this sector of population can be implemented such as the Dementia Echo programme in India. These courses can cut across national boundaries when provided using online resources (Nair et al., 2022). Mental health workforce is incomplete without nurses. Geriatric mental health nursing requires special training to address their specific needs. Such programmes should be put forth along with medical programmes. Training of healthcare workers such as ASHAs is also an essential step to the early identification of geriatric mental health problems.

5.5 *Policy Development and Implementation*

In 2002, the United Nations agreed upon the Madrid International Plan of Action on Ageing (MIPAA), which focused on three priority areas for "Building a Society for All Ages." One of these priorities is advancing health and well-being. This plan offers strategies and assistance to governments to develop locally relevant policies and decisions aimed at enhancing the health of the older adults. MIPAA acknowledges the mental well-being, emotional security, and psychological challenges faced by older adults. A review of current implementation suggests that little has been accomplished concerning these aspects in South Asia (Parry et al., 2018).

Mental health policies and programmes are currently operational in India, Pakistan, Nepal, and Sri Lanka; however, these policies are outdated and do not adequately fulfil the mandates set by MIPAA (Dey et al., 2019). Government policy must also transition from a healthcare model to a health promotion model that prioritises community-based services. Implementation efforts should concentrate on establishing non-profit, non-governmental partnerships with appropriate organisations. Intersectoral coordination, especially with agencies managing finance, media, and sanitation for the older adults, should be encouraged.

5.6 *Research*

There is a critical need to enhance the capacity for mental health research within South Asia (Sharma & Razzaque, 2017). In response, mental health leaders from various countries established the International Mental Health Development Group (IMHDG) to explore international collaborations aimed at improving public mental healthcare. The main objective was to identify underexplored research areas in South and East Asia and to foster partnerships among regional centres and beyond (Svob et al., 2024). It focuses on six key areas: public mental health; child and adolescent mental health; management of mental health comorbidity; collaboration with organisations; capacity building; and the advancement of previous initiatives. While some of these efforts may enhance the public mental health of older individuals, there is an urgent need for increased emphasis on geriatric psychiatry to align initiatives with the swiftly changing regional demographics.

5.7 *Strengthening Family and Caregiver Support*

In the absence of established social protection systems in South Asian countries, older individuals depend on their families for their well-being and care needs (Burholt et al., 2020). Policies designed to enhance family support can significantly improve the mental health of older age groups. Such policies can be implemented in countries that mandates the essential role of caretaking for the older adults. Measures such as financial incentives to caregivers of patients with dementia, establishing respite care for caregivers and patients as well as regular psychoeducational programmes conducted by community health workers and doctors can enhance caregiver support (Shaji & Reddy, 2012).

One essential and often overlooked aspect of family support is the lack of awareness regarding mental health issues among the older adults. Particularly in South Asian countries, mental health problems in older adults are often regarded as a normal reaction to ageing or attributed to various cultural phenomena. A nationwide or regional awareness programme, implemented through public or NGO channels, is a suggestion that could be easily carried out and would hasten the early identification and management of mental health issues of the older adults by educating family members (Koly et al., 2022).

Family therapy sessions that specifically target symptoms such as problematic behaviour and agitation in cases of dementia are another essential and necessary component. Since medical management alone is insufficient to address the behavioural and psychological symptoms of dementia, particular issues should be addressed in family therapy sessions, and access to such services is crucial (Kafczyk & Hämel, 2023). To strengthen support for families and caregivers, it is essential to incorporate family-based decision-making into the medical curriculum and training of healthcare professionals. This is crucial as families bear the burden of care and provide support to older adult patients. By considering the opinions and concerns of caregivers and making shared decisions regarding patient management, one can bolster their morale and establish a rapport that facilitates the long-term management of these cases. Therefore, this type of family-shared decision-making should be a key aspect of training doctors for geriatric mental healthcare (Carbonell et al., 2020; Naveen et al., 2020).

5.8 *Civic Engagement and Shared Decision-Making*

Civic engagement (CE) is a process through which people become actively and genuinely involved in the planning, development, and delivery of services, as well as in taking action to bring about change (James et al., 2020). It is a key focus of the WHO strategy to strengthen global health systems and is particularly important for the evolving mental health systems in low- and middle-income countries in South Asia.

Shared decision-making is a crucial aspect of CE, where the involvement of service users is sought in planning mental healthcare (James & Quirk, 2017). Peer support, involving individuals with personal experiences of mental health issues in service delivery, constitutes another form of CE (Chinman et al., 2015). In Western nations, CE has demonstrated promise and now constitutes an important aspect of mental health policy and research. However, it remains an underexplored area in the South Asian context due to various socio-cultural and economic factors (James et al., 2020).

Older adult mental health service users, backed by NGOs, families, and other support systems, can engage in the CE process to develop a suitable and acceptable treatment approach (Zavala et al., 2023). Theoretically, this aligns with the cultural values of the region, wherein elders are consulted on important matters, and it would also foster a sense of autonomy among the older adult service users.

6 Conclusion

Geriatric mental health is a growing public health challenge in South Asia. While some progress has been made, significant gaps remain in service delivery, policy implementation, and awareness. By integrating mental health into primary care, leveraging technology, and investing in research, South Asian nations can improve the quality of life for older adults. Collaboration between governments, international agencies, and civil society is essential to create a sustainable, inclusive mental healthcare system.

References

Aekwarangkoon, S., & Noonil, N. (2020). Effects of grandchildren's love language program on depression among Thai older adults. *Walailak Journal of Science and Technology (WJST), 17*(9), 924–932.

Afghanistan, U. (2024, November 5). *Mental Health Assessment—UNFPA Afghanistan 2024*. UNFPA Afghanistan. https://afghanistan.unfpa.org/en/publications/mental-health-assessment-unfpa-afghanistan-2024

Afshar, S., Roderick, P. J., Kowal, P., Dimitrov, B. D., & Hill, A. G. (2015). Multimorbidity and the inequalities of global ageing: A cross-sectional study of 28 countries using the World Health Surveys. *BMC Public Health, 15*, 1–10.

Arafat, S. M. Y., & Mazumder, A. H. (2025). Geriatric Psychiatry in Bangladesh: Current status and ways ahead. In *Geriatric Psychiatry in South Asia. Edi N Kar, SK Kar, SMY Arafat*. Springer Nature. https://doi.org/10.1007/978-981-96-7469-5_2

Arafat, S. M. Y., Mazumder, A. H., & Maruf, M. M. (2024). Geriatric psychiatry in Bangladesh. In S. M. Y. Arafat (Ed.) *Mental health in Bangladesh*. Springer. https://doi.org/10.1007/978-981-97-0610-5_18

Arokiasamy, P., Uttamacharya, U., Jain, K., Biritwum, R. B., Yawson, A. E., Wu, F., Guo, Y., Maximova, T., Espinoza, B. M., & Salinas Rodríguez, A. (2015). The impact of multimorbidity on adult physical and mental health in low-and middle-income countries: What does the study on global ageing and adult health (SAGE) reveal? *BMC Medicine, 13*, 1–16.

Berkman, L. F., Sekher, T., Capistrant, B., & Zheng, Y. (2012). Social networks, family, and care giving among older adults in India. In *Aging in Asia: Findings from new and emerging data initiatives*. National Academies Press (US).

Bhamani, M. A., Karim, M. S., & Khan, M. M. (2013). Depression in the elderly in Karachi, Pakistan: A cross sectional study. *BMC Psychiatry, 13*(1), 181. https://doi.org/10.1186/1471-244X-13-181

Bishwajit, G., O'Leary, D. P., Ghosh, S., Yaya, S., Shangfeng, T., & Feng, Z. (2017). Physical inactivity and self-reported depression among middle- and older-aged population in South Asia: World Health Survey. *BMC Geriatrics, 17*(1), 100. https://doi.org/10.1186/s12877-017-0489-1

Bloom, D. E., & Luca, D. L. (2016). Chapter 1—The global demography of aging: Facts, explanations, future. In J. Piggott & A. Woodland (Eds.), *Handbook of the economics of population aging* (Vol. 1, pp. 3–56). North-Holland. https://doi.org/10.1016/bs.hespa.2016.06.002

Bohra, N., Sharma, I., Srivastava, S., Bhatia, M. S., Chaudhuri, U., Parial, S., Sharma, A., & Kataria, D. (2015). Violence against women. *Indian Journal of Psychiatry, 57*(Suppl 2), S333-338. https://doi.org/10.4103/0019-5545.161500

Bulut, S. (2022). The positive correlation between well-being and religious practices & spirituality in the period of late adulthood. *Current Research in Psychology and Behavioral Science (CRPBS), 3*, 1–3. https://doi.org/10.54026/CRPBS/1057

Burholt, V., Maruthakutti, R., & Maddock, C. A. (2020). A cultural framework of care and social protection for older people in India. *GeroPsych.*

Cadeddu, C., Ianuale, C., & Lindert, J. (2015). Public mental health. In S. Boccia, P. Villari, & W. Ricciardi (Eds.), *A systematic review of key issues in public health* (pp. 205–221). Springer International Publishing. https://doi.org/10.1007/978-3-319-13620-2_12

Carbonell, Á., Navarro-Pérez, J.-J., & Mestre, M.-V. (2020). Challenges and barriers in mental healthcare systems and their impact on the family: A systematic integrative review. *Health & Social Care in the Community, 28*(5), 1366–1379. https://doi.org/10.1111/hsc.12968

Chakrapani, V., & Bharat, S. (2023). Mental health in India: Sociocultural dimensions, policies and programs—An introduction to the India Series. *SSM Mental Health, 4*. https://doi.org/10.1016/j.ssmmh.2023.100277

Chatterjee, S., Chowdhary, N., Pednekar, S., Cohen, A., Andrew, G., Andrew, G., Araya, R., Simon, G., King, M., Telles, S., Verdeli, H., Clougherty, K., Kirkwood, B., & Patel, V. (2008). Integrating evidence-based treatments for common mental disorders in routine primary care: Feasibility and acceptability of the MANAS intervention in Goa, India. *World Psychiatry, 7*(1), 39–46. https://doi.org/10.1002/j.2051-5545.2008.tb00151.x

Cheng, S.-T., & Heller, K. (2009). Global aging: Challenges for community psychology. *American Journal of Community Psychology, 44*(1–2), 161–173. https://doi.org/10.1007/s10464-009-9244-x

Chinman, M., Oberman, R. S., Hanusa, B. H., Cohen, A. N., Salyers, M. P., Twamley, E. W., & Young, A. S. (2015). A cluster randomized trial of adding peer specialists to intensive case management teams in the Veterans Health Administration. *The Journal of Behavioral Health Services & Research, 42*(1), 109–121. https://doi.org/10.1007/s11414-013-9343-1

Chokkanathan, S., Natarajan, A., & Mohanty, J. (2014). Elder abuse and barriers to help seeking in Chennai, India: A qualitative study. *Journal of Elder Abuse & Neglect, 26*(1), 60–79. https://doi.org/10.1080/08946566.2013.782786

Chomik, R., & Piggott, J. (2015). Population ageing and social security in Asia. *Asian Economic Policy Review, 10*(2), 199–222.

Chou, Y.-H., Lin, C., Lee, S.-H., Chang Chien, Y.-W., & Cheng, L.-C. (2023). Potential mobile health applications for improving the mental health of the elderly: A systematic review. *Clinical Interventions in Aging, 18*(null), 1523–1534. https://doi.org/10.2147/CIA.S410396

Coelho-Júnior, H. J., Calvani, R., Panza, F., Allegri, R. F., Picca, A., Marzetti, E., & Alves, V. P. (2022). Religiosity/spirituality and mental health in older adults: A systematic review and meta-analysis of observational studies. *Frontiers in Medicine (Lausanne), 9*, 877213. https://doi.org/10.3389/fmed.2022.877213

Cuijpers, P., Heim, E., Abi Ramia, J., Burchert, S., Carswell, K., Cornelisz, I., Knaevelsrud, C., Noun, P., van Klaveren, C., & van't Hof, E. (2022). Effects of a WHO-guided digital health intervention for depression in Syrian refugees in Lebanon: A randomized controlled trial. *PLoS Medicine, 19*(6), e1004025.

Dahal, M., Dhakal, S., Khanal, S., Baral, K., & Mahaseth, S. (2021). Linkage of depression with elder abuse among institutionalized older persons in Kathmandu Valley, Nepal. *Psychiatry Journal, 2021*, 5546623. https://doi.org/10.1155/2021/5546623

Dayani, K., Zia, M., Qureshi, O., Baig, M., & Sabri, T. (2024). Evaluating Pakistan's mental healthcare system using World Health Organization's assessment instrument for mental health system (WHO-AIMS). *International Journal of Mental Health Systems, 18*(1), 32. https://doi.org/10.1186/s13033-024-00646-6

Dey, S., Mellsop, G., Diesfeld, K., Dharmawardene, V., Mendis, S., Chaudhuri, S., Deb, A., Huq, N., Ahmed, H. U., Shuaib, M., & Khan, F. R. (2019). Comparing legislation for involuntary admission and treatment of mental illness in four South Asian countries. *International Journal of Mental Health Systems, 13*(1), 67. https://doi.org/10.1186/s13033-019-0322-7

Dhimal, M., Dahal, S., Adhikari, K., Koirala, P., Bista, B., Luitel, N., Pant, S., Marahatta, K., Shakya, S., Sharma, P., Ghimire, S., Gyanwali, P., Ojha, S. P., & Jha, A. K. (2022). A nationwide prevalence of common mental disorders and suicidality in Nepal: Evidence from National Mental Health Survey, 2019–2020. *Journal of Nepal Health Research Council, 19*(4), 740–747. https://doi.org/10.33314/jnhrc.v19i04.4017

Edirisinghe, P. A., Paranitharn, P., Perera, W. N., & Williams, S. S. (2014). Elder abuse among outpatient department attendees in a tertiary care hospital in Sri Lanka. *Ceylon Medical Journal, 59*(3), 84–89. https://doi.org/10.4038/cmj.v59i3.6527

Funk, M., & Pathare, S. (2003). *Organization of services for mental health* (Vol. 2). World Health Organization.

Giebel, C., Shrestha, N., Reilly, S., White, R. G., Zuluaga, M. I., Saldarriaga, G., Liu, G., Allen, D., & Gabbay, M. (2022). Community-based mental health and well-being interventions for older adults in low-and middle-income countries: A systematic review and meta-analysis. *BMC Geriatrics, 22*(1), 773.

Gilleard, C. (2023). Revisiting the social construction of old age. *Ageing and Society*, 1–14. https://doi.org/10.1017/S0144686X23000570

Gyeltshen, K., Chhetri, B., & Gyeltshen, D. (2024). Delivery of mental health services in Bhutan: Challenges and way forward. *Public Health Challenges, 3*. https://doi.org/10.1002/puh2.211

Hossain, M. K., Islam, M. N., Uddin, M. T., & Hossain, M. S. (2024). Understanding the impact of socioeconomic and health factors on geriatric depression: A comparative study in rural and urban Bangladesh. *Health Science Reports, 7*(2), e1849. https://doi.org/10.1002/hsr2.1849

Jacob, M. E., Abraham, V. J., Abraham, S., & Jacob, K. (2007). The effect of community based daycare on mental health and quality of life of elderly in rural south India: A community intervention study. *International Journal of Geriatric Psychiatry: A Journal of the Psychiatry of Late Life and Allied Sciences, 22*(5), 445–447.

James, K., Brooks, H., Susanti, H., Waddingham, J., Irmansyah, I., Keliat, B. A., Utomo, B., Rose, D., Colucci, E., & Lovell, K. (2020). Implementing civic engagement within mental health services in South East Asia: A systematic review and realist synthesis of current evidence. *International Journal of Mental Health System, 14*, 17. https://doi.org/10.1186/s13033-020-00352-z

James, K., & Quirk, A. (2017). The rationale for shared decision making in mental health care: A systematic review of academic discourse. *Mental Health Review Journal, 22*(3), 152–165.

Kabir, R., Isigi, S. S., & Candussi, C. (2024). Public mental health and access to mental health services in South Asia. In S. M. Y. Arafat & S. K. Kar (Eds.), *Access to mental health care in South Asia: Current status, potential challenges, and ways out* (pp. 229–243). Springer Nature Singapore. https://doi.org/10.1007/978-981-99-9153-2_11

Kafczyk, T., & Hämel, K. (2023). Primary mental healthcare for older people in India: Between stigmatization and community orientation. *Discover Mental Health, 3*(1), 14. https://doi.org/10.1007/s44192-023-00040-7

Karim, M. E., Islam, R., Mazumder, A. H., & Arafat, S. M. Y. (2024). Community psychiatry in Bangladesh: Development and current status. In S. M. Y. Arafat (Ed.), *Mental health in*

Bangladesh: From Bench to Community (pp. 129–137). Springer Nature Singapore. https://doi.org/10.1007/978-981-97-0610-5_8
Kathriarachchi, S. T., Seneviratne, V. L., & Amarakoon, L. (2019). Development of mental health care in Sri Lanka: Lessons learned. *Taiwanese Journal of Psychiatry, 33*(2), 55–65. https://doi.org/10.4103/tpsy.Tpsy_15_19
Kaur, H., Sivakumar, T., Manikappa, S. K., & Sarkar, S. (2023). The conundrum of geriatric public mental health in India: Initiatives and the road ahead. *Indian Journal of Social Psychiatry, 39*(4), 312–315. https://doi.org/10.4103/ijsp.ijsp_276_23
Khan, A., Toor, R., & Amjad, Q. (2018). Assessment and management of geriatric care in Pakistan. *Journal of Gerontology & Geriatric Research, 7*. https://doi.org/10.4172/2167-7182.1000488
Ko, H. J., & Youn, C. H. (2011). Effects of laughter therapy on depression, cognition and sleep among the community-dwelling elderly. *Geriatrics & Gerontology International, 11*(3), 267–274. https://doi.org/10.1111/j.1447-0594.2010.00680.x
Kohli, N., Chawla, S. K., Banerjee, A., & Srinete, T. P. (2020). Ageing in developing societies: Issues and challenges. *Psychology and Developing Societies, 32*(2), 153–175. https://doi.org/10.1177/0971333620943408
Koly, K. N., Abdullah, R., Shammi, F. A., Akter, T., Hasan, M. T., Eaton, J., & Ryan, G. K. (2022). Mental health and community-based rehabilitation: A qualitative description of the experiences and perspectives of service users and carers in Bangladesh. *Community Mental Health Journal, 58*(1), 52–66. https://doi.org/10.1007/s10597-021-00790-0
Kosberg, J. I., Lowenstein, A., Garcia, J. L., & Biggs, S. (2003). Study of elder abuse within diverse cultures. *Journal of Elder Abuse & Neglect, 15*(3–4), 71–89. https://doi.org/10.1300/J084v15n03_05
Mahapatra, P., & Seshadri, S. (2024). Mental health in India: Evolving strategies, initiatives, and prospects. *Lancet Regional Health Southeast Asia, 20*, 100300. https://doi.org/10.1016/j.lansea.2023.100300
Malhotra, R., Chan, A., & Ostbye, T. (2010). Prevalence and correlates of clinically significant depressive symptoms among elderly people in Sri Lanka: Findings from a national survey. *International Psychogeriatrics, 22*(2), 227–236. https://doi.org/10.1017/s1041610209990871
Manandhar, K., Risal, A., Shrestha, O., Manandhar, N., Kunwar, D., Koju, R., & Holen, A. (2019). Prevalence of geriatric depression in the Kavre district, Nepal: Findings from a cross sectional community survey. *BMC Psychiatry, 19*(1), 271. https://doi.org/10.1186/s12888-019-2258-5
Masaki, K., & Tshering, J. (2021). Exploring the origins of Bhutan's gross national happiness. *Journal of South Asian Development, 16*(2), 273–292. https://doi.org/10.1177/09731741211039049
Matthews, N. R., Porter, G. J., Varghese, M., Sapkota, N., Khan, M. M., Lukose, A., Paddick, S.-M., Dissanayake, M., Khan, N. Z., & Walker, R. (2023). Health and socioeconomic resource provision for older people in South Asian countries: Bangladesh, India, Nepal, Pakistan and Sri Lanka evidence from NEESAMA. *Global Health Action, 16*(1), 2110198. https://doi.org/10.1080/16549716.2022.2110198
Mazumder, H., Faizah, F., Gain, E. P., Sharmin Eva, I., Ferdouse Mou, K., Saha, N., Rahman, F., Das, J., Islam, A. M. K., Nesa, F., & Hossain, M. M. (2023). Effectiveness of mental health interventions for older adults in South Asia: A scoping review. *PLoS ONE, 18*(7), e0287883. https://doi.org/10.1371/journal.pone.0287883
Mirza, A., & Singh, N. (2019). PERSPECTIVES: Mental health policy in India: Seven sets of questions and some answers. *The Journal of Mental Health Policy and Economics, 22*(1), 25–37.
Mubeen, S. M., Henry, D., & Nazimuddin Qureshi, S. (2012). Prevalence of depression among community dwelling elderly in Karachi, Pakistan. *Iran Journal of Psychiatry Behavioral Sciences, 6*(2), 84–90.
Murad, S., & Siraj, S. (2024). Bridging the void: Unraveling mental health policies for the older adults in Pakistan's tapestry—A literature review. *Journal of Clinical Psychology and Neurology.*
Murthy, R. S. (2015). Mental health programs at community level in South Asian countries: Progress, problems and prospects. In J. K. Trivedi & A. Tripathi (Eds.), *Mental health in South Asia:*

Ethics, resources, programs and legislation (pp. 155–190). Springer Netherlands. https://doi.org/10.1007/978-94-017-9017-8_10

Nair, S., Sinha, P., Chand, P., Sahu, P., Gorthi, N. V., Varghese, M., & Sivakumar, P. T. (2022). Extension for community healthcare outcomes based telementoring of physicians for dementia-effectiveness in India. *Front Psychiatry, 13*, 869685. https://doi.org/10.3389/fpsyt.2022.869685

Naveen, K. H. S., Goel, A. D., Dwivedi, S., & Hassan, M. A. (2020). Adding life to years: Role of gender and social and family engagement in geriatric depression in rural areas of Northern India. *Journal of Family Medicine and Primary Care, 9*(2), 721–728. https://doi.org/10.4103/jfmpc.jfmpc_1019_19

Noreen, N., Abdullah, M., & Lalani, N. (2022). Geriatric care in Pakistan: Current realities and way forward. *Pakistan Journal of Public Health, 11*, 214–219. https://doi.org/10.32413/pjph.v11i4.872

Pandya, A., Shah, K., Chauhan, A., & Saha, S. (2020). Innovative mental health initiatives in India: A scope for strengthening primary healthcare services. *Journal of Family Medicine and Primary Care, 9*(2), 502–507. https://doi.org/10.4103/jfmpc.jfmpc_977_19

Parry, J., Um, J., & Zaidi, A. (2018). Monitoring active ageing in the Asia-Pacific region: Recommendations for future implementation of the MIPAA.

Patel, M., Mantri, N., Joshi, N., Jain, Y., Goel, A. D., Gupta, M., Srinivasan, S., Yadav, V., Joshi, V., Singh, K., & Bhardwaj, P. (2024). Is anxiety a public health problem among older adults in India: Results from a systematic review and meta-analysis. *Journal of Family Medicine and Primary Care, 13*(7), 2545–2554. https://doi.org/10.4103/jfmpc.jfmpc_1664_23

Paul, R., Muhammad, T., Rashmi, R., Sharma, P., Srivastava, S., & Zanwar, P. P. (2023). Depression by gender and associated factors among older adults in India: Implications for age-friendly policies. *Science and Reports, 13*(1), 17651. https://doi.org/10.1038/s41598-023-44762-8

Philip, S., Gajera, G., Nirisha, P. L., Sivakumar, P. T., Barikar, M. C., Panday, P., Patley, R., Chander, R., Sinha, P., Basavarajappa, C., Manjunatha, N., Kumar, C. N., & Math, S. B. (2021). Future-proofing geriatric mental health care services in India: Training and policy directions. *Indian Journal of Psychological Medicine, 43*(5_suppl), S134–S141. https://doi.org/10.1177/02537176211032342

Prince, M., Livingston, G., & Katona, C. (2007). Mental health care for the elderly in low-income countries: A health systems approach. *World Psychiatry, 6*(1), 5. https://pmc.ncbi.nlm.nih.gov/articles/PMC1810377/pdf/wpa060005.pdf

Rai, Y., Gurung, D., & Gautam, K. (2021). Insight and challenges: Mental health services in Nepal. *BJPsych International, 18*(2), E5. https://doi.org/10.1192/bji.2020.58

Rajapakshe, O. B. W., Sivayogan, S., & Kulatunga, P. M. (2019). Prevalence and correlates of depression among older urban community-dwelling adults in Sri Lanka. *Psychogeriatrics, 19*(3), 202–211. https://doi.org/10.1111/psyg.12389

Rajasuriya, M., Hewagama, M., Ruwanpriya, S., & Wijesundara, H. (2021). Community-based psychiatric services in Sri Lanka: A model by WHO in the making. *Consort Psychiatry*, *2*(4), 40–52. https://doi.org/10.17816/cp106

Rajkumar, R. P. (2024). Access to mental health care in South Asia: Variations of challenges and ways forward. In S. M. Y. Arafat & S. K. Kar (Eds.), *Access to mental health care in South Asia: Current status, potential challenges, and ways out* (pp. 155–196). Springer Nature Singapore. https://doi.org/10.1007/978-981-99-9153-2_9

Rana, A. M., Wahlin, Å., Lundborg, C. S., & Kabir, Z. N. (2009). Impact of health education on health-related quality of life among elderly persons: Results from a community-based intervention study in rural Bangladesh. *Health Promotion International, 24*(1), 36–45.

Rangarajan, S. K., Sivakumar, P. T., Manjunatha, N., Kumar, C. N., & Math, S. B. (2021). Public health perspectives of geriatric mental health care. *Indian Journal of Psychological Medicine, 43*(5 Suppl), S1-s7. https://doi.org/10.1177/02537176211047963

Saha, S., Chauhan, A., Hamlai, M., Saiyad, V., Makwana, S., Shah, K., & Pandya, A. (2021). Unique collaboration of modern medicine and traditional faith-healing for the treatment of mental illness: Best practice from Gujarat. *Journal of Family Medicine and Primary Care, 10*(1), 521–526. https://doi.org/10.4103/jfmpc.jfmpc_979_19

Semrau, M., Lempp, H., Keynejad, R., Evans-Lacko, S., Mugisha, J., Raja, S., Lamichhane, J., Alem, A., Thornicroft, G., & Hanlon, C. (2016). Service user and caregiver involvement in mental health system strengthening in low- and middle-income countries: Systematic review. *BMC Health Services Research, 16*, 79. https://doi.org/10.1186/s12913-016-1323-8

Sengupta, P., & Benjamin, A. I. (2015). Prevalence of depression and associated risk factors among the elderly in urban and rural field practice areas of a tertiary care institution in Ludhiana. *Indian Journal of Public Health, 59*(1), 3–8. https://doi.org/10.4103/0019-557x.152845

Shaji, K. S., & Reddy, M. S. (2012). Caregiving: A public health priority. *Indian Journal of Psychological Medicine, 34*(4), 303–305. https://doi.org/10.4103/0253-7176.108191

Sharma, M., & Razzaque, B. (2017). Research capacity strengthening in South Asia: Based on the experience of South Asian Hub for Advocacy, Research and Education on Mental Health (SHARE). *Global Mental Health, 4*, e9.

Shoib, S., Hussaini, S. S., Nazari, S. K., & Saeed, F. (2024). Mental healthcare in Afghanistan. In S. M. Y. Arafat & S. K. Kar (Eds.), *Access to mental health care in South Asia: Current status, potential challenges, and ways out* (pp. 17–27). Springer Nature Singapore. https://doi.org/10.1007/978-981-99-9153-2_2

Srivastava, S. (2021). Geriatric mental health issues from India. In M. K. Shankardass (Ed.), *Ageing issues in India: Practices, perspectives and policies* (pp. 301–309). Springer Singapore. https://doi.org/10.1007/978-981-16-5827-3_17

Srivastava, S., & Muhammad, T. (2020). Violence and associated health outcomes among older adults in India: A gendered perspective. *SSM Population Health, 12*, 100702. https://doi.org/10.1016/j.ssmph.2020.100702

Svob, C., Lemon, C. A., & Bonomo, Y. A. (2024). Public health and mental health in the south and east of Asia: Review of opportunities for collaborative research and public health action. *Asian Journal of Psychiatry, 92*, 103886. https://doi.org/10.1016/j.ajp.2023.103886

Talpur, A., Ryan, T., Ali, P., & Hinchliff, S. (2018). Elder mistreatment in South Asian communities: a review of the literature. *The Journal of Adult Protection, 20*. https://doi.org/10.1108/JAP-06-2018-0011

Torous, J., Bucci, S., Bell, I. H., Kessing, L. V., Faurholt-Jepsen, M., Whelan, P., Carvalho, A. F., Keshavan, M., Linardon, J., & Firth, J. (2021). The growing field of digital psychiatry: Current evidence and the future of apps, social media, chatbots, and virtual reality. *World Psychiatry, 20*(3), 318–335.

Votruba, N., Ziemann, A., Grant, J., & Thornicroft, G. (2018). A systematic review of frameworks for the interrelationships of mental health evidence and policy in low- and middle-income countries. *Health Research Policy and System, 16*(1), 85. https://doi.org/10.1186/s12961-018-0357-2

WHO. (2017). *Global action plan on the public health response to dementia 2017–2025*. World Health Organization.

WHO. (2021). *Nepal—WHO special initiative for mental health*. World Health Organization. https://www.who.int/initiatives/who-special-initiative-for-mental-health/nepal

WHO. (2022). *Nepal—WHO special initiative for mental health situational assessment*. W. H. Organization. https://www.who.int/publications/m/item/Nepal_country_assessment_SIMH_2022

WHO. (2023). Mental health of older adults. *WHO Newsroom*. https://www.who.int/news-room/fact-sheets/detail/mental-health-of-older-adults

Zavala, G. A., Jennings, H. M., Afaq, S., Alam, A., Ahmed, N., Aslam, F., Arsh, A., Coales, K., Ekers, D., Nabi, M., Naz, A., Shakur, N., Siddiqi, N., Wright, J. M., & Kellar, I. (2023). Effectiveness and implementation of psychological interventions for depression in people with non-communicable diseases in South Asia: Systematic review and meta-analysis. *International Journal of Mental Health, 52*(3), 260–284. https://doi.org/10.1080/00207411.2023.2202431

Preventing Mental Illnesses in Old Age: Strategies and Evidence

Sarmishtha Bhattacharyya, Susan Mary Benbow, and Sathyan Soundararajan

Abstract The population of South Asia is ageing. This chapter reviews complex and interrelated risk factors influencing mental ill health and cognitive disorders in older adults, and highlights modifiable biopsychosocial factors. There is evidence supporting ways in which older adults' health can be promoted but more research is needed in low- and middle-income countries. Nevertheless, much can be done to improve the mental, cognitive, and physical health of South Asian older adults at a number of levels, including international and national strategies and interventions, as well as regional, local, and community interventions, and lifestyle changes at a family and individual level. A multi-level approach is essential.

Keywords Ageism · Dementia · Depression · Health Promotion · Nutrition · Social Isolation · South Asia

1 Introduction: The Context

The global population is ageing. In 2020, one billion people in the world were aged 60 years or over, and that number will nearly double between 2015 and 2050, from 12% of the total population to 22%. By 2030, it is predicted that one in six people in the world will be aged 60 years or older (World Health Organization, 2024a).

South Asia consists of a group of eight countries, most of which are classified as low- and middle-income countries (LAMIC) with heterogeneous culture, language, and religious needs. They are Bangladesh, Bhutan, India, Pakistan, Nepal, and Sri

The original version of the chapter has been revised. A correction to this chapter can be found at https://doi.org/10.1007/978-981-96-7469-5_13

S. Bhattacharyya · S. M. Benbow
University of Chester, Chester, UK

S. Bhattacharyya (✉) · S. Soundararajan
Betsi Cadwaladr University Health Board, Wales, UK
e-mail: drsharmib@gmail.com

N. Kar et al. (eds.), *Geriatric Psychiatry in South Asia*, South Asian Perspectives in Mental Health and Psychology , https://doi.org/10.1007/978-981-96-7469-5_11

Lanka, with Afghanistan and the Maldives being considered part of South Asia as well. The population of these countries is predicted to age rapidly, with the proportion of the "oldest old" (those people aged 80 years and over) increasing from the present 8% of the older population to 10% in 2025, and further increasing to 15% in 2050 (Mujahid & Siddhisena, 2009). Given that more than 23% of the world population lives in South Asian (Hossain et al., 2020) coupled with population ageing, the burden of mental ill health represents a considerable challenge now and for the future. Policies and programmes in South Asian countries will therefore have to address this change and increasingly focus on disability and long-term care. Evidence suggests that there will be more women in the older population, a change which will bring its own challenges. Mujahid and Siddhisena (2009) highlight that older women in South Asian countries are more vulnerable than older men, as a higher proportion of older women are "single" (unmarried, divorced, or widowed) and face a higher incidence of disability with fewer opportunities for productive employment. They are also financially less secure and have less access to means of care and support in illness and disability. An increase in older adults in rural areas also has significant implications in relation to accessing mental health or other services which may be more accessible in big cities. Different South Asian countries also have differing numbers of older adults and need to tailor policies to projected population changes in order to prevent mental illness in their older populations.

Older people may possess protective factors for good mental health, but many face numerous risk factors, including loneliness/social isolation, poor physical health, comorbidities, sensory losses, complex health states associated with ageing (e.g. frailty, falls) and, in some cases, poverty and racism (Centre for Mental Health and Age UK, 2024). The mental health needs of older adults are often complicated by multiple physical health issues, and mental illness still carries a stigma, possibly more so in South Asian countries and communities than in developed countries. Of older adults, around a quarter experiences mental health problems, with the commonest being depression, dementia, and anxiety. In addition, one older adult in six experiences abuse, sometimes from their own family members/carers (Yon et al., 2017). Mental disorders amongst older adults account for 10.6% of the total years lived with disability for this age group (World Health Organization, 2023a).

2 Prevalence of Mental Illness in Older Adults

Mental health problems affect 5–7% of those aged over 60, with depression and dementia the most common. Anxiety follows close behind and affects 3.8% of older adults. Edwards et al. (2023) reviewed the literature on the prevalence of depression in LMIC and found that rates of depression are similar in older people in LMIC compared to high-income countries, but that mental healthcare resources are more limited in the former, suggesting a large potential treatment gap.

Another study (Tiwari et al., 2012) found that mental illnesses were very common amongst residents of old age homes with a higher prevalence in residential homes than found in the community. Physical problems were also more common. Possible factors in this include significantly more psychological stressors, negligible family support, lack of medical (physical/mental) care and facilities, the restricted environment of old age homes, selection (people with mental illness may be more likely to move into a home), and financial constraints.

2.1 *Prevalence of Dementia in Older Adults*

The World Health Organization (2023b) reports that there are more than 55 million people with dementia across the globe and that a majority (60%) live in low- and middle-income countries. Ten million new people are affected each year. It is estimated that Alzheimer's disease is the most common dementia condition, probably contributing to around two-thirds of cases.

Alzheimer's disease and other dementias are ranked seventh in the top ten causes of death across the world, and are a source of disability and dependency: they affect women disproportionately (World Health Organization, 2024b). The cost of dementia to global economies is considerable, both in terms of formal and informal care, and was estimated at 1.3 trillion US dollars in 2019 (World Health Organization, 2023b). Informal care by family and friends accounts for around half the costs, and the burden of care falls disproportionately on women carers.

A recent article by Palliyaguru et al. (2024), which is still in pre-print, highlights the expanding older adult population in South Asian countries and the challenges that individuals and governments face since ageing remains the strongest risk factor for developing dementia. Unfortunately, even though the burden of dementia is high, it appears that health policy, research, and awareness do not adequately address these challenges in these countries.

3 Risk Factors Influencing Mental Health in Older Adults

Many factors have been shown to affect the mental health of older adults, and there are commonalities between factors influencing mental health and those influencing cognitive function. Table 1 summarises physical, psychological, and social factors that have a role. Genetic, environmental, and lifestyle factors may contribute, and there is evidence that many environmental and lifestyle factors can be changed or managed to improve mental health in older adults. It has been some years now since the Foresight Mental Capital and Well-being Project Report (2008) was published, but its synthesis of the trajectory of mental capital through life was ahead of its time and is still relevant today. It sets out factors affecting health across the life course and emphasises the roles of both physical and mental activity, social engagement and interventions, both dietary and medicinal, in later life.

Table 1 Some of the factors that increase risk of poor mental and cognitive health outcomes in later life

Physical factors	Psychological factors	Social factors
• Genetic predispositions	• Loneliness	• Poverty/financial constraints
• Lack of activity/exercise	• Lack of mental activity	• Ageism
• Poor general health	• Retirement	• Racism
• Decreased mobility/falls	• Loss of role in later life	• Abuse from family/carers
• Complex comorbidities	• Personality factors	• Institutional abuse/ageism
• Frailty	• Internalised ageism	• Lack of healthcare resources
• Poor nutrition	• Coping mechanisms	• Lack of family support
• Medication affecting cognition & mood	• Adverse life events/ trauma	• Lack of social engagement
• Sensory losses—hearing, sight		• Low educational attainment
• Lifestyle factors, smoking, alcohol		• Poor housing
• Poor sleep hygiene		• Low value attributed to older adults
		• Social isolation

Physical health and physical activity/exercise benefit mental health. Being physically active, through regular exercise, household chores, or other activities, helps maintain and improve strength and balance, prevent, or delay heart disease, diabetes, and other disorders and also improves mood, and reduces depression. US federal guidelines (US Centers for Disease Control & Prevention, 2024) recommend that adults aged 65 and over (just like their younger counterparts) engage in at least 150 min (2.5 h) each week of physical activity in addition to muscle-strengthening activities and balance exercises.

Loneliness and isolation remain significant issues for older adults across the world. South Asian communities often support their elders and often live with them. However, given the Westernisation of societies across developing countries, loneliness and isolation may become a more significant issue in future.

Smoking has been highlighted as a risk factor for higher levels of isolation and loneliness. Philip and co-workers (2022) found that, compared to non-smokers, smokers were more likely to be lonely and socially isolated and to have less contact with family and friends: this could be associated with an increased risk of mental health problems, including anxiety and depression.

A longitudinal study from China (Ao et al., 2021) reinforces concern about the health risks from indoor and ambient air pollution. Pollution has the potential to further burden global economic development by adversely affecting the mental health of older adults, particularly in respect of depressive symptomatology.

Further, it is known that sensory loss can affect mental health. Kiely et al. (2013) noted the role that dual sensory loss (visual and auditory) has to play in relation to decreased mental health, particularly the risk of developing depression, and suggest this should be an area for targeted interventions and rehabilitation.

Some of the interventions referred to could be regarded as new learning and some might be regarded as introducing potential lifestyle changes. The time period of follow up and whether changes are maintained is an important consideration, also the issue of what interventions would be appropriate in terms of a person's cultural background and available resources. Most of the literature originates from high-income countries and there is much overlap with factors that impact adversely on cognitive health.

4 Risk Factors for Developing Dementia

Considerable research has been carried out in recent years with regard to risk factors for dementia and what might be done to prevent dementia conditions. In 2020, the Lancet Commission (Livingstone et al., 2020) published a report on dementia prevention, intervention, and care with recommendations for improvements in education, healthcare, nutrition, and lifestyle modifications. The report identified 12 potentially modifiable risk factors for dementia. These include lack of education and awareness of dementia, hypertension, hearing impairment, obesity, smoking, depression, physical inactivity, social isolation, diabetes, excessive alcohol consumption, traumatic brain injury, and air pollution. Interestingly, the report found that these risk factors potentially account for up to 40% of cases of dementia worldwide. In 2024 an updated report was published (Livingstone et al., 2024) and added two more potentially modifiable risk factors, untreated visual loss and low-density lipoprotein (LDL) cholesterol. The modifiable risk factors support the importance of public health policy in emphasising lifestyle modifications, as well as childhood education, as important factors in improving cognitive health in all countries, and some of these would have an important role in low- and middle-income countries, such as those in South East Asia.

With regard to young-onset dementia, modifiable risk factors include lower levels of educational attainment, low socio-economic status, heavy alcohol use, and compromised cardiovascular health (Cations et al., 2019). These should be key targets for prevention or delay of young-onset dementia in South Asian countries.

It is relevant in connection with physical health to note that some commonly prescribed medications are thought to carry risks for mental health, for example antihistamines and antipsychotic drugs which increase anticholinergic burden. It has been suggested that high anticholinergic burden is associated with cognitive decline and dementia in older adults (Fox, 2014 in a review of 46 studies). However, Taylor-Rowan and colleagues (2022) carried out a Cochrane review and were unable to draw any clear conclusions regarding risk of accelerated cognitive deterioration amongst older adults with dementia or mild cognitive impairment.

Hypertension and diabetes affect both cognitive and physical function in older adults and, therefore, remain significant risk factors for developing both cognitive and other mental illnesses. There is also enough research to evidence the development of depression in people with diabetes; however, further research is needed to determine whether cardiovascular risk modification may help prevent the decline in both cognitive and functional performance amongst older adults (Kuo et al., 2005). Research shows that treating people in early (rather than later) adulthood for cardiovascular risk factors could preserve health in later life (Yaffe et al., 2021). Risk factors associated with worse cognitive health later in life include higher body mass index, fasting glucose, and systolic blood pressure. Obesity is a risk factor for heart disease that is associated with poorer cognitive health (Ma et al., 2020). Put simply, research supports the saying that what's good for the heart is good for the brain.

Research on modifying cardiovascular risk factors links with the possible role of a healthy diet in maintaining cognitive health. Marchand and Jensen (2017) reviewed a number of studies and concluded that eating a healthy balanced diet over a long period of time (probably at least five years) helps maintain cognition. Such a diet will consist of fruits and vegetables; whole grains; lean meats (e.g. fish or poultry); and seafoods/fish. Other possible components of a diet aiming to maintain brain health are low-fat or non-fat dairy products, controlled portion sizes, and drinking enough water and other fluids, whilst cutting down or avoiding red meats and sweets. There is interest in the possible benefit of a Mediterranean diet in lowering dementia risk. Another diet (Barnes et al., 2023), called MIND (a combination of the Mediterranean diet and Dietary Approaches to Stop Hypertension, referred to as DASH) has been regarded as promising with regard to reducing the risk of Alzheimer disease and slowing rate of cognitive decline (Liu et al., 2021). A physiological decline in food intake in older adults may lead to nutritional deficiencies, which are risk factors for chronic diseases and other health problems (Kaur et al., 2019). Harbottle (2019) suggests that nutritional vulnerability increases in older adults for various reasons, not just due to the physiological impact of ageing but also social and economic challenges. Overall diet quality may impact mood, whilst on the other hand, depression and anxiety may reduce intake and exacerbate symptoms. Zhou et al (2023) concluded in a systematic review on nutrition and healthy ageing in Asia that that the likelihood of healthy ageing in late life was positively increased by a higher consumption of healthy foods, such as vegetables, fruits, fish, nuts, legumes, tea, milk, and dairy, at midlife, and also by greater adherence to dietary patterns with high diversity scores or high total antioxidant capacities. Moreover, improving diet quality in midlife had a positive impact in later life. Nutrition is therefore an important factor affecting quality of life in older adults, possibly more so in low- and middle-income countries, and has an important role in maintaining physical, mental, and cognitive health.

Similarly, there is evidence to support the role of mental and social activity in maintaining cognitive health. Staying engaged in meaningful activities in later life brings important benefits. Krell-Roesch and colleagues (2019) in the US studied 2000 cognitively intact people in the community aged 70 and older over a median of 5 years and found that engaging in mentally stimulating activities was associated with a decreased risk of mild cognitive impairment. Examples of mentally stimulating activities include reading, crafting, computer activities, and social activities. One study

(Park et al., 2013) found that older adults who learned quilting or digital photography had more memory improvement than those who socialised or engaged in less cognitively demanding activities. What constitutes a mentally stimulating activity is likely to be influenced by cultural setting. Dodge and colleagues in the US (2023) studied 186 participants aged 75 and older using semi-structured conversations over the internet with trained interviewers in a randomised controlled trial. This was an intensive programme involving conversations four times each week for six months then twice weekly for the following six months. They concluded that regular stimulating internet-based conversations could reduce dementia risk by decreasing social isolation. It is debatable how this could be extrapolated into an effective practical intervention, but the principle of alleviating social isolation amongst older adults is an important one. Park and colleagues (2013) perhaps took a more practical approach to social engagement: they analysed data from more than 7000 participants aged 65 and older and found that high levels of social engagement, including visiting neighbours and doing volunteer work, was associated with better cognitive health.

A study in the Netherlands by Deckers et al. (2024) highlighted the importance of a multidomain approach to prevent cognitive decline and dementia. Their study combined seven lifestyle interventions: these addressed physical, cognitive, and social activity, counselling with regard to diet/nutrition and sleep, and the management of cardiovascular risk factors and stress. They suggest for the future combining lifestyle changes with pharmacological treatments, possibly in addition to using new technologies.

In a systematic review on emerging trends in cognitive impairment and dementia in older adults in Asia, Islam et al. (2024) emphasise the limited data available from Southeast, South, and Central Asia and that comprehensive data is needed to help address the growing burden of dementia in South Asian countries. Ravindranath and Sundarakumar (2021) reviewed the literature in relation to dementia epidemiology and risk factors, particularly in the Indian population. They note that further work needs to be done to implement public policies that address these risk factors and that increasing life span will have implications for the growing burden of dementia. Known vascular risk factors in this population include obesity, diabetes, and hypertension. They argue the importance of community-based multimodal interventions, adapted to the sociocultural context, that target vascular risks, diet, and levels of physical activity.

5 Factors Affecting Mental and Cognitive Health Are Interrelated

Ageism and discrimination against older adults remain real issues across the world. It is important to embed dignity in the care of older people due to their multiple interdependent vulnerabilities encompassing physical health, mental health, and cognition.

Banerjee and colleagues (2021) highlight the role of addressing stigma and discrimination in individuals with mental illness, combatting ageism, preventing/managing elder abuse, and focusing on functional recovery and independence to improve mental health and prevent mental illness in older adults. Elder abuse remains a significant psychological risk factor which affects the mental and cognitive health of older adults. Tackling these risk factors and boosting protective factors on an individual and collective level has the potential to increase well-being in later life and prevent or stop the escalation of mental health problems.

Evidence suggests that 1 in 6 people aged 60 years and over experience some form of abuse in the community, and the rate is higher in institutions such as nursing homes and long-term care facilities (World Health Organization, 2024; Yon et al., 2017). The rate of abuse increased during the COVID-19 pandemic. Abuse in older adults can have serious and significant consequences for physical and mental health, but also brings financial and social consequences, including physical injuries, premature mortality, depression, cognitive decline, financial devastation, and early placement in nursing homes. The World Health Organization (2023) notes that abuse of older people is predicted to increase as a consequence of rapid population ageing. Policymakers and care providers must therefore be aware of this and develop strategic plans to identify and eliminate abuse of older adults in the community and in institutions to prevent the associated mental health deterioration.

Loneliness and social isolation amongst older adults remain significant risk factors for developing mental health conditions and deteriorating cognitive function. Mukku and co-workers (2018) carried out a review that found that continued employment or a planned schedule of voluntary work can promote mental health in older adults in India. Although the paper suggests that the effects of retirement may be culture-specific, there are a few studies from India which suggest lower self-esteem, low mood, physical health, and financial insecurity as mental health consequences of retirement. There is also evidence that mental health problems can increase on relocation to a care home. An Indian study (Gurappu et al., 2024) emphasises the need for staff in care homes to be better educated about caregiving skills to enable older adults to experience better social support and quality of life. Supporting group-based activities and encouraging contact with family members and friends help to reduce loneliness.

Alcohol remains a modifiable risk factor for both cognitive decline and depression in older adults. The Lancet Commission report (2020) recommends that drinking fewer than 21 units of alcohol per week reduce dementia risk. Notably, some other studies mentioned in this report suggest the threshold should be lower than that. The report also suggests that psychosocial interventions for alcohol use disorders are effective and helpful in preventing dementia and that these interventions should become more available. There is evidence that recovery from alcohol-related brain damage is possible, and therefore timely and effective early intervention for alcohol reduction is an important individual lifestyle change as well as being amenable to interventions at collective and governmental levels (Visontey et al., 2020).

Smoking remains another potentially modifiable risk factor for increased mental health problems in older adults, as it contributes to higher levels of isolation and loneliness (Philip et al., 2022). Smokers were more likely to be lonely and socially isolated and to have less contact with family and friends, which leads to an increased risk of mental health problems, including anxiety and depression.

6 Mental Health Promotion in Later Life

Mental health promotion and prevention are important across the life course and are at least as important for older adults as for those earlier in life. The aim is to support healthy ageing as far as possible, both for people who are regarded as healthy and for those who have physical and mental health challenges. Figure 1 shows an older adult at the centre of a number of different levels, illustrating that interventions/strategies can be planned and implemented at each level.

At an international and national level, strategies and interventions aim to support and create physical and social environments that nurture and support well-being,

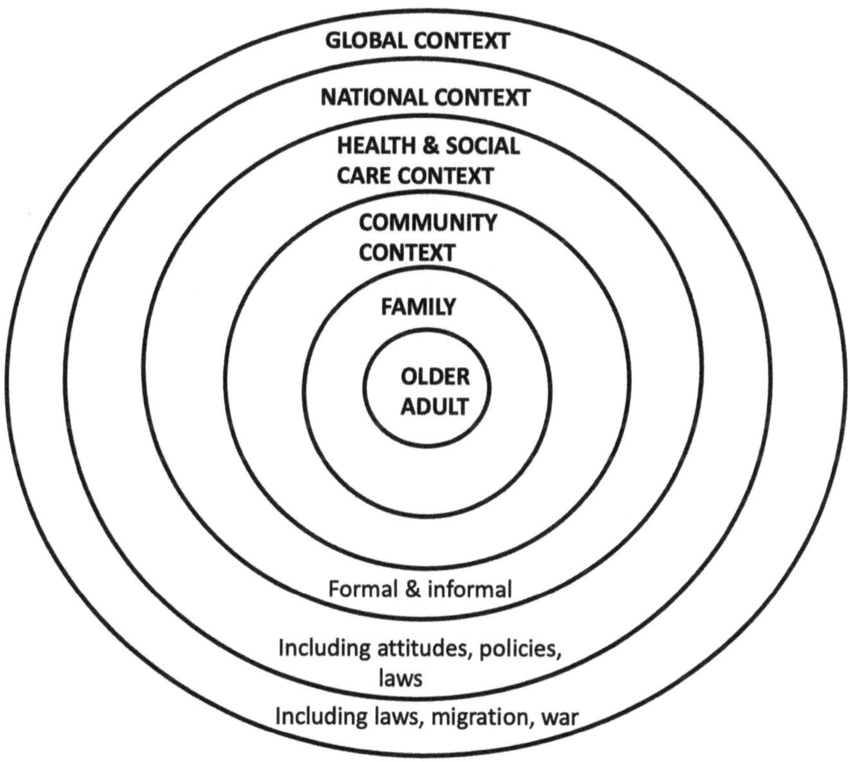

Fig. 1 The individual and their mental health shown at the centre of multiple levels of influence—Interventions to promote mental health can be designed for each, some, or all of these levels

enabling older people to make healthy choices in life and to do what is important to them and those close to them (irrespective of comorbidities and losses in capacity). Table 2 sets out national and international interventions that contribute to promoting mental well-being in later life. These are wide-ranging and, in general, promote both mental and physical health. They target policy-making at all levels, from changes involving international cooperation (such as decreasing air pollution across the globe) through measures to promote financial security for older adults and carers and changes in health and social care to eliminate ageism and stigma and better educate the workforce. At a societal level, this will include anti-discrimination policies and laws, educational interventions, and facilitating intergenerational activities. The fact that health promotion in older adults is not currently prioritised is likely to be the result of ageism at all the levels shown in Fig. 1; including both systemic ageism, which leads to a lack of health and well-being support and missed opportunities (Centre for Mental Health and Age UK, 2024), and internalised ageism, which may lead older adults to regard themselves and their peers as of lesser priority in terms of their health and lifestyles (Marques et al., 2020). The result is what the Centre for Mental Health and Age UK report describes as: "normalis(ing) poor mental health and prevent(ing) both help-seeking and offers of support". At an international and national level opportunities are missed in the planning of health services and prioritisation of resources.

Table 3 sets out interventions to promote mental well-being in later life at an individual, family and community level. Suragarn and co-workers (2021) highlight the importance of intergenerational and community-orientated approaches, particularly in mitigating social isolation and low mood and providing interest and stimulation. Example interventions include befriending initiatives, community and support groups, social skills training, creative arts groups, leisure and education services, and volunteering programmes. At the level of health and social care services and in their local community, older people are too often excluded from services and support that could help them to stay healthier and active for longer and to enjoy a happier later life. Within the family, and also for older individuals themselves, low expectations of health and activity may normalise poor mental health and the futility of seeking help. Interventions in all these areas are important to make a difference.

How changes are made will differ depending on context and available resources. Kafczyk and Hämel (2023) examined primary mental healthcare for older people in India and argue the case for comprehensive mental healthcare close to home (an argument that might be usefully made in higher income countries too). Some of the basic principles are family participation, community involvement at all levels, early access to care, respect for societal values, cultural sensitivity, and education. Integration of care services is an important aspiration: Kafczyk and Hämel (2023) address the important roles of community health workers in supporting family participation, encouraging early access to mental healthcare, and contributing to empowering communities, families, and older people through mental health education.

Palliyagaru et al. (2024) looked into six behavioural, metabolic, and environmental risk factors, which included low physical activity, tobacco use, alcohol use, obesity, hypertension, and air pollution. They also looked at three disease risk factors,

Table 2 Publications that support national and international level interventions

Author/s	Year	Country (focus/origin)	Type of publication	Recommendations drawn from the publication NOTE: these are the recommendations the authors draw from the papers
Age UK	2024	UK	Independent charity briefing document	• National Health Service & higher education to train up workforce—skills, knowledge, understanding • Organisations responsible for primary care services to relate service provision to prevalence data and involve older adults in service design • Adequate continuing funding for voluntary and community organisations supporting older adults' mental health • Increased sustainable research funding for this area
Ao et al.	2021	China	Research using data from the China Health and Retirement Longitudinal Study	• Measures to decrease ambient air pollution e.g. use of fossil fuels • Measures to decrease indoor pollution e.g. improving electricity and gas infrastructure, controls on cigarette smoking
Cations et al.	2019		Review	• Target poor educational attainment, low socio-economic status, heavy alcohol use, poor cardiovascular status to delay onset of dementia in under 65s
Deckers et al.	2024	The Netherlands	Research—1210 adults aged 60–79 with risk factors for cognitive decline	• Further research into multidomain lifestyle interventions in combination with nutritional products and/or pharmacological interventions • Public education regarding lifestyle factors related to cognitive decline • Improved management of cardio-vascular risk factors by health service providers

(continued)

Table 2 (continued)

Author/s	Year	Country (focus/origin)	Type of publication	Recommendations drawn from the publication NOTE: these are the recommendations the authors draw from the papers
Gurrapu et al.	2024	India	Research involving 40 residents of 4 care homes	• Policies to improve social engagement and prevent loneliness in care homes • Training of staff in care homes
Huang	2019	Taiwan	Analysis of World Values Survey dataset across 5 Asian societies	• Government policies to encourage older adults to volunteer, particularly active volunteering in self-help and cultural organisations
Kafczyk & Hamel	2023	India	Research article—analysis of interviews with stakeholders	• Tackle old age mental health stigmatisation (e.g. public education, information initiatives) • Develop age-appropriate care approaches • Provision of supportive services for communities/families, e.g. outreach community health workers • Financial support for carers
Kalaria et al.	2024	Low- and Middle-Income Countries	Symposium on dementia and brain ageing in low- and middle-income countries:	• Rethink a global approach to dementia • Population-level risk reduction strategies for dementia • Nutritional and psychosocial interventions to promote brain health • Improved professional and public education • Interventions to promote cardiovascular health • Resource health and social care services to meet population needs • Promote research in Low- and Middle-Income Countries
Kaur et al.	2019	India	Narrative review	• Public education regarding role of nutrition in late life mental health promotion • Availability of dietary supplements

(continued)

Table 2 (continued)

Author/s	Year	Country (focus/ origin)	Type of publication	Recommendations drawn from the publication NOTE: these are the recommendations the authors draw from the papers
Krell-Roesch et al.	2019	USA	A prospective cohort study	• Association between quantity and quality of mentally stimulating activities and a decreased risk of incident MCI
Kuo et al.	2005	USA	Research using data obtained from longitudinal study	• Policies to improve identification and management of high-risk patients with diabetes and hypertension to help prevent or delay the development of cognitive and functional decline
Lancet Commission	2020		Evidence-based report on dementia prevention and care	• Policies to improve treatment of hypertension (all ages) • Policies to reduce hearing loss by protecting ears from excessive noise exposure (all ages) • Policies to reduce exposure to air pollution and second-hand tobacco smoke (all ages) • Policies to prevent head injury (e.g. in sports such as football, boxing (all ages)) • Policies/programmes to reduce alcohol use • Policies/programmes to reduce smoking/prevent smoking uptake • Provide all children with primary and secondary education • Programmes to reduce obesity (and hence diabetes) • Programmes to encourage physical activity (all ages)

(continued)

Table 2 (continued)

Author/s	Year	Country (focus/ origin)	Type of publication	Recommendations drawn from the publication NOTE: these are the recommendations the authors draw from the papers
Liu et al.	2021	USA	Multicentre, randomised controlled trial	• The MIND dietary pattern is tailored for brain health by targeting the intake of food components that reflect scientific findings linking nutrition and dementia • Limiting the intake of foods that are unhealthy for the brain
Philip et al.	2022	UK	Cohort study	• Policies to improve psychoeducation on smoking to prevent poor health and premature mortality via well-known direct and indirect tobacco-related pathways, but also to decrease social isolation and loneliness
Marchand and Jensen	2017	BOSTON USA	Dietary patterns and Cognitive health—A review of the literature	• Healthy dietary patterns, including a variety of fruits and vegetables, whole grains, and fish/seafood and avoiding red and processed meats and sweets • The Mediterranean Diet has been shown to be beneficial in maintaining cognitive health and in preventing cognitive decline, including MCI and AD
Mukku et al.	2018	India	Literature review	• Social security measures • Retirement planning • Planned schedule of activities post-retirement including voluntary work
Taylor-Rowan et al.	2022	UK	Prospective and retrospective longitudinal cohort and case-control observational studies	• Caution when prescribing anticholinergic medications in a cognitively impaired population due to higher risk of mortality for people with a high anticholinergic burden

(continued)

Table 2 (continued)

Author/s	Year	Country (focus/origin)	Type of publication	Recommendations drawn from the publication NOTE: these are the recommendations the authors draw from the papers
US Federal guidelines		USA		• All adults at least 150 min physical activity/week (all ages)
Vishwakarma et al.	2023	India	Review	• Improve financial support to elders/social security • Put in place measures to combat abuse and abandonment of elders • Availability of counselling • Public education regarding obesity and exercise • Relevant screening to improve physical health • Expand geriatric psychiatry
Visontay et al.	2020	n/a	Review	• Importance of timely and effective early intervention as recovery from Alcohol-related brain damage is possible • Substitution of parenteral thiamine is a well-established treatment in Wernicke-Korsakoff syndrome • Thiamine may have a role in preventing the incidence of dementia in those with alcohol use disorders

(continued)

Table 2 (continued)

Author/s	Year	Country (focus/origin)	Type of publication	Recommendations drawn from the publication NOTE: these are the recommendations the authors draw from the papers
World Health Organization	2023	n/a	Online Factsheet	• Measures to decrease the financial insecurity of older adults • Action to ensure safe accessible housing, public buildings, and transport for older adults • Social support for older adults and carers • Policies to discourage/decrease smoking (all ages) • Policies to reduce alcohol use (all ages) • Programmes to encourage physical activity in later life • Programmes to support vulnerable/at-risk groups in later life • Programmes to support good nutrition in later life/those at-risk

(continued)

Table 2 (continued)

Author/s	Year	Country (focus/ origin)	Type of publication	Recommendations drawn from the publication NOTE: these are the recommendations the authors draw from the papers
Yaffe et al.	2021	USA	A Pooled Cohort Study	• Policies to decrease increasing trends in diabetes and obesity even in early adulthood due to significant public health implications for cognitive health • Young adulthood represents a time for intervention and an opportunity for widespread public health education regarding the importance of heart health to brain health
Yon et al.	2017	UK	Meta-analysis	• The health sector has an important role to prevent, raise awareness of, and provide evidence-based guidance for healthcare practitioners to respond to elder abuse, particularly on psychological and financial abuse, which are more prevalent • Investment in developing and assessing elder abuse interventions must be a public health priority to help to reduce the effect of elderly abuse worldwide

namely diabetes mellitus, depression, and hearing loss. They concluded that, although research priorities identified are focused on prevention, reduction of dementia risk, delivery and quality of life, and care for people with dementia and their caregivers, the South Asian region appears to lack policies and protocols owing to poor prioritisation of dementia as a public health concern.

One of the difficulties in planning a comprehensive health promotion strategy for older adults is that much of the existing research has been carried out in the context of developed economies. The principles of effective strategies can however be extrapolated to low- and middle-income countries and used to tailor strategies to that particular area whilst more research is needed to add to the knowledge base.

Table 3 Publications that support individual, family, and community-level interventions

Author/s	Year	Country (if applicable)	Type of publication	Recommendations drawn from the publication NOTE: These are the recommendations the authors draw from the papers
Deckers et al.	2024	The Netherlands	Research—1210 adults aged 60–79 with risk factors for cognitive decline	• Lifestyle changes may prevent or slow cognitive decline including: exercise, cognitive training, advice regarding sleep, nutrition and stress management and social activities
Dodge et al.	2023	USA	Research involving 186 participants aged 75 and older	• Regular online conversations were found to improve cognitive function
Gurrapu et al.	2024	India	Research involving 40 residents of 4 care homes	• Family education on the importance of continued engagement with elders who move into care homes
Huang	2019	Taiwan	Analysis of the World Values Survey dataset across 5 Asian societies	• Educate families and individuals about the benefits of volunteering
Krell-Roesch et al.	2019	USA	A prospective cohort study	• Engaging in a higher number of activities, particularly in late life, appears to be more strongly associated with a decreased risk of incident MCI as compared to engaging in only 1 or 2 activities
Kafczyk & Hamel	2023	India	Research article—analysis of interviews with stakeholders	• Encourage families to seek help/access services

(continued)

Table 3 (continued)

Author/s	Year	Country (if applicable)	Type of publication	Recommendations drawn from the publication NOTE: These are the recommendations the authors draw from the papers
Kiely et al.	2013	Australia	Research analysis of longitudinal data from 1611 people aged 65–103	• Improve access to visual and auditory aids • Educate and encourage people in use of aids
Mazumder et al.	2023	Bangladesh	Scoping review of mental health interventions	• Beneficial interventions for older adult mental health were: • Meditative movement • Behavioural/ occupational/ learning-based interventions • Technology-based interventions • Music therapy • "New healthcare" initiatives
Mukku et al.	2018	India	Literature review	• Public education regarding the value of engaging in activities including voluntary work post-retirement

(continued)

Table 3 (continued)

Author/s	Year	Country (if applicable)	Type of publication	Recommendations drawn from the publication NOTE: These are the recommendations the authors draw from the papers
Park et al.	2013	USA	Research involving 259 participants aged 60–90	• Engagement in "novel cognitively challenging activities" improved memory
Suragarn et al.	2021	Thailand/USA	Literature review	• Methods of enhancing social connection and mitigating social isolation amongst older adults: o Intergenerational connections o Ageing-friendly communities o Community-based group physical activities o Use of technology to connect with others

7 What Can We Do?—Individuals, Communities, and Governments

In the UK, Age UK commissioned the Centre for Mental Health (2024) to explore evidence relating to mental health in later life. The resulting report shows the pressing need to challenge ageism relating to mental health in any healthcare system. It acknowledges the importance of identifying the risk factors which contribute to deteriorating mental health and combatting stigma and ageism in society to promote better mental health in older adults. Older people have strengths and can contribute significantly, psychologically, physically, and financially to society. It is, therefore, important to work collaboratively with older adults to tackle discrimination and educate on modifiable risk factors to boost mental and physical health. Many of the recommendations suggested by the report are relevant, not just to the UK, but worldwide, particularly in South Asian countries. The report highlights the need to tackle ageism and discrimination both at an individual level and in the development of appropriate health and care systems. It also shows the lack of national strategy or blueprint in the UK and across the globe to prevent mental ill health in later life. It is important to acknowledge the complex interaction of physical and mental health, and promoting both will help promote mental health and well-being for those in later life. This will involve person-centred and holistic approaches to mental health so that no one's needs are overlooked or inadequately met: the principles of holistic care and prevention are applicable generally to all countries, irrespective of culture and language. There is no one-size-fits-all model for promoting mental health in later life. Prevention of mental ill health in late life involves acknowledging that older adults have an important role to play in society and that having meaningful roles and opportunities is beneficial for both older adults' mental and physical health and for society as a whole. Positive social connections, including face-to-face contact and safe supportive networks, can boost mental health but may also help in the early identification of risks, including the risk of elder abuse. There are myths about older adults and digital technology, and the use of such technology could enhance positive connections.

An Indian review paper highlights the high morbidity and mortality rates associated with depression, particularly in older adults: Vishwakarma and co-workers (2023) pointed out that they found no precise guidelines in India for routine screening for depression and suggested that the Government of India should launch several measures to improve the health of older people. The National Programme for Health Care of the Senior is mentioned as a relatively new initiative, which combined two previous strategies, the Maintenance and Welfare of Parents and Senior Citizens Act and the National Policy on Older Persons. These included free and exclusive senior-only medical facilities provided by the public health delivery system and other preventive, promotional, and curative treatment interventions. Although in India, the Parents and Senior Citizens Act 2007 is in place, older people may still be abandoned, so strict and mandatory sentences are necessary for those who abuse and abandon older people. Hence, some policies and strategies are already in place, but more focus is needed on preventative measures, and policies need to be developed around identified modifiable risk factors.

In 2022, a symposium was held on dementia and brain ageing in low- and middle-income countries (Kalaria et al., 2024). This symposium noted that two-thirds of persons with dementia live in low- and middle-income countries, yet research and costs are skewed towards high-income countries. Dementia prevalence will double in low- and middle-income countries where socio-economic disparities are high, and this will have a significant effect on the mental health of older adults. A multi-faceted approach is needed, including designing and promoting national dementia plans to address the challenges in low- and middle-income countries.

Air pollution remains an important modifiable risk factor for cognitive decline and policies are needed to reduce air pollution in South Asian countries. Alongside this public health measures for early identification of physical illnesses such as hypertension, diabetes, obesity are vital, as all of these have an effect on cognition and mental health. Regular hearing and vision check-ups in older adults are essential and could be supported by government initiatives and individual effort: the public health message for this age group must be that individuals and families should be aware of the consequences of dual sensory loss.

Social contact, positive connections, and acknowledging the role of older adults in society are all positive boosts to mental health in older adults. In addition, some older adults have caring responsibilities which may be a risk factor for poor mental health. There is therefore a need to acknowledge those in a caring role and provide adequate education and support, both on an individual basis and from a public health perspective. Huang (2019) highlighted the association of volunteering with the well-being of older people in rapidly ageing Asian societies. Huang's study not only identifies the types of volunteer work that most effectively enhance the well-being of older adults but suggests that volunteer work might help the transition to retirement and older age with better well-being, as well as helping ageing societies alleviate their labour shortage problems by involving productive older people.

8 Where Next?

This chapter covers evidence and strategies for interventions in older adults to prevent and reduce mental health problems, including cognitive issues. It is clear that there is a complex mix of physical, mental, and psychological issues which may contribute to mental health and cognitive problems in older adults and that there are modifiable factors which need to be considered, sometimes much earlier in life, to prevent decline at a later stage. Unfortunately, most evidence for prevention and potential interventions rely on work done in high-income countries, and more South Asian research is needed. Although the message is similar for all the South Asian countries, it needs to be interpreted in the context of the culture, language, and religious characteristics of that region. Nevertheless, some broad conclusions can be drawn.

We identified biological, psychological, and social factors and evidence and strategies to modify risks. Risk modification is multi-tiered at individual, collective, public health, and governmental levels. Palliyaguru et al. (2024) found that there are very few resources dedicated to dementia care and research in South Asia, in spite of the high burden of dementia in some of the countries; hence, policies and protocols need to be developed to address the known modifiable risk factors and prevent dementias. The authors also highlight the lack of good quality data needed to inform healthcare service development in these countries and that underdiagnosis and/or underreporting remains a challenge.

Biological risk factors, including controlling diabetes and managing hypertension, are factors which need individual involvement, healthcare services, and public health initiatives. Psychoeducation on diabetes and hypertension is important for the individual, however, effective public health programmes through health centres, with routine monitoring of blood pressure and blood sugar, require governmental initiatives if the health of the general population is to improve. Nutrition and lifestyle modification are important factors: healthy diet, physical exercise, and smoking cessation are all modifiable risk factors and need to be targeted by government and public health measures. At the same time, evidence argues that targeting one risk factor in isolation is unlikely to be sufficient: risk factors are interlinked, and programmes and policies need to target several together if population health is to improve.

Alcohol consumption is another biological risk factor and related to socio-economic status as well as mental health. Evidence shows that excess alcohol use causes mental health and cognitive issues (Visontay et al., 2020). Knodel and Pothisiri (2021) carried out a comparative analysis of smoking and drinking behaviours in older adults in three South Asian countries and suggest successful reduction in smoking and alcohol can be achieved by antidrinking and other relevant campaigns. Limiting the availability of alcohol and tobacco, perhaps by higher pricing and public education to prevent early use, are public health initiatives by which governments may reduce alcohol and tobacco consumption and thereby improve mental health.

Interestingly, air pollution has been found to be a significant risk factor in poor mental health and poor physical health, which itself can impact mental health (Ao et al., 2021). A recent paper by Shaw et al. (2024) based in India implies particular policy implications for India with regard to indoor air pollution. It suggests that India has some of the highest global burden of disease attributable to air pollution and that indoor air pollution is a relatively unaddressed but important factor: a significant number of the population, especially in the North, East, and North Eastern parts of India, use unhealthy cooking fuels, burn various household products, and smoke tobacco. This risk factor clearly needs global and individual government initiatives to reduce air pollution. Many South Asian countries are seeking solutions and have set targets to achieve National Ambient Air quality standards. India, for example, has a National Clean Air programme, which involves targets to address this issue.

Psychosocial risk factors such as loneliness, social isolation, and elder abuse all need interventions at several levels if mental health is to improve in future. The starting point is raising awareness around ageism and age discrimination, emphasising dignity and how older adults contribute to society. Most older adults continue to have roles where they contribute to society emotionally, financially, and sometimes in the form of active engagement in employment or volunteering. Retirement brings consequences such as loss of role, which may contribute to poorer mental health. Communities and governments need to eliminate ageism and discrimination in societies and continue to encourage older adults to have meaningful roles within their communities.

Public education on the mental health consequences of loneliness and isolation is essential if the mental health of older adults is to improve. Elder abuse remains a significant problem, often hidden and something that individuals, families and society are embarrassed to acknowledge. However, it is common, and carers, attendants, and the general public require education to identify and prevent it. Most South Asian countries have significant older populations, but, although previously a value-based system respected older family members, societal changes have led to nuclear families, with little contact or support for older adults: this may be contributing to psychological and financial abuse. The role of governments is to have stringent legislation to identify and punish those committing these kinds of abuses. Such abuse has significant impacts on mental health, and a society which supports older adults to live free from abuse will have better outcomes.

Mujahid and Siddhisena (2009) make several overarching recommendations including good quality and relevant data collection; social and welfare support; encouraging easy access to community-based care especially both physical and mental healthcare; dispelling myths and misconceptions about the older population;

recognising older adults' contribution to society, and promoting respect for older generations. Poverty, available and accessible healthcare, supportive community-based care, and gainful employment for older adults are additional potentially modifiable factors which impact on both physical and mental health of older adults. These are all interrelated and promote both mental health and physical health in older adults, preventing mental illness in older adults.

9 Conclusions

The starting point for any strategy for prevention of mental illness in older adults should be in eliminating ageism and discrimination in society, since it has a significant effect on mental health in older adults in a variety of ways. A generic systematic review of prevalence of mental disorders in South Asia (Naveed et al., 2020) suggests that although there is a high burden of mental disorders in these countries, challenges remain with regard to associated stigma and underreporting or under-identification of such disorders. Mental health is not always a health priority in these countries and hence there is under-utilisation coupled with poor availability of mental health services. This predicts a higher need for multi-level multi-pronged interventions engaging local, national, regional, and international stakeholders. Individuals, communities, and governments all have roles in supporting and developing strategies to prevent mental health and cognition in older adults from deteriorating. To improve the mental health of the older population multi-tiered approaches will be necessary, targeting a number of potentially modifiable risk factors.

References

Ao, C.-K., Dong, Y., & Kuo, P.-F. (2021). Industrialization, indoor and ambient air quality, and elderly mental health. *China Economic Review, 69*(69), Article 101676. https://doi.org/10.1016/j.chieco.2021.101676

Banerjee, D., Rabheru, K., Ivbijaro, G., & Mendonca Lima, C. A. de. (2021). Dignity of Older Persons with Mental Health Conditions: Why Should Clinicians Care? *Frontiers in Psychiatry, 12*(1). https://doi.org/10.3389/fpsyt.2021.774533

Barnes, L. L., Klodian Dhana, Liu, X., Carey, V. J., Ventrelle, J., Johnson, K., Hollings, C. S., Bishop, L., Laranjo, N., Stubbs, B. J., Reilly, X., Agarwal, P., Zhang, S., Grodstein, F., Tangney, C. C., Holland, T. M., Aggarwal, N. T., Konstantinos Arfanakis, Martha Clare Morris, & Sacks, F. M. (2023). Trial of the MIND Diet for Prevention of Cognitive Decline in Older Persons. *The New England Journal of Medicine, 389*(7). https://doi.org/10.1056/nejmoa2302368

Cations, M., Withall, A., & Draper, B. (2019). Modifiable risk factors for young onset dementia. *Current Opinion in Psychiatry, 32*(2), 138–143. https://doi.org/10.1097/yco.0000000000000475

CDC. (2024, April 19). *What You Can Do to Meet Physical Activity Recommendations*. Physical Activity Basics. https://www.cdc.gov/physical-activity-basics/guidelines/index.html

Deckers, K., Zwan, M. D., Soons, L. M., Waterink, L., Beers, S., Sofie van Houdt, Berrit Stiensma, Kwant, J. Z., Sophie, Rachel, Jurgen, Oosterman, J. M., de, A., van, Yannick Vermeiren, Oude,

R. C., Smidt, N., Broersen, L. M., Sietske A. M. Sikkes, & Aarts, E. (2024). A multidomain lifestyle intervention to maintain optimal cognitive functioning in Dutch older adults—Study design and baseline characteristics of the FINGER-NL randomized controlled trial. *Alzheimer's Research & Therapy, 16*(1). https://doi.org/10.1186/s13195-024-01495-8

Dodge, H. H., Yu, K., Wu, C.-Y., Pruitt, P. J., Asgari, M., Kaye, J. A., ... & Ellis, A. (2023). Internet-Based conversational engagement randomized controlled clinical trial (I-CONECT) among socially isolated adults 75+ years old with normal cognition or mild cognitive impairment: Topline results. *The Gerontologist, 64*(4). https://doi.org/10.1093/geront/gnad147

Edwards, N., Walker, S., Paddick, S.-M., Prina, A. M., Chinnasamy, M., Reddy, N., Mboya, I. B., Mtei, M., Varghese, M., Nakkasuja, N., Guerra, M., Sapkota, N., & Dotchin, C. (2023). Prevalence of depression and anxiety in older people in low- and middle- income countries in Africa, Asia and South America: A systematic review and meta-analysis. *Journal of Affective Disorders, 325*(325), 656–674. https://doi.org/10.1016/j.jad.2023.01.068

Foresight Mental Capital and Wellbeing Project (2008). *Final Project report*. The Government Office for Science, London. Retrieved December 5, 2024, https://assets.publishing.service.gov.uk/media/5a7c59eced915d6969f44488/mental-capital-wellbeing-report.pdf

Fox, C., Smith, T., Maidment, I., Chan, W.-Y., Bua, N., Myint, P. K., Boustani, M., Kwok, C. S., Glover, M., Koopmans, I., & Campbell, N. (2014). Effect of medications with anti-cholinergic properties on cognitive function, delirium, physical function and mortality: A systematic review. *Age and Ageing, 43*(5), 604–615. https://doi.org/10.1093/ageing/afu096

Government Office for Science, London. (2008). *Mental Capital and Wellbeing: Making the most of ourselves in the 21st century Final Project Report*. https://assets.publishing.service.gov.uk/media/5a7c59eced915d6969f44488/mental-capital-wellbeing-report.pdf

Gurrapu, R., Ammapattian, T., & Antony, S. (2024). Perceived social support, loneliness, and depression among elderly living in old-age homes. *Journal of Family Medicine and Primary Care, 13*(3), 864–868. https://doi.org/10.4103/jfmpc.jfmpc_799_23

Huang, L.-H. (2019). Well-being and volunteering: Evidence from aging societies in Asia. *Social Science & Medicine, 229*, 172–180. https://doi.org/10.1016/j.socscimed.2018.09.004

Harbottle, L. (2019). The effect of nutrition on older people's mental health. *British Journal of Community Nursing, 24*(Sup7), S12–S16.

Hossain, M. M., Purohit, N., Sultana, A., Ma, P., McKyer, E. L. J., & Ahmed, H. U. (2020 June). Prevalence of mental disorders in South Asia: An umbrella review of systematic reviews and meta-analyses. *Asian Journal of Psychiatry, 51*, Article 102041. https://doi.org/10.1016/j.ajp.2020.102041

Huang, L. H. (2019 May). Well-being and volunteering: Evidence from aging societies in Asia. *Social Science and Medicine, 229*, 172–180. https://doi.org/10.1016/j.socscimed.2018.09.004

Iskander-Reynolds, A. (2024). *Mental health in later life understanding needs, policies and services in England*. https://www.centreformentalhealth.org.uk/wp-content/uploads/2024/03/CentreforMH_MentalHealthInLaterLife-1.pdf

Islam, B., Li, T., Xu, M., Yang, D., Lv, H., Gassara, G., Ibrahim, T. I., Radman, B. A., & Wang, J. (2024). Emerging trends in cognitive impairment and dementia among older populations in Asia: A systematic review. *Journal of Global Health, 14*, 04233.

Kafczyk, T., & Hämel, K. (2023). Primary mental healthcare for older people in India: Between stigmatization and community orientation. *Discover Mental Health, 3*(1), 14. https://doi.org/10.1007/s44192-023-00040-7

Kalaria, R., Maestre, G., Mahinrad, S., Acosta, D. M., Akinyemi, R. O., Alladi, S., … & Ismail, O. (2024). The 2022 symposium on dementia and brain aging in low- and middle-income countries: Highlights on research, diagnosis, care, and impact. *Alzheimer's & Dementia: The Journal of the Alzheimer's Association, 20*(6), 4290–4314. https://doi.org/10.1002/alz.13836

Kaur, D., Rasane, P., Singh, J., Kaur, S., Kumar, V., Mahato, D. K., Dey, A., Dhawan, K., & Kumar, S. (2019). Nutritional interventions for elderly and considerations for the development of geriatric foods. *Current Aging Science, 12*(1), 15–27. https://doi.org/10.2174/18746098126661905211 10548

Kiely, K. M., Anstey, K. J., & Luszcz, M. A. (2013). Dual Sensory Loss and Depressive Symptoms: The Importance of Hearing, Daily Functioning, and Activity Engagement. *Frontiers in Human Neuroscience, 7*. https://doi.org/10.3389/fnhum.2013.00837

Knodel, J., & Pothisiri, W. (2021). Smoking and drinking behaviors among older adults: A comparative analysis of three Southeast Asian countries. *Journal of Cross-Cultural Gerontology, 36*(4), 369–386.

Krell-Roesch, J., Syrjanen, J. A., Vassilaki, M., Machulda, M. M., Mielke, M. M., Knopman, D. S., Kremers, W. K., Petersen, R. C., & Geda, Y. E. (2019). Quantity and quality of mental activities and the risk of incident mild cognitive impairment. *Neurology, 93*(6), e548–e558. https://doi.org/10.1212/wnl.0000000000007897

Kuo, H.-K., Jones, R. N., Milberg, W. P., Tennstedt, S., Talbot, L., Morris, J. N., & Lipsitz, L. A. (2005). Effect of Blood Pressure and Diabetes Mellitus on Cognitive and Physical Functions in Older Adults: A Longitudinal Analysis of the Advanced Cognitive Training for Independent and Vital Elderly Cohort. *Journal of the American Geriatrics Society, 53*(7), 1154–1161. https://doi.org/10.1111/j.1532-5415.2005.53368.x

Liu, X., Morris, M. C., Dhana, K., Ventrelle, J., Johnson, K., Bishop, L., Hollings, C. S., Boulin, A., Laranjo, N., Stubbs, B. J., Reilly, X., Carey, V. J., Wang, Y., Furtado, J. D., Marcovina, S. M., Tangney, C., Aggarwal, N. T., Arfanakis, K., Sacks, F. M., & Barnes, L. L. (2021). Mediterranean-DASH Intervention for Neurodegenerative Delay (MIND) study: Rationale, design and baseline characteristics of a randomized control trial of the MIND diet on cognitive decline. *Contemporary Clinical Trials, 102*(102), Article 106270. https://doi.org/10.1016/j.cct.2021.106270

Livingston, G., Huntley, J., Liu, K. Y., Costafreda, S. G., Selbæk, G., Alladi, S., Ames, D., Banerjee, S., Burns, A., Brayne, C., Fox, N. C., Ferri, C. P., Gitlin, L. N., Howard, R., Kales, H. C., Kivimäki, M., Larson, E. B., Nakasujja, N., Rockwood, K., … Mukadam, N. (2024). Dementia prevention, intervention, and care: 2024 report of the Lancet standing Commission. *Lancet (London, England), 404*(10452), 572–628. https://doi.org/10.1016/S0140-6736(24)01296-0

Livingston, G., Huntley, J., Sommerlad, A., Ames, D., Ballard, C., Banerjee, S., Brayne, C., Burns, A., Cohen-Mansfield, J., Cooper, C., Costafreda, S. G., Dias, A., Fox, N., Gitlin, L. N., Howard, R., Kales, H. C., Kivimäki, M., Larson, E. B., Ogunniyi, A., & Orgeta, V. (2020). Dementia prevention, intervention, and care: 2020 report of the lancet commission. *The Lancet, 396*(10248), 413–446. https://doi.org/10.1016/S0140-6736(20)30367-6

Ma, Y., Ajnakina, O., Steptoe, A., & Cadar, D. (2020). Higher risk of dementia in English older individuals who are overweight or obese. *International Journal of Epidemiology*, *49*(4). https://doi.org/10.1093/ije/dyaa099

Marchand, N. E., & Jensen, M. K. (2017). The role of dietary and lifestyle factors in maintaining cognitive health. *American Journal of Lifestyle Medicine, 12*(4), 268–285. https://doi.org/10.1177/1559827617701066

Marques, S., Mariano, J., Mendonça, J., De Tavernier, W., Hess, M., Naegele, L., Peixeiro, F., & Martins, D. (2020). Determinants of ageism against older adults: A systematic review. *International Journal of Environmental Research and Public Health, 17*(7), 2560. https://doi.org/10.3390/ijerph17072560

Mazumder, H., Faizah, F., Gain, E. P., Sharmin Eva, I., Ferdouse Mou, K., Saha, N., Rahman, F., Das, J., Islam, A. M. K., Nesa, F., & Hossain, M. M. (2023). Effectiveness of mental health interventions for older adults in South Asia: A scoping review. *PLoS ONE, 18*(7), Article e0287883. https://doi.org/10.1371/journal.pone.0287883

Mujahid G, Siddhisena K.A.P. (2009). Demographic Prognosis For South Asia: A future of rapid ageing. South_ Asia.pdf. Last Accessed December 16, 2024.

Mukku, S. S. R., Harbishettar, V., & Sivakumar, P. T. (2018). Psychological morbidity after job retirement: A review. *Asian Journal of Psychiatry, 37*, 58–63. https://doi.org/10.1016/j.ajp.2018.08.003

Naveed, S., Waqas, A., Chaudhary, A. M. D., Kumar, S., Abbas, N., Amin, R., Jamil, N., & Saleem, S. (2020). Prevalence of common mental disorders in South Asia: A systematic review and meta-regression analysis. *Frontiers in Psychiatry, 11*, Article 573150.

Office of disease prevention and health promotion. (2020). *Current Dietary Guidelines | odphp.health.gov*. Health.gov. https://odphp.health.gov/our-work/nutrition-physical-activity/dietary-guidelines/current-dietary-guidelines

Pandey, N., Tiwari, S., & Singh, I. (2012). Mental health problems among inhabitants of old age homes: A preliminary study. *Indian Journal of Psychiatry, 54*(2), 144. https://doi.org/10.4103/0019-5545.99533

Park, D. C., Lodi-Smith, J., Drew, L., Haber, S., Hebrank, A., Bischof, G. N., & Aamodt, W. (2013). The impact of sustained engagement on cognitive function in older adults. *Psychological Science, 25*(1), 103–112. https://doi.org/10.1177/0956797613499592

Palliyaguru, D. L., Palliyaguru, N., Texiera, C. V. L., Armstrong, N. M., Liyanage, S., Senarath, U., Arambepola, C., Jayasinghe, S., Dalpatadu, C- la. (2024). Status, determinants and risk factors of all cause dementia in South Asia: Findings from a preliminary analysis of global health data. medRxiv 2024.03.06. 24303854: https://doi.org/10.1101/2024.03.06.24303854

Philip, K. E., Bu, F., Polkey, M. I., Brown, J., Steptoe, A., Hopkinson, N. S., & Fancourt, D. (2022). Relationship of smoking with current and future social isolation and loneliness: 12-year follow-up of older adults in England. *The Lancet Regional Health—Europe, 14*(14), Article 100302. https://doi.org/10.1016/j.lanepe.2021.100302

Ravindranath, V., & Sundarakumar, J. S. (2021). Changing demography and the challenge of dementia in India. *Nature Reviews. Neurology, 17*, 747–758.

Shaw, S., Kundu, S., Chattopadhyay, A., et al. (2024). Indoor air pollution and cognitive function among older adults in India: A multiple mediation approach through depression and sleep disorders. *BMC Geriatrics, 24*, 81.

Suragarn, U., Hain, D., & Pfaff, G. (2021). Approaches to enhance social connection in older adults: An integrative review of literature. *Aging and Health Research, 1*(3). https://doi.org/10.1016/j.ahr.2021.100029

Taylor-Rowan, M., Kraia, O., Kolliopoulou, C., Noel-Storr, A. H., Alharthi, A. A., Cross, A. J., Stewart, C., Myint, P. K., McCleery, J., & Quinn, T. J. (2022). Anticholinergic burden for prediction of cognitive decline or neuropsychiatric symptoms in older adults with mild cognitive impairment or dementia. *Cochrane Database of Systematic Reviews, 2022*(8). https://doi.org/10.1002/14651858.cd015196.pub2

Tiwari, S. C., Pandey, N. M., & Singh, I. (2012 April). Mental health problems among inhabitants of old age homes: A preliminary study. *Indian J Psychiatry., 54*(2), 144–148.

US Centers for Disease Control and Prevention. (2024). *What you can do to meet physical activity recommendations*. Retrieved from December 5, 2024, https://www.cdc.gov/physical-activity-basics/guidelines/index.html

Visontay, R., Rao, R. T., & Mewton, L. (2020). Alcohol use and dementia. *Current Opinion in Psychiatry, Publish Ahead of Print*. https://doi.org/10.1097/yco.0000000000000679

Vishwakarma, D., Gaidhane, A., & Bhoi, S. R. (2023). Depression and Its Associated Factors Among the Elderly Population in India: A Review. *Cureus, 15*(6). https://doi.org/10.7759/cureus.41013

World Health Organisation. (2017, December 7). *Global action plan on the public health response to dementia 2017–2025*. https://www.who.int/publications/i/item/global-action-plan-on-the-public-health-response-to-dementia-2017---2025

World Health Organisation. (2023a, March 15). *Dementia*. World Health Organization. https://www.who.int/news-room/fact-sheets/detail/dementia

World health Organisation. (2023b, October 20). *Mental health of older adults*. https://www.who.int/news-room/fact-sheets/mental-health-of-older-adults

World Health Organization. (2019). *Risk reduction of cognitive decline and dementia: WHO guidelines*. https://www.who.int/publications/i/item/risk-reduction-of-cognitive-decline-and-dementia

World Health Organization. (2024a, August 7). *The top 10 causes of death*. World Health Organization; World Health Organization. https://www.who.int/news-room/fact-sheets/detail/the-top-10-causes-of-death

World Health Organization. (2024b, October 1). *Ageing and Health*. World Health Organization. https://www.who.int/news-room/fact-sheets/detail/ageing-and-health

Yaffe, K., Vittinghoff, E., Hoang, T., Matthews, K., Golden, S. H., & Hazzouri, A. Z. A. (2021). Cardiovascular risk factors across the life course and cognitive decline: A pooled cohort study. *Neurology, 96*(17), e2212–e2219. https://doi.org/10.1212/WNL.0000000000011747

Yon, Y., Mikton, C. R., Gassoumis, Z. D., & Wilber, K. H. (2017). Elder abuse prevalence in community settings: A systematic review and meta-analysis. *The Lancet Global Health, 5*(2), e147–e156. https://doi.org/10.1016/s2214-109x(17)30006-2

Zhou, Y. F., Song, X. Y., Pan, A., & Koh, W. P. (2023). Nutrition and healthy ageing in Asia: A systematic review. *Nutrients, 15*(14), 3153.

Policies, Programs, and Action Plans in Geriatric Mental Health in South Asia

Nilamadhab Kar, Sanhita Bhattacharya, and Shreyan Kar

Abstract Matching with the growing population of older adults in South Asian countries, the number of people having health-related problems, including mental illnesses, needing medical treatment, care, and support is increasing. Depression and dementia are common concerns, along with suicide. Financial problems, high cost of care, lack of support, lack of availability of appropriate professional care, and struggles associated with informal family caregiving are some of the contributing factors. The increased need for old-age mental healthcare is well reported, and countries have developed various policies, and programs to support older adults, along with different laws to protect their interests. However, the gaps in the needs and available supportive facilities are obvious and the specific support for the mental health-related concerns of older adults is minuscule in most areas. Lack of appropriate resources, manpower, and training are obvious reasons, which need to be addressed as a priority by the countries, to avoid the situation becoming a crisis.

Keywords Older adults · Geriatric health service · Geriatric nursing · Mental health · Geriatric psychiatry · Health planning · Legislation

---

N. Kar (✉) · S. Bhattacharya · S. Kar
Department of Psychiatry, Black Country Healthcare NHS Foundation Trust, Wolverhampton, UK
e-mail: n.kar@nhs.net

N. Kar
Research Institute in Health Sciences, University of Wolverhampton, Wolverhampton, UK

Faculty of Contemplative and Behavioural Sciences, Sri Sri University, Govindpur, India

N. Kar et al. (eds.), *Geriatric Psychiatry in South Asia*, South Asian Perspectives in Mental Health and Psychology , https://doi.org/10.1007/978-981-96-7469-5_12

1 Introduction

Countries in South Asia, namely Afghanistan, Bangladesh, Bhutan, India, Maldives, Nepal, Pakistan, and Sri Lanka, have been experiencing an increase in the population of older adults for many years at an unprecedented rate, bringing forth complex challenges related to geriatric mental health. Old age is associated with higher morbidity and care needs. Besides health, economic, family, interpersonal, and social factors become different with changing dynamics in old age. Issues of loneliness, lack of social interaction, bereavement, poor healthcare access, elder abuse, and caregiving issues gain prominence. In addition, various old age-related illnesses lead to frailty and an increased need for specialist care, which often is not available in developing economies. With countries in the region at varying levels of economic development and healthcare infrastructure, the need for targeted policies, programs, and action plans to support older adults has never been more pressing.

This chapter explores the current landscape of geriatric mental health initiatives across South Asia, highlighting national strategies, government policies, financial support mechanisms, and legal frameworks in place to address the mental well-being of older adults. It examines how different nations are responding to the unique needs of their ageing populations. Although the information on specific focus on old-age mental health services in many countries is meagre, we have tried to provide other supportive services that would suggest the level of preparedness with various concerns affecting the mental health of older adults.

While some countries have established robust healthcare policies and financial assistance programs, others face significant barriers due to political instability, resource constraints, or deeply rooted sociocultural factors. The analysis presented in this chapter underscores the importance of multi-sectoral collaboration, evidence-based policymaking, and sustainable action plans to ensure that older adults receive the care, dignity, and support they deserve. By presenting different national approaches, identifying gaps, and drawing on best practices, this chapter aims to contribute to the ongoing discourse on geriatric mental health in South Asia. It serves as a foundation for future policy recommendations and program development, advocating for a comprehensive and inclusive approach to aging and mental healthcare in the region.

It is essential that robust planning is in place for managing old age-related mental health issues. This would involve mental health promotion, efforts to support positive mental health, anticipating common psychological stress in old age and preparing for it, availability of appropriate treatment for mental illness of old age, etc. Major areas that need to be looked into are health (promotion, specific protection, and maintenance), illness prevention and management, financial security, family, interpersonal, and social activities, as all of these can influence mental health. In addition, remaining active, participating in various activities till late into the age, and contributing to the society may contribute to positive mental health in older adults.

Supporting the mental health of older adults can not only be achieved by top-down policies, programs, and laws by the states but also by the efforts of individuals themselves, their families, and the communities they live in. All these need to be structured at multiple levels and domains. It should start early in life, at various levels of individuals, families, communities, and governments with specific interventions in different domains (Fig. 1). The aim should be to maintain independent living as long as possible, taking care of oneself.

2 Individual Level

Individuals need to plan for their old age, which would include financial support, healthcare connectedness, etc. Often, it does not dawn on the people until a life event such as retirement, the onset of an illness, or a functional disability late in

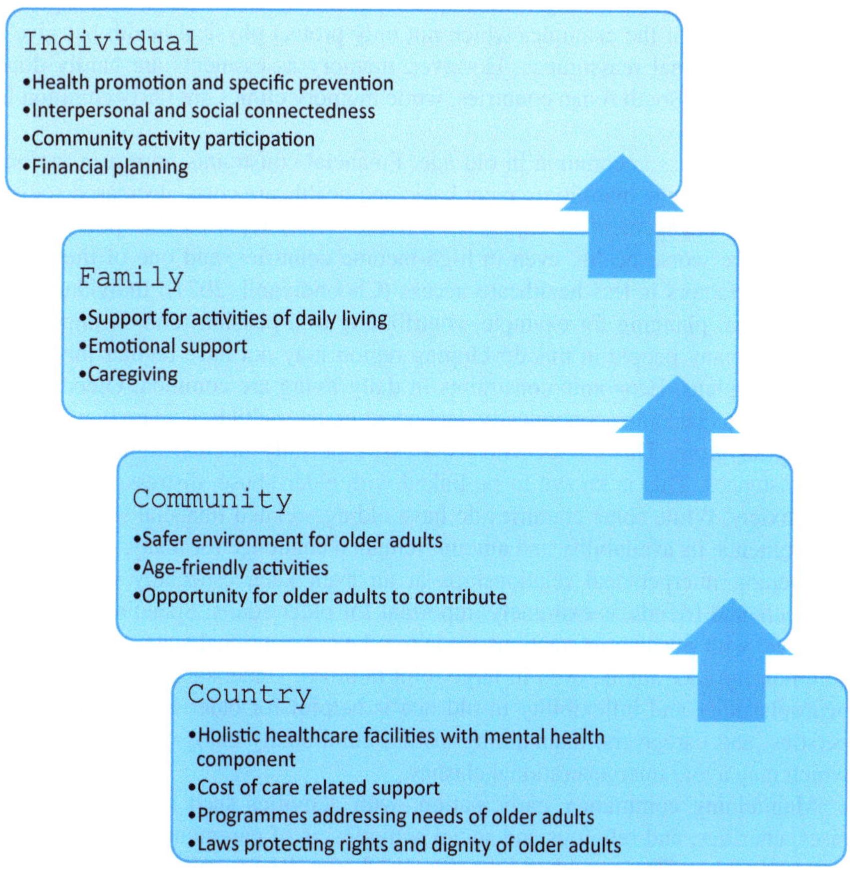

Fig. 1 A comprehensive structure of levels and domains for supporting positive mental health in old age

life. Although starting the old-age care plan after an event may appear rather late, it is still appropriate to refocus and plan at any age.

Multi-morbidity is common in old age, with both physical and mental health issues (Kar, Das et al., 2019) and physical illness contributes significantly to psychological distress. Health promotion and specific prevention, e.g. of nutritional deficiency, are essential components of sound mental health in older adults. Illnesses are associated with pain and distress, negatively impacting life in general and mental health in particular. Often, in old age, these are associated with mobility problems, frailty, and other disabilities. As health plays an intricate role in life satisfaction and happiness (Kar, 2023b), approaches to improve health, and prevent illnesses and disabilities, are important as well as having appropriate financial planning for the cost of treatment and care in old age.

A healthy body is an essential component of a healthy mind. Practising regular physical activity and remaining active are essential. Specific protection, e.g. flu vaccination and nutritional supplement; routine health screening such as cervical smear tests, mammograms, prostrate specific antibody checks, and dental procedures are some of the examples which not only protect physical health but give a sense of emotional reassurance. However, memory assessments are hardly done when needed in South Asian countries, while memory clinics are fairly common in developed nations.

Financial stress is common in old age. Financial constraints impact in various ways, leading to the inability to meet basic and healthcare costs, decreased socialization, and engagement in enjoyable activities. It is reported that poorer individuals have worse health, even in high-income countries, and one of the major associated factors is less healthcare access (Choondiyanil, 2024). Individual old-age financial planning for example, contributing to a pension fund, is important. However, many people in this developing region may not have regular job-based retirement plans. Economic constraints in daily living are common. Older adults in these areas become economically dependent on their children when they are not earning anymore. This comes with its stress, especially in challenging economic circumstances. This is known to be linked with elder abuse, distress, depression, and anxiety. While some countries do have old age-related financial support from governments, its availability and amount remain a challenge for many.

Keeping interpersonal relationships at an even keel, especially with family members and friends, is extremely important for older adults. Spending time with someone with positive interactions leads to a better emotional state. Loneliness is common in older adults, even in large joint families. Understanding the changing neuroplasticity and inflexibility in old age is helpful for older adults, their close persons, and caregivers, maintaining lasting emotionally enjoyable relationships, which may avoid intergenerational clashes.

Maintaining community participation, with activities such as hobbies, exercises, charities, and religious and social activities, is of paramount importance for a healthy mind. These need to be gradually factored into while planning for old age. Finding out the local opportunities for such participation and blending these with personal interest is of utmost importance.

3 Family Level

The family in South Asian countries has been changing very fast for the last few decades, moving towards a more nuclear structure. However, while a lot of older adults are living with family, the proportion of living alone is growing. As most of the older adults are taken care of by their family members in South Asia, it is important to plan the process of care for the older adults in the family well in advance.

In the changing circumstances, there are emerging challenges of lack of time, caring expertise, or required skills. Professional or semi-professional care is often unavailable and is costly. A proportion of families in these countries struggle to support even the treatment costs of older adults. Besides activities of daily living, families provide support for specific illness-related disabilities, end-of-life care, and psychological support for stressful life events such as bereavement.

Families need support for caring for older adults. Caregiver issues such as burnout, the inability of the caregivers to do a job outside the home, and caregivers' stress leading to elder abuse have become common. These issues do not seem to be addressed currently in many regions of South Asia. It has become a necessity to think about how the care of the older adults in the family can be planned and how the family can support and be supported in their effort of caring for the older family member.

4 Community Level

The community has a great role in supporting the older adults locally. Social activities were the most cited reason for happiness in older adults, following family/friends, travelling, reading and writing, meeting people, etc. (Kar et al., 2023). Social connectedness and being generous have been linked to happiness (Kar, 2023b). Involving older adults in social activities, and creating opportunities and avenues for them is essential.

Creating old age-friendly settings in social areas, footpaths, parks, shopping malls, office spaces, etc. is essential to help older adults socialize and deal with loneliness. There can be many examples, such as walking groups, clubs, social organizations, combined religious or spiritual activities, choruses, etc. Religious and spiritual activities bring in meaningfulness. It is more important to create space and opportunity for older adults to participate and contribute to the community.

Major causes of psychological stress for older adults originate from a lack of respect and unacceptable behaviour of younger people in public places. Although there are protective safeguards and laws, many of these concerns are not reported, and the laws are not enforced (Kar et al., 2019). Besides the effective implementation of the laws, policies, and programs from the authorities, there is a need for culture change, with public education and persistent effort. Non-governmental organizations (NGOs) or community organizations have a major role in supporting older adults locally. Many such organizations are active in South Asian countries.

5 Country Level

Countries in South Asia have various policies and programs to support healthcare and other needs of older adults, and laws protecting their rights (Arafat & Kar & Arafat, 2025; Khan et al., 2025; Mazumder, 2025; Sharma et al., 2025; Vidya & Kumar, 2025; Wickramasinghe & Gunathilake, 2025). A summary of these supportive arrangements is presented here. Recent studies suggest that healthcare, long-term old-age care, welfare, and social security of older persons are the critical domains (Mohan et al., 2025), that need to be addressed through appropriate policies.

5.1 Afghanistan

The old-age population of Afghanistan has largely been overlooked amid the ongoing conflicts and economic hardships. Although comprehensive data are lacking, estimates suggest that around 3.7% of the population is above 65 (Wikipedia, 2025). Afghanistan's worsening economic crisis has marginalized the needs of older individuals (Ruttig, 2023). Older adults in Afghanistan face severe difficulties due to the lack of essential services such as healthcare, old-age care facilities, and financial support. Government efforts to support older individuals remain inadequate. Temporary assistance programs for impoverished older adults have been ineffective due to their limited scope and short duration. Many older adults without family support are forced to perform physically demanding labour despite their age and declining health. Due to economic instability, many families find it difficult to provide adequate support to the older members. While retired government employees receive pensions, these benefits reach only a small portion of the older adult population (Ehsan, 2023).

There is another concern that a large proportion of people in Afghanistan are displaced (UNHCR, 2020), either internally or as refugees, and older adults face additional challenges because of displacement (Age International, 2021). Many lack legal documentation, preventing them from accessing healthcare, housing, and financial aid. Being separated from family and community support leaves them isolated and struggling in unfamiliar environments. This is associated with massive psychological stress for older adults.

Access to mental healthcare in Afghanistan remains limited, especially for older adults. Mental health services are often inaccessible, particularly in rural

Table 1 Policies, programs, and laws for older adults in Afghanistan

Categories	Examples
Policies	Emergency relief prioritization for older adults Accessibility standards for public buildings
Programs	Pension allocation for older adults
Laws	Legal protections for older adults Prison release for elderly individuals

areas. Afghanistan has a National Strategy for Mental Health (NSMH) (Ministry of Public Health, 2019), integrated mental health services into the Basic Package of Healthcare Services (BPHS); however, mental health problems are widespread (Alemi et al., 2023). The worsened state of mental health concerns for older persons was highlighted during the COVID-19 pandemic (Hall & International, 2020).

Afghanistan's legal system includes provisions to protect older individuals from discrimination (Table 1). The Afghan Constitution mandates government support for older individuals, disabled persons, and vulnerable groups (Constitute, 2004). Laws also allow prisoners aged 65 and older to be released under specific conditions. Additionally, there are established guidelines for construction standards to improve accessibility for older individuals and people with disabilities.

In 2009, the Afghan government proposed a home-based elder care program (Ruttig, 2023), and in 2010, the Afghan Red Crescent Society suggested creating retirement homes (Ehsan, 2023); however, reportedly, these initiatives were not implemented. With limited health facilities, there is hardly any specific support for the mental health problems of older adults in Afghanistan (Kar & Arafat, 2025).

Despite these challenges, older adults in Afghanistan are generally well-respected within society. Community members often assist them in public spaces, and emergency relief efforts prioritize older adults. However, without a structured support system, many continue to struggle with daily living issues.

5.2 *Bangladesh*

Bangladesh is undergoing a significant demographic transformation, with the older adult population increasing rapidly (Arafat et al., 2024). This increase in population presents considerable challenges, particularly in healthcare, social welfare, and policy adaptation (Khan & Leeson, 2006). There is mounting pressure on healthcare infrastructure, pension systems, and social services to meet the needs of older adults. Bangladesh has developed many policies, programs, and legal frameworks to safeguard the rights and well-being of older citizens (Table 2).

Bangladesh has made notable strides in recognizing the rights of its older citizens. There are policies such as the Old Age Allowance Program (OAAP) (Khoda & Kröger, 2024), and the Population Policy (2012). The National Policy on Older Persons (2013) focuses on securing the dignity, participation, self-dependence, and

Table 2 Policies, programs, and laws for older adults in Bangladesh

Categories	Examples
Policies	National Policy on Older Persons (2013) National Committee on Older Persons (2017) National Mental Health Policy (2019) National Mental Health Strategic Plan (2020–2030)
Programs	National Social Security Strategy (NSSS) Old-Age Allowance (OAA) Allowance for Freedom Fighters Allowance for Widow and Husband Deserted Women Social Security Policy Support (SSPS) Programme Vulnerable Groups' Feeding Widow, Deserted, and Destitute Women Allowances
Laws	Maintenance of Parents Act (2013) Probin Unnayan Foundation Act (2017) The Mental Health Act (2018)

(Dana et al., 2023; Government of Bangladesh, 2021, 2025a, 2025b; Poutiainen, 2023)

overall well-being of older individuals in society (Dana et al., 2023). The National Committee on Older Persons (2017) is responsible for overseeing the implementation of policies and initiatives aimed at the older adult population.

Bangladesh tries to safeguard the constitutional and legal rights of older adults. The Maintenance of Parents Act (2013) mandates that children provide financial support to their old parents, ensuring they are not left destitute (Yasmin, 2019). Additionally, the Probin Unnayan Foundation Act (2017) is a draft law focused on advancing the welfare of the older adult population (Poutiainen, 2023).

As Bangladesh's old-age population continues to grow, mental health issues among older adults have become an increasing concern. There are many research reports suggesting the prevalence of mental illnesses among older adults in Bangladesh (Arafat & Mazumder, 2025). However, mental health services remain critically underfunded (Moyna et al., 2024). The Mental Health Act (2018) and the National Mental Health Policy (2019) aim to improve mental health services across the country, but implementation remains slow, and funding for mental health is disproportionately low. The National Mental Health Strategic Plan (2020–2030) outlines a roadmap for improving mental health services, but resource constraints and lack of political support hinder the progress (National Institute of Mental Health, 2022). While these approaches are gaining roots, the focus on geriatric mental health at present is gradually improving in Bangladesh.

5.3 Bhutan

It needs to be highlighted that Bhutan has a high Gross National Happiness score, which has been increasing over the years (Karma et al., 2023). Bhutan is set to transition into an ageing society by 2027, with the older adult population reaching 7.4% of the total population, increasing to approximately 13.4% by 2047 (National Statistics Bureau, 2019). These projections also indicate that by 2047, one in ten Bhutanese will be over 65 years old, and one in five will be over 60 (Namgay, 2024). Currently, older citizens, especially in rural areas, face challenges such as poor health, homelessness, food insecurity, and financial instability (Dorji et al., 2017a, 2017b). There are reports of depression, anxiety, insomnia, memory decline, and dementia being common in older persons in Bhutan (Dorji et al., 2017a, 2017b; KGUMSB, 2023).

Bhutan is developing various policies and programs to support older adults (Table 3). Bhutan has the National Policy for Senior Citizens of Bhutan (NPSCB) to create a more inclusive society where older adults can live meaningful, dignified, and healthy lives (Laabar & Dema, 2023; Royal Society for Senior Citizens, 2019). The Royal Society for Senior Citizens (RSSC) has been instrumental in developing the policy, which proposes nine key interventions, including improving social support, economic security, health services, and old age-friendly infrastructure. The NPSCB 2023 includes nine key interventions aimed at creating a supportive environment for older citizens. These are improving family and social support systems, ensuring economic security, enhancing health and well-being, providing old age-friendly infrastructure and public services, promoting multigenerational bonding, ensuring safety, increasing media accessibility, researching on ageing, and providing engagement opportunities for retirees. The policy promotes collective responsibility, emphasizing that while the government provides resources and policies, implementation would depend on civil society, local communities, and the private sector. In addition, NGOs would play a role in supporting vulnerable groups, including persons with disabilities, while the Royal Bhutan Police would protect senior citizens from abuse and violence.

Bhutan's National Mental Health Program, established in 1997, integrates mental health services into primary healthcare, though resource shortages remain a challenge (Pelzang, 2012). The COVID-19 pandemic exacerbated mental health concerns, prompting government interventions such as medicine delivery and tele-counselling (Tsheten et al., 2023). There has been some training on old-age psychiatry for mental health professionals in Bhutan in the recent past (KGUMSB, 2023). At present, there is inadequate information about specific provisions for older adult mental health services (Kar & Arafat, 2025). However, it is expected through the health component of the NCSCB geriatric care and support will be enhanced. Through these measures, Bhutan aims to ensure a dignified, healthy, and secure life for its old-age population.

Table 3 Policies, programs, and laws for older adults in Bhutan

Categories	Examples
Policies	National policy for senior citizens of Bhutan (NPSCB) 2023
Programs	Family and Social Support Royal Society for Senior Citizens National Elderly Care Programme
Laws	Right to health and social care

5.4 India

The government of India has implemented various policies and programs to support the healthcare, financial security, and legal rights of older adults. With the increasing number of older citizens, efforts have been made to address their health, social welfare, and financial stability (Table 4). There are several national and state initiatives to provide comprehensive mental healthcare and assistance to older adults in India.

The National Programme for Health Care of the Elderly (NPHCE) was launched to address the growing healthcare needs of India's ageing population (Government of India, 2010; Vaishnav et al., 2022). The program aims to provide accessible, affordable, and specialized healthcare services for older citizens at various levels of the healthcare system. With a focus on both preventive and promotive care, it seeks to ensure the overall well-being of older individuals by integrating geriatric healthcare facilities within the existing medical infrastructure.

The primary objective of NPHCE is to establish comprehensive healthcare services for older adults across district hospitals, community health centres, primary health centres, and sub-centres. Through the State Health Society, these facilities offer dedicated medical services that are either free or highly subsidized (Directorate General of Health Services, 2011). The program is designed

Table 4 Policies, programs, and laws for older adults in India

Categories	Examples
Policies	National policy on older persons (NPOP) Varishta Mediclaim Policy
Programs	The National Programme for Health Care of the Elderly (NPHCE) National Programme for Palliative Care (NPPC) Integrated Programme for Senior Citizens, 2020 Atal Vayo Abhyuday Yojna (AVYAY), 2020 Varishta Pension Bima Yojana (VPBY) Pradhan Mantri Jan Arogya Yojana (PMJAY) Senior Citizen's Welfare Fund Indira Gandhi National Old Age Pension Scheme (IGNOAPS) National Programme for Health Care of the Elderly (NPHCE) National Social Assistance Programme, NSAP, 1995 Central Sector Scheme of Integrated Programme for Senior Citizens (IPSrC), 1992 State Action Plan for Senior Citizens (SAPSrC) National Mental Health Programme, NMHP, 1982
Laws	The Maintenance and Welfare of Parents and Senior Citizens Act, 2007 (MWPS) Indian Penal Code: provisions to deal with crime against older adults Mental Healthcare Act, 2017 (MHCA) The Rights of Persons with Disabilities Act, 2016 (RPWD) The Legal Services Authority Act, 1987 The Indian Succession Act, 1925

(Girdhar et al., 2019; Government of India, 2010, 2022, 2025b; NHRC, 2020; Sastry et al., 2024; Thomas & Dasgupta, 2024)

to strengthen the availability of preventive, promotive, curative, and rehabilitative care for older citizens. As part of the initiative, district hospitals have dedicated geriatric outpatient departments (OPDs) and 10-bed geriatric wards to cater to older patients requiring specialized treatment. Community health centres are expected to operate bi-weekly geriatric clinics, addressing common health concerns among older adults. Primary health centres conduct weekly geriatric clinics, ensuring continued medical attention for ageing individuals in smaller towns and rural areas. At the sub-centre level, the program provides assistive devices such as hearing aids, walking sticks, and other essential mobility aids to support independent living for older adults (Government of India, 2025a; Vaishnav et al., 2022). However, there is limited information about the ground-level reality of the effective implementation of this program.

In addition to NPHCE, there are several other initiatives. The Varishtha Mediclaim Policy covers essential medical expenses, including medicines, blood transfusions, ambulance charges, and diagnostic tests for older adults (IRDAI, 2021). *Rashtriya Vayoshri Yojana* (RVY), provides free physical aids and assistive living devices to older citizens Below the Poverty Line (BPL) category (Government of India, 2019b; Sastry et al., 2024). Through this scheme, eligible beneficiaries receive essential equipment such as hearing aids, wheelchairs, walking sticks, and artificial limbs, helping them maintain mobility and independence. This program is entirely funded by the Government of India, ensuring that economically disadvantaged older individuals receive the necessary support.

The Pradhan Mantri Jan Arogya Yojana (PMJAY), a part of the *Ayushman Bharat scheme*, offers annual health coverage of up to a fixed limit per family, including older persons (Government of India, 2019a). This program is crucial in reducing the financial burden of healthcare costs, particularly for older citizens. By covering expenses related to hospitalizations and specialized treatments, PMJAY provides a safety net for older adults in need of critical healthcare services.

The number of older people with depression and dementia is increasing in India (Girdhar et al., 2019). Besides mental illness, a considerable proportion of the Indian old-age population experiences negative expressed emotions, abuse, and neglect (Girdhar et al., 2019). Specific old-age mental healthcare is scarce, so also trained professionals for geriatric care. There has been an initiative to provide mental healthcare for older adults through geriatric telepsychiatry services, using telephone and video-based support (Sivakumar et al., 2020). Specific guidelines for the practices of geriatric telepsychiatry have been developed.

Mental health remains a crucial aspect of old-age care, and the government has introduced policies to address this concern. The Mental Healthcare Act, of 2017, recognizes the rights of individuals with mental health conditions, including dementia and depression (Government of India, 2017; Sivakumar et al., 2019). The act prohibits forced institutionalization and ensures the autonomy of older patients in making healthcare decisions.

To enhance caregiving support, the National Institute of Social Defence (NISD) conducts training programs for caregivers and healthcare workers, equipping them with essential skills for geriatric care (National Institute of Social Defence, 2020).

Additionally, the National Helpline for Senior Citizen, Elderline helpline (14,567) provides 24/7 assistance to older adults facing abuse, neglect, or mental health challenges, offering them immediate support and legal aid (Sastry et al., 2024).

The Indian legal framework includes several provisions to safeguard the rights of older adults. The Maintenance and Welfare of Parents and Senior Citizens Act, enacted in 2007 (Government of India, 2007), mandates financial and emotional support for older individuals by their families. It allows older adults to seek maintenance from their children through legal tribunals (Issac et al., 2021). Further legal protection is provided through the Indian Penal Code, which includes provisions to penalize crime against older adults. The National Policy for Older Persons (NPOP), introduced in 1999 and updated in 2011, ensures income security, healthcare access, shelter, and welfare measures for older citizens, thereby addressing their fundamental needs (Ministry of Social Justice, 2011; Rajan & Mishra, 2011).

Despite these efforts, many older citizens remain unaware of available programs. There is also a shortage of trained professionals working for older adults, where access to healthcare is limited. The urban–rural divide further complicates old-age care, as healthcare and social services are more accessible in urban areas, leaving rural older citizens with limited resources. There are many old-age care homes mushrooming at present; however, there are concerns too, that require in-depth research (Augustine et al., 2020).

Old-age psychiatry services are gradually increasing in India and this is available at various levels (Vidya & Kumar, 2025). However further strengthening the infrastructure, improving awareness, and increasing investment in mental health services are needed. Ensuring equal access to these programs across all regions remains a significant challenge.

5.5 *Maldives*

In recent years, the Maldives has experienced a significant rise in life expectancy, contributing to a growing older adult population. Presently, 8.3% are above 60 years old (HelpAge International, 2023). Projections indicate that by 2050, this figure will increase to approximately 12%, and by 2054, 14% of the population will be older persons, emphasizing the importance of sustainable ageing strategies (Maldives Bureau of Statistics, 2024). Maldives has started a few such programs.

Maldives has a National Elderly Policy (Table 5), and the National Elderly Action Plan which focuses on addressing the social and economic challenges faced by older adults, improving their well-being and protection, and encouraging their active participation in society (Ministry of Gender, Family & Social Services, 2017).

Various programs in the Maldives to support older persons include 'Home for Persons with Special Needs', 'Bedridden Program' focusing on providing basic healthcare services for bedridden patients above 65 years, social worker support for the attendance to cases related to older persons' neglect and abuse, pension

Table 5 Policies, programs, and laws for older adults in Maldives

Categories	Examples
Policies	National Elderly Policy Mental health policy: National Centre for Mental Health and Mental Health Bill Strategic Action Plan (SAP) Ranveyla: Promote healthy ageing Pension policy: State-funded pension
Programs	Ijthimaee Badhahi Madhadhuverin (IBAMA) Initiative Aasandha: State-funded insurance scheme Elderly Village Community Social Groups
Laws	National Human Rights Action Plan (NHRAP)

(National Bureau of Statistics, 2019). Ranveyla Campaign is a nationwide effort promoting healthy ageing by emphasizing balanced nutrition, mental well-being, and increasing awareness about pension schemes. *Aasandha Scheme* provides state-funded health insurance, ensuring universal healthcare access for all Maldivians, including older persons. The Elderly Village Initiative focuses on creating residential, daycare, and nursing care facilities aimed at improving the well-being, independence, and recreational opportunities of older persons. Community Social Groups (CSGs) offer localized social protection by identifying at-risk older individuals in partnership with UNICEF (National Bureau of Statistics, 2019). Presently, the Home for People with Special Needs (HPSN) serves as the sole state facility for older persons, primarily catering to those with mental health conditions.

Maldives has a Mental Health Policy that includes plans to establish a National Mental Health Centre and propose a mental health bill aimed at enhancing services and protections (Ministry of Health, 2017). Though there is limited focus and facilities at present on old-age mental health services (Kar & Arafat, 2025), it is expected that emphasis will gradually grow.

5.6 *Nepal*

Nepal is experiencing significant changes in its population structure. According to the 2021 census, older adults constitute 10.2% of the population (National Statistics Office, 2023). With increasing life expectancy, the number of older adults is growing, creating new social and healthcare challenges (Chalise et al., 2022).

In Nepal, the state-funded healthcare program (2004), and '*Aarogya Ashram*' (2010) aim to support older citizens (Table 6). Since 2019, the government has focused on equitable healthcare through the National Health Policy, the Fifteenth Plan (2019/2020–2024/2025), and the Gender Equality and Social Inclusion (GESI) Strategy. These initiatives aim to improve healthcare access, promote

Table 6 Policies, programs, and laws for older adults in Nepal

Categories	Examples
Policies	Geriatric Health Service Strategy, (GHSS), 2021 National Health Policy, the Fifteenth Plan (2019/20–2024/25)
Programs	State-funded Healthcare Program (2004) Aarogya Ashram (2010) National Health Insurance Programme (2017)
Laws	Senior Citizens Act, 2006

healthy ageing, strengthen community support, and ensure gender-equitable services (Ministry of Health & Population, 2020).

Healthcare services are provided by both public and private institutions, including hospitals, primary health centres, and clinics. The Constitution guarantees free basic healthcare for all citizens, supported by the National Health Insurance Program (NHIP), introduced in 2017 (Kandel, 2018). The NHIP enrolment is voluntary, providing free basic healthcare services such as outpatient visits, emergency care, and selected medications. For older adults, the government covers enrolment costs fully and offers an additional amount for healthcare expenses; however, there have been many challenges in implementation (Khanal et al., 2023).

The Geriatric Health Service Strategy (GHSS) of 2021 focuses on establishing the foundation for geriatric healthcare through assessments, capacity-building, and institutional development. It guarantees free healthcare for marginalized individuals aged 60 and above, those aged 65 and older with disabilities or mental illnesses, and all individuals aged 70 and above (Ministry of Health & Population, 2022). It also provides subsidies for chronic conditions such as Alzheimer's, Parkinson's, cancer, and heart disease. The GHSS emphasizes education, awareness, and training. Public health campaigns aim to inform older persons about their rights, while caregivers and healthcare workers receive training to improve home and institutional care. Strengthening health data systems helps identify healthcare needs and barriers, while efforts to provide free treatment for chronic conditions ensure better access to essential services.

Financial frameworks are being developed to allocate resources for geriatric care, while medical professionals receive specialized training to bridge the gap in expertise. Social health insurance is being strengthened by improving hospital capacities, encouraging enrolment, and developing sustainable financing models. Integrating geriatric healthcare into the national system remains a priority, with collaboration across sectors playing a crucial role in shaping policies (Paneru et al., 2022).

Despite progress, Nepal faces several challenges in old-age mental healthcare. Many studies highlight the prevalence of mental illnesses and the service gaps (Sharma et al., 2025). There are reports of a higher prevalence of depression and feelings of loneliness (Maharjan et al., 2024; Risal et al., 2024). Many older adults are unaware of free healthcare services, and some prefer traditional healing practices, limiting the use of medical care. Healthcare facilities are concentrated in urban areas, requiring rural residents to travel long distances. Public hospitals often face medicine shortages and long wait times, pushing many towards expensive private providers (Dhakal et al., 2024).

Nepal has a limited workforce for geriatric care (Dhakal et al., 2024; Shrestha, 2013), with only a few geriatricians, trained geriatric nurses, and inadequate focus on training in geriatric care. Infrastructure for rehabilitation, palliative care, and assisted living is nearly non-existent (Joshi, 2023). The country faces a shortage of specialized care facilities, with older adults often deprived of basic healthcare services due to the lack of trained professionals and dedicated institutions (Basnet et al., 2023). Similarly, there are no specific old-age mental health services, and most of these are taken care of by mainstream psychiatric services (Risal et al., 2024).

Nepal is working to improve its healthcare system to meet the needs of its ageing population. While policies and programs have been introduced, challenges such as workforce shortages, infrastructure gaps, and lack of awareness remain. Continued government efforts, better implementation of policies, and increased investment in healthcare capacity are necessary.

5.7 Pakistan

Pakistan's older adult population over 60 years of age increased by 75.1% between 1990 and 2012 and is expected to be 11% of the population in 2025 (Jalal & Younis, 2014). The increasing older adult population has led to many challenges in physical and mental healthcare. Access to healthcare remains one of the most pressing concerns in the current system in Pakistan. With only a few geriatric healthcare facilities available, most older individuals rely on general healthcare services, often lacking the necessary geriatric expertise (Noreen et al., 2021).

Mental health problems, including depression and anxiety, are highly prevalent among older persons in Pakistan (Bhamani et al., 2013). Studies indicate that rural areas report higher levels of depression due to poverty, lack of healthcare access, and cultural stigmas surrounding mental health (Noreen et al., 2021). Social isolation and neglect are also significant concerns, particularly for those living alone or in rural areas.

Older persons in Pakistan often face financial dependency due to inadequate pension schemes and limited employment opportunities. The decline of extended family structures further aggravates this dependency, as urbanization and nuclear family setups reduce the traditional support systems for older persons. Cases of elder abuse and neglect, ranging from emotional to financial exploitation, are increasingly reported, necessitating societal awareness campaigns and stricter legal protections.

Pakistan has introduced many policies and initiatives to address the needs and welfare of older persons and to protect their rights and well-being (Table 7).

Table 7 Policies, programs, and laws for older adults in Pakistan

Categories	Examples
Policies	National Policy, 1999 Islamabad Bill, 2019 Senior Citizen Bill, 2007
Programs	Relief Package for Older Adults, 2004
Laws	Parental Protection Ordinance, 2021 The Maintenance and Welfare of Parents and Senior Citizens Act

The National Policy on Elderly Health (1999) marked a significant step towards improving healthcare for older adults (Social Protection Resource Centre, 2022). It sought to train primary healthcare providers in gerontology and set up a multi-tiered system of care. The policy also emphasized the need for dental and domiciliary care for older adults. However, the implementation of this policy has faced many challenges, leading to uneven results across the country.

In 2004, the government introduced a Relief Package for Older People, aiming to address the essential health and social needs of older citizens (Social Protection Resource Centre, 2022). A key feature of the package was raising awareness among younger generations about respecting older persons. Its reach was limited due to a lack of proper dissemination and inadequate funding, which prevented it from achieving its full potential.

There are different acts, including the Maintenance and Welfare of Old Parents and Senior Citizens Act, for the support of older adults (Government of Pakistan, 2019). The Senior Citizens Bill (2007) was introduced, proposing a wide range of benefits for older citizens, including discounts on public transportation, tax exemptions, free access to recreational spaces, and priority services in banks and hospitals (Social Protection Resource Centre, 2022). This bill provided a strong foundation for older persons' welfare, but its passage and enforcement have been delayed multiple times, hindering its effectiveness. In 2021, the Parental Protection Ordinance was passed to ensure that parents have the right to continue living in their homes, even if those homes are owned or rented by their children (Government of Pakistan, 2021). This ordinance also imposed penalties for neglect or eviction, aiming to reinforce families' responsibility towards their older members. There is an Islamabad Bill, 2019 which advocates establishing for council, old-age home, and senior card for healthcare, travel discounts, and legal protection for old parents.

Despite these efforts, gaps remain in policy implementation, healthcare access, and social protection, due to limited funding primarily and scant awareness (Khan et al., 2025). Adequate provision of mental health issues remains a concern in Pakistan, and targeted mental health policies for older adults are not available (Murad & Siraj, 2024).

5.8 Sri Lanka

The older adult population in Sri Lanka is increasing faster than any other South Asian Country; the proportion was 6.6% in 1981, and 12.4% in 2012 and is expected to reach 21.1% by 2050 (Perera, 2017). With the life expectancy of males and females around 72 and 79 years, respectively, society must adapt to support an increasing number of older adults. The old-age dependency ratio has increased to 20 per 100 working-age individuals in 2012 (Perera, 2017). This demographic shift presents significant challenges for healthcare, social security, and community-based old-age care systems, along with age-related mental health concerns.

The Sri Lankan government has taken steps to address the well-being of older citizens (Table 8). Home Care Services have been introduced, delivering medical, nutritional, and general assistance directly to older adults who face challenges in mobility, making access to medical care more difficult (Samaraweera & Maduwage, 2016). Healthy Lifestyle Centres (HLCs) emphasize preventive healthcare, and Public Health Nursing Officers deliver community-based palliative care. Additionally, Day Centres for Elders offer opportunities for social engagement and structured activities (Government of Sri Lanka, 2025). For those requiring specialized medical attention, Geriatric Care Units in hospitals focus on age-related health issues, while Healthy Lifestyle Centres (HLCs) promote preventive care and early screening for non-communicable diseases. Complementing these efforts, Public Health Nursing Officers provide community-based support, including palliative and preventive care (Samaraweera & Maduwage, 2016; Watt et al., 2014).

In 2000, Sri Lanka enacted the Protection of Elders Rights Act (Government of Sri Lanka, 2000). This legislation led to the establishment of the National Council and Secretariat for Elders, ensuring that older persons could live with dignity and independence while receiving essential protections. Building upon this, the National Charter for Senior Citizens, introduced in 2006, emphasized the integration of

Table 8 Policies, programs, and laws for older adults in Sri Lanka

Categories	Examples
Policies	National Elderly Healthcare Policy (2017)
Programs	National Charter for Senior Citizens (2006) Day Centres for Elders Elder Identity Cards Financial Assistance Community Committees Home Care Services Geriatric Care Units Healthy Lifestyle Centres (HLCs) Public Health Nursing Officers Elder-Friendly Community Centres Private-sector nursing homes, and elder homes Pension schemes
Laws	Protection of Elders Rights Act (2000)

old-age care into national development policies (Ministry of Social Services & Social Welfare, 2006). It recognized older adults as valuable contributors to society and aimed to ensure their voices were heard in policymaking. Further reinforcing this commitment, the National Elderly Healthcare Policy of 2017 was designed to address age-specific health concerns. This policy placed a strong emphasis on preventive healthcare and ensured that older individuals had access to personalized, comprehensive medical services (Samaraweera & Maduwage, 2016).

Sri Lanka's approach to geriatric care extends far beyond legal frameworks; it actively fosters social, financial, and healthcare support systems to improve the quality of life for older adults. At the heart of this effort are Day Centres for the Elderly, which are vibrant community spaces where older persons can engage in recreational, social, and physical activities, helping to combat isolation and enhance overall well-being. To further empower older adults, the government introduced Elder Identity Cards, granting access to healthcare discounts, priority services, and financial aid, making essential services more affordable and accessible (Perera, 2017).

Beyond government initiatives, NGOs and private enterprises have stepped in to bridge gaps in geriatric care. Sarvodaya has established old-age homes that offer a holistic approach to ageing, combining spiritual well-being through meditation, physical fitness programs, and on-site medical clinics (Samaraweera & Maduwage, 2016). The private sector has also stepped in with Home-Based Nursing Services, employing professional caregivers to provide personalized, flexible home care (Samaraweera & Maduwage, 2016). Meanwhile, private old-age homes cater to those seeking long-term residential care, particularly among higher-income groups.

Despite these efforts, significant challenges remain (Wickramasinghe & Gunathilake, 2025). Health inequalities persist, with gaps between healthy and unhealthy life expectancy, highlighting an urgent need for better preventive and rehabilitative care. Particularly vulnerable groups are older women, those in poverty, those with limited pension access, and those without adequate financial support. The shrinking caregiver pool poses a serious concern, as migration and declining birth rates reduce the availability of younger caregivers. Regulatory monitoring for old-age care facilities remains weak, raising questions about the quality of care provided in certain old-age homes and services. Geriatric mental health services such as old-age psychiatry, memory clinics, and dementia care homes are still evolving.

6 Focus Areas Relating to Older Adults with Mental Illnesses

6.1 *Dementia*

Although a large proportion of patients with dementia live in South Asian countries, there is limited information about their experience, the concerns of their caregivers who are mostly family members, and the services available for their management and care. Lack of information, misinformation, and stigma are commonly reported (Hossain et al., 2020), suggesting the need for specific actions. There are many studies on accessing and using dementia services by South Asian patients living in different countries; which highlighted various areas such as lack of awareness about dementia and local services, stigma, and linguistic and culture-related barriers in communication and decision-making (Giebel et al., 2015). Lack of resources for dementia care is another major concern (Ali et al., 2023).

There are specific suggestions for dementia prevention (Livingston et al., 2024), and many of these are extremely relevant for South Asian countries. For example, improving the scope of providing education early in life, and reducing the number of traumatic brain injuries, specifically related to traffic accidents and unsafe working conditions, air pollution, especially in major cities, smoking, and high alcohol consumption should be some of the immediate priorities.

Delays in dementia diagnosis are common in South Asian countries, and in fact, a considerable proportion is not diagnosed. There is low awareness among the public and even among medical professionals, and a shortage of specialist services (Shaji & Dias, 2006; Thomas et al., 2024). Post-diagnostic care facilities for dementia patients are also limited and costly. Only India and Nepal among South Asian countries offer some financial assistance to people with dementia (Matthews et al., 2023). Dementia care homes are emerging in some parts of South Asian countries but all countries have disproportionately low numbers of old-age care homes (Matthews et al., 2023). However, considering the enormity of the needs and inability of average citizens to afford institutional care (Shaji & Dias, 2006); more appropriate local solutions are to be explored in these countries rather than following Western models.

Community-based dementia care models are essential, including home-based care, which can be supported through various methods such as telehealth and online training of the informal caregivers, besides local health services (Balouch et al., 2021; Thomas & Dasgupta, 2024). However, these approaches need further exploration. The lack of research in the areas of effective care provision for dementia patients in South Asian countries is clearly evident (Abdullah et al., 2023).

6.2 *Carers' Concerns*

Most old-age patients with mental illness, including dementia, are taken care of by their family members as informal caregivers in South Asian countries (Shaji & Dias, 2006; Thomas et al., 2024; Watt et al., 2014). Caring is enjoyable, however, it can be psychologically stressful for family caregivers, at high intensities, in challenging clinical conditions, when there is no respite (Kar, 2024; Watt et al., 2014), and is associated with a subjective burden (Rathnayake et al., 2025). Caregivers of older adults with mental illness face enormous challenges, with little awareness of the illness, lack of knowledge about care methods, no training opportunities or supportive mechanisms, and financial challenges.

Burnout, anxiety, and depression in caregivers are common (Shaji & Dias, 2006). A study in India reported that challenges in caregiving for older persons with mental illnesses were financial, hampered leisure activity of family caregivers, psychological stress, and mental health problems such as depression (Kar, 2021). In most situations, the caregivers have to travel long distances to access care (Mahanta et al., 2022). In Pakistan, the reasons for the massive burden on family caregivers have been identified as the shrinking of family structure, industrialization, poverty, and the prevalence of chronic illnesses among older adults (Noreen et al., 2021). Although there are schemes to support older adults by the states, they are either inadequate or not accessed (Poutiainen, 2023; Shaji & Dias, 2006).

6.3 Mental Capacity of Older Adults and Decisions Making

Many psychiatric illnesses in old age along with physical illnesses may affect the mental capacity to decide regarding the treatment and decisions in other areas of life. One of the frequently assessed areas in old-age psychiatry is the decision-making capacity of older persons regarding their treatment. There are specific laws in different developed countries such as the UK, protecting the interests and rights of older adults who lack mental capacity. Information about such specific laws is lacking in the South Asian countries. India does not have specific laws related to mental capacity (Dalvi et al., 2023); which is covered in other acts such as Mental Healthcare Act (MHCA), 2017 (Namboodiri, 2019). In most situations, family members or the next of kin take the treatment and other decisions. The specific aspect of mental capacity to decide regarding treatment needs to be clearer in legislation and the information should be available to the clinicians explicitly to be used in clinical practice. There is a need for adequate training for professionals working in geriatric mental health and other related fields in this area.

6.4 Role of NGOs

The NGOs and professional bodies contribute massively to the actual service or development of supportive facilities for mental illnesses in old age. They can contribute meaningfully to the policies and programs of the states. A few examples are Alzheimer and Related Dementia Society of India, Geriatric Psychiatry Specialty section of the Indian Psychiatric Society, Indian Association of Geriatric Mental Health, Geriatric Care and Research Organisation (GeriCaRe), India; Sangath, India; Nepalese Society for Gerontology and Geriatrics; Bangladesh Association for the Aged and Institute of Geriatric Medicine (Khoda & Kröger, 2024), Sarvodaya, Sri Lanka; South Asian Mental Health Initiative & Network,

HelpAge International, etc. (Girdhar et al., 2019). Supporting the NGOs to build their capacity, and expertise through training and regional cooperation, sharing experience and expertise is expected to be helpful in old-age mental healthcare.

7 Reflections About the Current State of Old-age Mental Healthcare

Like other areas of the world, the older adult population of South Asian countries is also increasing. Higher longevity can be a positive factor in utilizing the expertise of older persons to strengthen society in various ways, including the economy (Tripathy & Kar, 2022), and older persons are useful resources for the country (Ray et al., 2018). The old age-related mental health concerns in these countries are increasing too, however, there is a lack of focus on the mental health of the older adults. There has been general progress in healthcare infrastructure, policies, and legal framework, however, specific support for old-age mental healthcare is at a low level (Kar, 2023a). These could be due to multiple factors, such as non-recognition, inadequate emphasis or prioritization in policies and programs, lack of resources, and trained professionals. Besides, old-age mental health issues get sidetracked among the more pressing healthcare-related issues of the general population.

The countries in South Asia have adopted diverse strategies to support the mental health needs of the population and most of the old age-related mental healthcare is presumed to be covered through these systems, without any specific measures in most regions. Healthcare access, especially in rural areas, is inadequate, and mental health services remain underfunded. Improving the availability, accessibility, and affordability of physical and mental healthcare along with social care is the need of the hour.

The financial dependency of older adults on family persists due to insufficient financial support. Most countries try to provide financial support for the healthcare of older persons; however, its awareness, utilization, and availability remain a concern. Financial hardship for day-to-day living including care in old age remains a challenge for most of the population in these countries. Some regions have financial support such as old-age allowance or pension, and healthcare-related insurance, which are covered by the countries.

Although most of the older persons in these countries are still being cared for by their family members, there are brewing concerns. Traditional family support systems are also weakening due to constantly increasing nuclear family structures and youth migration, leaving many older individuals without adequate care or a system to provide the care. Fast-changing societies, urbanization, and economy-related movements have weakened the family support systems as well, leaving many older adults without caregivers.

Many local, national, and international NGOs are working for old age-related concerns in these countries, however, their reach and effectiveness in real-life scenarios and crises for individual older adults or their families are not clear. Similarly, community-driven initiatives are supporting older adults in their access to support systems and social engagement.

In addition, inadequate awareness, misinformation, and stereotypical thinking about old age also impede the effective care of older adults. Mental health stigma prevents older individuals from seeking and receiving appropriate care. Although the exact number of professional experts available for geriatric care is not clear, the available multidisciplinary workforce is low, especially for mental health issues. There is inadequate input in undergraduate medicine, nursing and allied healthcare courses (Matthews et al., 2023), and hardly any postgraduate training program.

Despite policies, it has been observed that resource and manpower constraints hinder their effective implementation. Budget shortages, lack of coordination among agencies, and weak administrative frameworks limit the effective utilization of the policies and ground-level progress. Legislative measures to safeguard the rights and dignity of older adults are available in many countries, but their implementation and effectiveness at the ground level remain a concern. Limited awareness of rights and services further restricts access to essential support. Specifically, elder abuse and neglect lack strict regulations.

8 Action Plans

Based on the currently available information, there is assurance that the focus on the needs of older adults in South Asian countries is developing; however, this needs to be more robust, and the planning, programs, and laws should be active at the ground level. There should be specific supporting structures and methods of providing help to older adults without any struggle for them, as only goodwill gestures would not help. The focus areas where actions should be taken based on the current understanding of the needs of older adults in South Asian countries are given in Box 1.

Box 1 Summary of focus areas for action for geriatric mental healthcare

1. Prioritize mental health in healthcare policies and strategies
2. Improve the availability of appropriate care for older adults
3. Financial support for the healthcare of older adults
4. Support for family caregivers
5. Develop a multidisciplinary workforce
6. Support for NGOs working for older adults
7. Evidence-based policies and their implementation
8. Legislative measures to safeguard the rights and dignity of older adults

It is essential to explore the unmet healthcare needs, especially for the mental health problems of older adults, and arrange appropriate support. Related to this are the specific care needs of older adults with mental illnesses and the caregivers' concerns, especially of the family informal caregivers. End-of-life care support for families with older adults, especially those with mental health difficulties, is almost not available in these developing countries.

There is a massive rural–urban divide in these countries regarding healthcare accessibility, availability, and affordability. Expanding rural healthcare facilities, integrating mental health services into primary care, and providing free treatment for chronic illnesses will improve old age-related health outcomes. The service gaps for the mental health concerns of older persons and their remedies should be looked into and addressed. There is a need for regular research in this area, matching the rise of the older adult population.

Despite the dwindling informal family caregiving system, families are still the first line of support for older persons in South Asian countries. There should be appropriate support, training, and respite facilities for the informal family caregivers of older adults with mental illnesses. Developing an old age-friendly safe environment, with a distinct place and respect for the older adults in the community, is of paramount importance. This will happen not just through appropriate safeguards and laws but also through the culture shift through public education.

There should be a focused approach to facilitate public and professional awareness about mental illnesses in older adults. There are shortages of trained professionals, and this requires training clinicians in different disciplines and carers in geriatric care; until that happens, appropriate task-shifting may address the gap (Thomas et al., 2024). Training healthcare professionals specifically for mental health issues in old age is also necessary.

Many traditional and cultural methods such as yoga and pranayama (Rawat et al., 2024), which have been practised in the region for a long period, need to be utilized more, which might help for physical and mental well-being. Spirituality has also been linked to happiness (Kar, 2023b); this is a commonly observable attribute in older persons. For this reason, these approaches need to be further facilitated and integrated as community measures in supporting older adults' mental health.

Financial struggles are commonly reported sources of stress for older persons. Comprehensive support for finances in old age is needed to reduce stress and specifically for the treatment of physical and mental illnesses, related disability, frailty, and care needs. Increased funding for healthcare and social security schemes in the budgetary provision is essential.

Despite available policies, programs, and laws related to old-age-specific support in South Asian countries, implementation challenges are obvious. Adequate policy execution, increased funding, and awareness initiatives are key to addressing these challenges effectively. However, the reasons for the inadequate implementation of existing supportive services need to be further ascertained regionally, and corrective measures should be put in place. Governments must enforce existing laws and review the effectiveness of existing comprehensive ageing policies and programs.

A multi-sectoral approach involving governments, NGOs, private organizations, and communities is crucial for holistic old-age care. Developing sustainable financial support schemes for older persons, fostering intergenerational programs, and launching awareness campaigns can enhance social and economic support. Strengthening NGOs and corporate involvement through corporate social responsibility programs will further improve the welfare of older adults. Multi-stakeholder task forces should oversee policy implementation and evaluation.

9 Conclusions

In the changing demographic scenarios, developing countries in South Asia need to plan, develop programs, create appropriate laws for supporting older adults, and implement these, as the requirements are growing fast. The focus areas are physical and mental health, financial security, old-age care-related resources, developing old age-friendly communities and environments, supporting their community participation, and protecting their rights. Old-age mental healthcare should be given due importance in these policies and programs, as at present there is a massive gap between the number of people requiring care and the available resources. Countries should prioritize that appropriate healthcare is available and affordable, provide funding for social care (e.g. family support or care-home placement for old age-related mental illnesses, community facilities for older adults), evaluate and address the changing needs of older adults, and ensure implementation of existing programs and laws at the grass-root level. Regional cooperation and sharing the knowledge base are expected to be helpful. Multilevel efforts involving governments, private organizations, NGOs, the local community, and families, are essential which are expected to improve the holistic health and quality of life of older adults.

Acknowledgements Geriatric care and research organization (GeriCaRe), India; Quality of Life Research and Development Foundation (QoLReF), India; the Institute of Insight, UK; Black Country Healthcare NHS Foundation Trust, UK.

References

Abdullah, J. M., Courtney-Pratt, H., Doherty, K., & Andrews, S. (2023). Needs of older people living with dementia in low and middle-income Asian countries: A scoping review. *Dementia (London, England), 22*(8), 1977–1993. https://doi.org/10.1177/14713012231198952

Age International. (2021). *Crisis in Afghanistan: The older people | Age International*. https://www.ageinternational.org.uk/news-stories/news/2021/crisis-in-afghanistan-helping-some-of-the-most-vulnerable-older-people/

Alemi, Q., Panter-Brick, C., Oriya, S., Ahmady, M., Alimi, A. Q., Faiz, H., Hakim, N., Sami Hashemi, S. A., Manaly, M. A., Naseri, R., Parwiz, K., Sadat, S. J., Sharifi, M. Z., Shinwari, Z., Ahmadi, S. J., Amin, R., Azimi, S., Hewad, A., Musavi, Z., & Ventevogel, P. (2023).

Afghan mental health and psychosocial well-being: Thematic review of four decades of research and interventions. *Bjpsych Open, 9*(4), Article e125. https://doi.org/10.1192/bjo.2023.502

Ali, S., Zehra, M., Fatima, T., & Nadeem, A. (2023). Advancing dementia care in Pakistan: Challenges and the way forward. *Frontiers in Dementia, 2*, 1241927. https://doi.org/10.3389/frdem.2023.1241927

Arafat, S. M. Y., & Mazumder, A. H. (2025). Geriatric psychiatry in Bangladesh: Current status and ways ahead. In Edi N. Kar, S. K. Kar, & S. M. Y. Arafat (Eds.), *Geriatric psychiatry in South Asia*. Springer Nature. https://doi.org/10.1007/978-981-96-7469-5_2

Arafat, S. M. Y., Mazumder, A. H., & Maruf, M. M. (2024). Geriatric psychiatry in Bangladesh. In S. M. Y. Arafat (Eds.), *Mental health in Bangladesh*. Springer. https://doi.org/10.1007/978-981-97-0610-5_18

Augustine, A., George, S., & CT, S. K. (2020). Life in old age homes: Reflections from God's own country, Kerala, India. *Journal of Geriatric Care and Research, 7*(2), 64–67.

Balouch, S., Zaidi, A., Farina, N., & Willis, R. (2021). Dementia awareness, beliefs and barriers among family caregivers in Pakistan. *Dementia (London, England), 20*(3), 899–918. https://doi.org/10.1177/1471301220915066

Basnet, S., Thapa, S., & Silwal, S. (2023). Common Health problems and Satisfaction of Health Services among Elderly in Nepal. *Nepal Medical Journal, 6*, 18–24. https://doi.org/10.37080/nmj.170

Bhamani, M. A., Karim, M. S., & Khan, M. M. (2013). Depression in the elderly in Karachi, Pakistan: A cross sectional study. *BMC Psychiatry, 13*(1), 181. https://doi.org/10.1186/1471-244X-13-181

Chalise, H., Bohora, P., & Khanal, T. (2022). Older people and social security system in Nepal. *Gerontol Geriatr Res, 8*(2), 1075.

Choondiyanil, A. (2024). Wealth and health inequality in the elderly: A narrative review of the challenges in an ageing UK population. *Journal of Geriatric Care and Research, 11*(2), 44–50.

Constitute. (2004). *Afghanistan 2004 Constitution—Constitute*. https://www.constituteproject.org/constitution/Afghanistan_2004

Dalvi, M. M., Mudholkar, S., & Dhadphale, M. (2023). Comparative analysis of mental capacity legislation within the Indian Mental Healthcare Act 2017 with the devolved nations of the United Kingdom. *Indian Journal of Psychiatry, 65*(8), 882–886. https://doi.org/10.4103/indianjpsychiatry.indianjpsychiatry_224_23

Dana, G. P. T., Hossain, A. H. M. K., & Hasan, S. (2023). Aging policy of Bangladesh: Issues and challenges for implementation. *Social Science Review, 40*(2), Article 2. https://doi.org/10.3329/ssr.v40i2.72207

Dhakal, U., Briceño, E., Sharma, U., Bogati, U., Sharma, A., Shrestha, L., Ghimire, D., & Mendes de Leon, C. F. (2024). Health care systems and policies for older adults in Nepal: New challenges for a low-middle income country. *Discover Public Health, 21*(1), 256. https://doi.org/10.1186/s12982-024-00382-9

Directorate General of Health Services. (2011). *Operational Guidelines: National Programme for Health Care of the Elderly (NPHCE)*. Government of India. https://mohfw.gov.in/sites/default/files/8324324521Operational_Guidelines_NPHCE_final.pdf

Dorji, L., Jamtsho, C., Norbu, T., & Bhujel, D. (2017). *Understanding the situation of elderly citizens in Bhutan*. National Statistics Bureau.

Dorji, N., Dunne, M. P., Seib, C., & Deb, S. (2017b). Quality of life among senior citizens in Bhutan. *Asia-Pacific Journal of Public Health, 29*(1), 35–46. https://doi.org/10.1177/1010539516685609

Ehsan, K. (2023, March 23). Poverty and old age: The struggle of Afghanistan's senior citizens. *KabulNow*. https://kabulnow.com/2023/03/poverty-and-old-age-the-struggle-of-afghanistans-senior-citizens/

Giebel, C. M., Zubair, M., Jolley, D., Bhui, K. S., Purandare, N., Worden, A., & Challis, D. (2015). South Asian older adults with memory impairment: Improving assessment and access to dementia care. *International Journal of Geriatric Psychiatry, 30*(4), 345–356. https://doi.org/10.1002/gps.4242

Girdhar, G., Sethi, S., Vaid, R. P., & Khurana, H. (2019). Geriatric mental health problems and services in India: A burning issue. *Journal of Geriatric Care and Research, 6*(1), 15–19.

Government of Bangladesh. (2021). *Office of the Chief Accounts Officer Pension and Fund Management*. https://www.pension.gov.bd/

Government of Bangladesh. (2025a). সমাজকলয্াণ মন্তর্ণালয়-গণপর্জাতন্তর্ী বাংলাদেশ সরকার. https://msw.gov.bd/

Government of Bangladesh. (2025b, February 6). *Social Security Policy Support (SSPS) Programme | An initiative of the Cabinet Division and the General Economics Division (GED), Bangladesh Planning Commission, Government of Bangladesh*. https://socialprotection.gov.bd/

Government of India. (2007). *Maintenance and Welfare of Parents and Senior Citizens Act, 2007*. Government of India. https://www.indiacode.nic.in/bitstream/123456789/6831/1/maintenance_and_welfare_of_parents_and_senior_citizens_act.pdf

Government of India. (2010). *National Programme for Health Care of the Elderly(NPHCE) | Ministry of Health and Family Welfare | GOI*. https://mohfw.gov.in/?q=major-programmes/Non-Communicable-Diseases/Non-Communicable-Diseases-1

Government of India. (2017). *Mental Healthcare Act, 2017*. http://indiacode.nic.in/handle/123456789/2249

Government of India. (2019a). *About PM-JAY - National Health Authority*. https://nha.gov.in/PM-JAY

Government of India. (2019b). *Rashtriya Vayoshri Yojana| National Portal of India*. https://www.india.gov.in/spotlight/rashtriya-vayoshri-yojana

Government of India. (2022). *National Programme for Health Care of the Elderly(NPHCE) | Ministry of Health and Family Welfare | GOI*. https://mohfw.gov.in/?q=major-programmes/Non-Communicable-Diseases/Non-Communicable-Diseases-1

Government of India. (2025a). *National Health Mission*. https://nhm.gov.in/

Government of India. (2025b). *National Programme for Palliative care (NPPC): National Health Mission*. https://nhm.gov.in/index1.php?lang=1&level=2&sublinkid=1047&lid=609

Government of Pakistan. (2019). *The maintenance and welfare of old parents and senior citizens Act*. https://www.senate.gov.pk/uploads/documents/1556601589_129.pdf

Government of Pakistan. (2021). *A Bill to provide for the protection of parents*. https://www.na.gov.pk/uploads/documents/1623253018_894.pdf

Government of Sri Lanka. (2000). *Protection of the Rights of Elders Act, No 9 of 2000*. https://stateminsamurdhi.gov.lk/web/images/content_image/pdf/legislation/profeld.pdf

Government of Sri Lanka. (2025). *Services for Elders*. Ministry of Rural Development, Social Security and Community Empowerment. https://stateminsamurdhi.gov.lk/web/index.php?Itemid=150&id=29&lang=en&option=com_content&view=article

Hall, S., & International, H. (2020, September 1). *The impact of COVID-19 on older persons; Afghanistan analytical brief* (Afghanistan). https://static1.squarespace.com/static/5cfe2c8927234e0001688343/t/5f857ce98108b70047c11831/1602583788535/Afghanistan-Analytical-Brief-September-2020.Pdf; https://www.ecoi.net/en/document/2052943.html

HelpAge International. (2023, January 8). *Maldives: Population Ageing - Policy case study*. HelpAge International. https://www.helpage.org/resource/maldives-population-ageing-policy-case-study/

Hossain, M., Crossland, J., Stores, R., Dewey, A., & Hakak, Y. (2020). Awareness and understanding of dementia in South Asians: A synthesis of qualitative evidence. *Dementia (London, England), 19*(5), 1441–1473. https://doi.org/10.1177/1471301218800641

IRDAI. (2021). *Varishtha Mediclaim Policy for Senior Citizens*. Insurance Regulatory and Development Authority of India (IRDAI). https://irdai.gov.in

Issac, T. G., Ramesh, A., Reddy, S. S., Sivakumar, P. T., Kumar, C. N., & Math, S. B. (2021). Maintenance and Welfare of Parents and Senior Citizens Act 2007: A critical appraisal.

Indian Journal of Psychological Medicine, 43(5 Suppl), S107–S112. https://doi.org/10.1177/02537176211043932
Jalal, S., & Younis, M. Z. (2014). Aging and elderly in Pakistan. *Ageing International, 39*(1), 4–12. https://doi.org/10.1007/s12126-012-9153-4
Joshi, P. R. (2023). *Taking care of Nepal's elderly*. Kathmandu Post. https://kathmandupost.com/columns/2023/09/25/taking-care-of-nepal-s-elderly
Kandel, N. (2018). Nepal Health Insurance Bill: Possible challenges and way forwards. *JNMA: Journal of the Nepal Medical Association, 56*(210), 633–639.
Kar, N. (2021). Family members as caregivers of older people with mental illness: Issues and interventions. *Journal of Geriatric Care and Research, 8*(1), 21–28.
Kar, N. (2023a). Ageing and care related issues: A focus on India. *Journal of Geriatric Care and Research, 10*(1), 1–2.
Kar, N. (2023b). Happiness and health: An intricate relationship. In S. Chetri, T. Dutta, M. K. Mandal, & P. Patnaik (Eds.), *Understanding happiness: An explorative view* (pp. 205–231). Springer Nature. https://doi.org/10.1007/978-981-99-3493-5_9
Kar, N. (2024). Taking care of elderly at home: Approaches for the family caregivers. *Journal of Geriatric Care and Research, 11*(1), 1–3.
Kar, S., Das, T., Mohapatra, P., Kar, B., Senapati, A., & Kar, N. (2019). Health concerns of older adults: Observations from a survey and Public Education Programme in Bhubaneswar, India. *Journal of the Indian Academy of Geriatrics, 15*, 10–16. https://doi.org/10.35262/jiag.v15i1.10-16
Kar, S. K., & Arafat, S. M. Y. (2025). Geriatric psychiatry in other South Asian countries: Afghanistan, Bhutan, the Maldives. In Edi N. Kar, S. K. Kar, & S. M. Y. Arafat (Eds.), *Geriatric psychiatry in South Asia*. Springer Nature. https://doi.org/10.1007/978-981-96-7469-5_7
Kar, S., Mahapatra, P. K., Rath, N., Kar, B., Das, T. K., & Kar, N. (2023). Survey of factors contributing to the happiness of older persons: A cross-sectional study of associated worries, anxiety, and depression. *Odisha Journal of Psychiatry, 19*(1), 14–19. https://doi.org/10.4103/OJP.OJP_19_23
Kar, S., Mohapatra, P., Kar, B., Senapati, A., Rath, N., Das, T., & Kar, N. (2019). Social security of elderly is at stake: Concerns raised by older adults from India. *Journal of Geriatric Care and Research, 6*, 64–68.
Karma, U., Alkire, S., Wangdi, K., & Zangmo, T. (2023). *GNH 2022*. Centre for Bhutan & GNH Studies.
KGUMSB. (2023). *Bhutan Old Age Psychiatry Education Program 2023 | Khesar Gyalpo University of Medical Sciences of Bhutan*. https://www.kgumsb.edu.bt/?p=238805; https://www.kgumsb.edu.bt/?p=238805
Khan, H. T. A., & Leeson, G. W. (2006). The demography of aging in Bangladesh: A scenario analysis of consequence. *Hallym International Journal of Aging, 8*(1), Article 1. https://doi.org/10.2190/HA.8.1.a
Khan, O., Sheikh, S., & Farooq, S. (2025). Geriatric psychiatry in Pakistan. In In Edi N. Kar, S. K. Kar, & S. M. Y. Arafat (Eds.), *Geriatric psychiatry in South Asia: Current status and ways ahead*. Springer Nature.
Khanal, G. N., Bharadwaj, B., Upadhyay, N., Bhattarai, T., Dahal, M., & Khatri, R. B. (2023). Evaluation of the National Health Insurance Program of Nepal: Are political promises translated into actions? *Health Research Policy and Systems, 21*(1), 7. https://doi.org/10.1186/s12961-022-00952-w
Khoda, Md. S. E., & Kröger, T. (2024). Policy-makers and population ageing in Bangladesh: A dearth of attention. *Journal of Population Ageing*. https://doi.org/10.1007/s12062-024-09452-x
Laabar, T. D., & Dema, P. (2023). Well-being of the elderly population: A multi-factorial approach. *The Druk Journal, 9*(1), 64–70.
Livingston, G., Huntley, J., Liu, K. Y., Costafreda, S. G., Selbæk, G., Alladi, S., Ames, D., Banerjee, S., Burns, A., Brayne, C., Fox, N. C., Ferri, C. P., Gitlin, L. N., Howard, R.,

Kales, H. C., Kivimäki, M., Larson, E. B., Nakasujja, N., Rockwood, K., & Mukadam, N. (2024). Dementia prevention, intervention, and care: 2024 report of the Lancet standing Commission. *The Lancet, 404*(10452), 572–628. https://doi.org/10.1016/S0140-6736(24)01296-0

Mahanta, D., Mohanty, N. G., Kar, S., Mohapatra, S., & Kar, N. (2022). Clinical profile and comorbidity of elderly patients presenting to a psychiatric outpatient unit of a tertiary care hospital in Odisha, India: A cross sectional study. *Journal of Geriatric Care and Research, 9*(2), 40–46.

Maharjan, S., Tiwari, N., Bista, S., & Basel, P. (2024). Prevalence of depressive symptoms and associated factors among older adults living in aged care homes of Kathmandu Metropolitan City, Nepal. *PLOS Global Public Health, 4*(11), Article e0003359. https://doi.org/10.1371/journal.pgph.0003359

Maldives Bureau of Statistics. (2024). *International Day of Older Persons*. Ministry of Housing, Land & Urban Development. https://statisticsmaldives.gov.mv/mbs/wp-content/uploads/2024/10/ElderlyPersonsDay2024-Eng.pdf

Matthews, N. R., Porter, G. J., Varghese, M., Sapkota, N., Khan, M. M., Lukose, A., Paddick, S.-M., Dissanayake, M., Khan, N. Z., & Walker, R. (2023). Health and socioeconomic resource provision for older people in South Asian countries: Bangladesh, India, Nepal, Pakistan and Sri Lanka evidence from NEESAMA. *Global Health Action, 16*(1), 2110198. https://doi.org/10.1080/16549716.2022.2110198

Mental Health Act, 2018, Laws of Bangladesh. http://bdlaws.minlaw.gov.bd/act-1273.html (accessed on February 23, 2025)

Ministry of Gender, Family & Social Services. (2017, October 1). *Maldives inaugurates first-ever National Elderly Policy*. https://gender.gov.mv/en/?p=1748

Ministry of Health. (2017). *National Mental Health Policy 2015–2025*. WHO Country Office for Maldives. https://health.gov.mv/storage/uploads/EoAjylw9/zae5c6sf.pdf

Ministry of Health and Population. (2020). *NHSSP: Nepal Health Sector Support Programme*. https://www.nhssp.org.np/about.html

Ministry of Health and Population. (2022). *Geriatric Health Service Strategy*. Government of Nepal, Ramshah Path, Kathmandu. https://www.nhssp.org.np/Resources/GESI/Geriatric%20health%20service%20strategy%20English%20version%20-%202022.pdf

Ministry of Public Health. (2019). *National Strategy for Mental Health 2019–2023*. Ministry of Public Health, Afghanistan. https://moph.gov.af/sites/default/files/2019-09/Mental%20Health%20Staregy%202019-2023.pdf

Ministry of Social Justice. (2011). *National Policy for Senior Citizens*. Government of India. https://socialjustice.gov.in/writereaddata/UploadFile/dnpsc.pdf

Ministry of Social Services and Social Welfare. (2006). *National Charter for Senior Citizens & National Policy for Senior Citizens*. Government of Sri Lanka. https://stateminsamurdhi.gov.lk/web/images/content_image/pdf/legislation/citizens_national_pfsc.pdf

Mohan, A., Jothikaran, T. A. J., Gudi, N. K. A. A., & Ashok, L. (2025). *Growing old before growing rich: A scoping review on ageing-related policy interventions from the WHO Southeast Asian Region, 15*. https://doi.org/10.1136/bmjopen-2023-079621

Moyna, S. A., Hasan, K., Kabir, K. H., Khan, Md. A., & Saha, S. K. (2024). Depressive symptoms among women in disaster-prone region in Bangladesh. *Journal of Affective Disorders Reports, 16*, Article 100762. https://doi.org/10.1016/j.jadr.2024.100762

Murad, S., & Siraj, S. (2024). Bridging the void: Unraveling mental health policies for the older adults in Pakistan's Tapestry- A literature review. *Journal of Clinical Psychology and Neurology, 2*(2), 1–4. https://doi.org/10.61440/JCPN.2024.v2.17

Namboodiri, V. (2019). Capacity for mental healthcare decisions under the Mental Healthcare Act. *Indian Journal of Psychiatry, 61*(Suppl 4), S676. https://doi.org/10.4103/psychiatry.IndianJPsychiatry_76_19

Namgay, T. (2024). *National policy for inclusive and caring future for senior citizens*. Kuensel Online. https://kuenselonline.com/national-policy-for-inclusive-and-caring-future-for-senior-citizens/

National Bureau of Statistics. (2019). *Population and Development in Maldives 2019*. Ministry of National Planning and Infrastructure, Male. https://statisticsmaldives.gov.mv/nbs/wp-content/uploads/2019/07/ICPD-25FINAL-1.pdf

National Institute of Mental Health. (2022). Policy Documents – NIMH. *Policy Documents*. https://nimh.gov.bd/english/policy-documents/

National Institute of Social Defence. (2020). *Old Age Care*. https://www.nisd.gov.in/old_age_training.html

National Statistics Bureau (Ed.). (2019). *Population projections Bhutan, 2017–2047*. National Statistics Bureau. https://bhutan.unfpa.org/sites/default/files/pub-pdf/Bhu_Pop_proj.pdf

National Statistics Office (Ed.). (2023). *National population and housing census 2021. Volume 01: National report* (Reprint). Government of Nepal, Office of the Prime Minister and Council of Ministers, National Statistics Office.

NHRC. (2020). *Rights of senior citizens*. National Human Rights Commission. https://nhrc.nic.in/sites/default/files/9%20Right%20of%20Senior%20Citizens_compressed.pdf

Noreen, N., Abdullah, M., & Lalani, N. (2021). Geriatric Care in Pakistan: Current Realities and Way Forward. *Pakistan Journal of Public Health, 11*(4), Article 4. https://doi.org/10.32413/pjph.v11i4.872

Paneru, D. P., Adhikari, C., Poudel, S., Adhikari, L. M., Neupane, D., Bajracharya, J., Jnawali, K., Chapain, K. P., Paudel, N., Baidhya, N., & Rawal, A. (2022). Adopting social health insurance in Nepal: A mixed study. *Frontiers in Public Health, 10*, Article 978732. https://doi.org/10.3389/fpubh.2022.978732

Pelzang, R. (2012). Mental health care in Bhutan: Policy and issues. *WHO South-East Asia Journal of Public Health, 1*(3), 339–346. https://doi.org/10.4103/2224-3151.207030

Perera, E. L. S. J. (2017). *Ageing population of Sri Lanka: Emerging issues, needs and policy implications*. United Nations Population Fund, Sri Lanka. https://srilanka.unfpa.org/sites/default/files/pub-pdf/UNFPA%20Ageing%20Monograph%20Report_0.pdf

Poutiainen, T. (2023, October 1). *Fulfilling social protection for older persons in Bangladesh | United Nations in Bangladesh*. https://bangladesh.un.org/en/248154-fulfilling-social-protection-older-persons-bangladesh, https://bangladesh.un.org/en/248154-fulfilling-social-protection-older-persons-bangladesh

Rajan, S. I., & Mishra, U. S. (2011). *The National Policy for Older Persons: Critical Issues in Implementation*. United Nations Population Fund (UNFPA).

Rathnayake, N., Kannangara, W., Abeygunasekara, T., De Zoysa, W., Palangasinghe, D., & Lekamwasam, S. (2025). Burden of caregivers of older people in Sri Lanka: An overlooked concern in the health care system. *BMC Geriatrics, 25*, 32. https://doi.org/10.1186/s12877-025-05681-7

Rawat, S., Chetri, S., & Kaushik, A. (2024). Well-being and happiness: The healing power of yoga. *Journal of Geriatric Care and Research, 11*(1), 12–15.

Ray, S., Suar, D., & Mukhopadhyay, S. (2018). Are senior citizens resources? A qualitative inquiry. *Journal of Geriatric Care and Research, 5*(2), 43–51.

Risal, A., Kunwar, D., & Shrestha, B. (2024). Mental health among the elderly in Nepal: Special emphasis on depression. *OBM Geriatrics, 8*(1), Article 1. https://doi.org/10.21926/obm.geriatr.2401268

Royal Society for Senior Citizens. (2019). *Launch the National Policy for Senior Citizens*. https://rssc.org.bt/our-programme-details/launch-the-national-policy-for-senior-citizens

Ruttig, T. (2023, March 23). *Poverty and old age: The struggle of Afghanistan's senior citizens*. Afghanistan Analysts Network - English. https://www.afghanistan-analysts.org/en/recommended-reading/poverty-and-old-age-the-struggle-of-afghanistans-senior-citizens/

Samaraweera, D., & Maduwage, S. (2016). Meeting the current and future health-care needs of Sri Lanka's ageing population. *WHO South-East Asia Journal of Public Health, 5*(2), 96. https://doi.org/10.4103/2224-3151.206259

Sastry, N. B., Vempadapu, M., & Sivananjiah, S. (2024). Toward adapting the UN's healthy aging agenda for India: Tailoring to unique historical context and traditions. *Frontiers in Public Health, 11*, 1346962. https://doi.org/10.3389/fpubh.2023.1346962

Shaji, K. S., & Dias, A. (2006). Dementia care in India: A progress report. *International Psychiatry, 3*(4), 9–10.

Sharma, P., Rijal, R., & Dhungel, O. (2025). Geriatric Psychiatry in Nepal. In *Geriatric Psychiatry in South Asia. Edi N Kar, SK Kar, SMY Arafat*. Springer Nature. https://doi.org/10.1007/978-981-96-7469-5_4

Shrestha, L. (2013). Geriatric health in Nepal: Concerns and experience. *Nepal Medical College Journal: NMCJ, 15*(2), 148–152.

Sivakumar, P. T., Mukku, S. S. R., Antony, S., Harbishettar, V., Kumar, C. N., & Math, S. B. (2019). Implications of Mental Healthcare Act 2017 for geriatric mental health care delivery: A critical appraisal. *Indian Journal of Psychiatry, 61*(Suppl 4), S763–S767. https://doi.org/10.4103/psychiatry.IndianJPsychiatry_100_19

Sivakumar, P. T., Mukku, S. S. R., Kar, N., Manjunatha, N., Phutane, V. H., Sinha, P., Kumar, C. N., & Math, S. B. (2020). Geriatric telepsychiatry: Promoting access to geriatric mental health care beyond the physical barriers. *Indian Journal of Psychological Medicine, 42*(5 Suppl), 41S-46S. https://doi.org/10.1177/0253717620958380

Social Protection Resource Centre. (2022). *Legislation for older people in Pakistan*. https://www.sprc.org.pk/wp-content/uploads/2022/03/SPRC-POLICY-BRIEF-updated.pdf

Thomas, P. T., Rajagopalan, J., Hurzuk, S., Ramasamy, N., Pattabiraman, M., De Poli, C., Lorenz-Dant, K., Comas-Herrera, A., & Alladi, S. (2024). Pathways to care for people with dementia in India: An exploratory study using case vignettes. *Dementia (London, England), 23*(3), 493–511. https://doi.org/10.1177/14713012231193081

Thomas, T., & Dasgupta, J. (2024). A narrative review of community-based dementia care in India: Experiences, challenges, and policy initiatives. *Current Opinion in Psychiatry, 37*(5), 370–375. https://doi.org/10.1097/YCO.0000000000000944

Tripathy, S., & Kar, S. K. (2022). Optimizing the economy by optimal use of longevity opportunity: Lesson for low-and middle-income countries. *Journal of Geriatric Care and Research, 9*(1), 7–9.

Tsheten, T., Chateau, D., Dorji, N., Pokhrel, H. P., Clements, A. C. A., Gray, D. J., & Wangdi, K. (2023). Impact of COVID-19 on mental health in Bhutan: A way forward for action. *The Lancet Regional Health - Southeast Asia, 11*, Article 100179. https://doi.org/10.1016/j.lansea.2023.100179

UNHCR. (2020). *Afghanistan—Internally displaced*. Global Focus. https://reporting.unhcr.org/afghanistan-internally-displaced-17

Vaishnav, L. M., Joshi, S. H., Joshi, A. U., & Mehendale, A. M. (2022). The National Programme for health care of the elderly: A review of its achievements and challenges in India. *Annals of Geriatric Medicine and Research, 26*(3), 183–195. https://doi.org/10.4235/agmr.22.0062

Vidya, K., & Kumar, P. (2025). Geriatric psychiatry in India. In Edi N. Kar, S. K. Kar, & S. M. Y. Arafat (Eds.), *Geriatric psychiatry in South Asia: current status and ways ahead*. Springer Nature.

Watt, M. H., Perera, B., Østbye, T., Ranabahu, S., Rajapakse, H., & Maselko, J. (2014). Caregiving expectations and challenges among elders and their adult children in Southern Sri Lanka. *Ageing and Society, 34*(5), 838–858. https://doi.org/10.1017/S0144686X12001365

Wickramasinghe, A., & Gunathilake, M. (2025). Geriatric psychiatry in Sri Lanka. In Edi N. Kar, S. K. Kar, & S. M. Y. Arafat (Eds.), *Geriatric psychiatry in South Asia: Current status and ways ahead*. Springer Nature.

Wikipedia. (2025). Demographics of Afghanistan. In *Wikipedia*. https://en.wikipedia.org/w/index.php?title=Demographics_of_Afghanistan&oldid=1273504351

Yasmin, S. (2019). The rights of parents to maintenance in Bangladesh: An overview of the Parents Maintenance Act, 2013. *Scholars International Journal of Law, Crime and Justice, 02*(10), 309–313. https://doi.org/10.36348/SIJLCJ.2019.v02i10.003

Correction to: Geriatric Psychiatry in South Asia

Nilamadhab Kar, Sujita Kumar Kar, and S. M. Yasir Arafat

Correction to:
N. Kar et al. (eds.), Geriatric Psychiatry in South Asia, South Asian Perspectives in Mental Health and Psychology, https://doi.org/10.1007/978-981-96-7469-5

In the original version of this book, an incorrect reference has been included in chapter 5, and the author name 'Betsi Cadwaladr' has been inadvertently added, which have now been corrected. The book and the chapters have been updated with the changes.

The updated versions of these Chapters can be found at
https://doi.org/10.1007/978-981-96-7469-5_5
https://doi.org/10.1007/978-981-96-7469-5_11

N. Kar et al. (eds.), *Geriatric Psychiatry in South Asia*, South Asian Perspectives in Mental Health and Psychology , https://doi.org/10.1007/978-981-96-7469-5_13